Imaging of Common Oral Cavity, Sinonasal, and Skull Base Pathology

Editor

DINESH RAO

ORAL AND MAXILLOFACIAL SURGERY CLINICS OF NORTH AMERICA

www.oralmaxsurgery.theclinics.com

Consulting Editor
RUI P. FERNANDES

August 2023 • Volume 35 • Number 3

ELSEVIER

1600 John F. Kennedy Boulevard • Suite 1800 • Philadelphia, Pennsylvania, 19103-2899

http://www.oralmaxsurgery.theclinics.com

ORAL AND MAXILLOFACIAL SURGERY CLINICS OF NORTH AMERICA Volume 35, Number 3
August 2023 ISSN 1042-3699, ISBN-13: 978-0-443-18262-4

Editor: John Vassallo; j.vassallo@elsevier.com
Developmental Editor: Jessica Nicole B. Cañaberal

Oral and Maxillofacial Surgery Clinics of North America (ISSN 1042-3699) is published quarterly by Elsevier Inc., 360 Park Avenue South, New York, NY 10010-1710. Months of issue are February, May, August, and November. Business and Editorial Offices: 1600 John F. Kennedy Blvd., Suite 1800, Philadelphia, PA 19103-2899. Periodicals postage paid at New York, NY and additional mailing offices. Subscription prices are $409.00 per year for US individuals, $785.00 per year for US institutions, $100.00 per year for US students/residents, $483.00 per year for Canadian individuals, $941.00 per year for Canadian institutions, $100.00 per year for Canadian students/residents, $535.00 per year for international individuals, $941.00 per year for international institutions and $235.00 per year for international students/residents. To receive student/resident rate, orders must be accompanied by name or affiliated institution, date of term, and the *signature* of program/residency coordinator on institution letterhead. Orders will be billed at individual rate until proof of status is received. Foreign air speed delivery is included in all *Clinics* subscription prices. All prices are subject to change without notice. **POSTMASTER:** Send address changes to *Oral and Maxillofacial Surgery Clinics of North America,* Elsevier Periodicals **Customer Service, 11830 Westline Industrial Drive, St. Louis, MO 63146. Tel: 1-800-654-2452 (U.S. and Canada); 314-447-8871 (outside U.S. and Canada). Fax: 314-447-8029. E-mail: journalscustomerservice-usa@elsevier.com (for print support); journalsonlinesupport-usa@elsevier.com (for online support).**

Reprints. For copies of 100 or more, of articles in this publication, please contact the Commercial Reprints Department, Elsevier Inc., 360 Park Avenue South, New York, NY 10010-1710. Tel.: 212-633-3874; Fax: 212-633-3820; Email: reprints@elsevier.com.

Oral and Maxillofacial Surgery Clinics of North America is covered in *MEDLINE/PubMed (Index Medicus)*, *Science Citation Index Expanded (SciSearch®)*, *Journal Citation Reports/Science Edition*, and *Current Contents®/Clinical Medicine*.

Contributors

CONSULTING EDITOR

RUI P. FERNANDES, MD, DMD, FACS, FRCS(Ed)
Clinical Professor and Chief, Division of Head and Neck Surgery, Program Director, Head and Neck Oncologic Surgery and Microvascular Reconstruction Fellowship, Departments of Oral and Maxillofacial Surgery, Neurosurgery, and Orthopaedic Surgery and Rehabilitation, University of Florida Health Science Center, University of Florida College of Medicine, Jacksonville, Florida, USA

EDITOR

DINESH RAO, MD
Associate Professor of Radiology and Neurosurgery, Director of Clinical Operations, Section Chief of Neuroradiology, Department of Radiology, UF Health Jacksonville, University of Florida, College of Medicine, Jacksonville, Florida, USA

AUTHORS

KWASI ADDAE-MENSAH, MD
Department of Radiology, Baylor College of Medicine, Houston, Texas, USA

AMIT AGARWAL, MD
Associate Professor, Department of Radiology, Mayo Clinic, Jacksonville, Florida, USA

YAHIA ALROHAIBANI, MD
Batterjee Medical College, Jeddah, Saudi Arabia

RICHARD D. BEEGLE, MD
AdventHealth Medical Group Radiology, Windermere, Florida, USA

CHRIS BELTRAN, PhD
Department of Radiation Oncology, Mayo Clinic, Jacksonville, Florida, USA

RITA BHATIA, MD
Associate Professor of Radiology, Department of Radiology, University of Miami Miller School of Medicine, Jackson Memorial Hospital, Miami, Florida, USA

ANTHONY BUNNELL, MD, DMD
Assistant Professor of Oral and Maxillofacial Surgery, Department of Oral and Maxillofacial Surgery, University of Florida, College of Medicine, Jacksonville, USA

YU CAI, MD, MS
Ascension Seton Medical Center Austin, Austin, Texas, USA

MARGARET N. CHAPMAN, MD
Department of Radiology, Virginia Mason Medical Center, Seattle, Washington, USA

BO CHEN, MD
Department of Diagnostic and Interventional Radiology, McGovern Medical School at the University of Texas HSC Houston, Houston, Texas, USA

JEANIE CHOI, MD
Associate Professor, Department of Neuroradiology, Division of Diagnostic Radiology, The University of Texas MD Anderson Cancer Center, Houston, Texas, USA

ROI DAGAN, MD, MS
Associate Professor, Department of Radiation Oncology, University of Florida College of Medicine, Jacksonville, FL, USA

JAMES MATTHEW DEBNAM, MD
Professor, Neuroradiology, The University of Texas MD Anderson Cancer Center, Houston, Texas, USA

MIGUEL FABREGA, MD
Department of Diagnostic and Interventional Imaging, McGovern Medical School at UTHealth Houston, Assistant Professor of Radiology, University of Texas at Houston, Houston, Texas, USA

ELLIOTT FRIEDMAN, MD
Department of Radiology, Houston Methodist Hospital, Houston, Texas, USA

ASHLEY GOAD, PA-C
Texas Children's Hospital, Houston, Texas, USA

NOELANI S. GONZALES, MS-IV
Nova Southeastern University, Dr. Kiran C. Patel College of Osteopathic Medicine, Fort Lauderdale, Florida, USA

MAURICIO HERNANDEZ, PhD
Department of Radiology, University of Florida, College of Medicine–Jacksonville, Jacksonville, Florida, USA

ADAM L. HOLTZMAN, MD
Assistant Professor, Department of Radiation Oncology, University of Florida College of Medicine, Jacksonville, Florida, USA

KUANG-CHUN JIM HSIEH, MD
Assistant Professor, Department of Radiology, Baylor College of Medicine, Houston, Texas, USA

DEREK HUELL, BS
Medical Student, New York University Grossman School of Medicine, New York, New York, USA

JOHN KIM, MD
Department of Radiology, University of Florida College of Medicine–Jacksonville, Jacksonville, Florida, USA; Department of Radiology, University of Michigan, Ann Arbor, Michigan, USA

MARCUS J. LACEY, MD
Department of Radiology, Virginia Mason Medical Center, Seattle, Washington, USA

KIM LEARNED, MD
Associate Professor, Department of Neuroradiology, Division of Diagnostic Radiology, The University of Texas MD Anderson Cancer Center, Houston, Texas, USA

VOLODYMYR MAYMESKUL, MD
Department of Radiology, University of Florida College of Medicine–Jacksonville, Jacksonville, Florida, USA

WILLIAM M. MENDENHALL, MD
Professor, Department of Radiation Oncology, University of Florida College of Medicine, Jacksonville, FL, USA

JOHN MURRAY, MD
Department of Radiology, Mayo Clinic, Jacksonville, Florida, USA

JOHN V. MURRAY JR, MD
Mayo Clinic, Jacksonville, Florida, USA

NATALYA NAGORNAYA, MD
Assistant Professor of Radiology, Department of Radiology, University of Miami Miller School of Medicine, Jackson Memorial Hospital, Miami, Florida, USA

JEET PATEL, MD
Department of Radiology, University of Florida College of Medicine–Jacksonville, Jacksonville, Florida, USA

DINESH RAO, MD
Associate Professor of Radiology and
Neurosurgery, Director of Clinical Operations,
Section Chief of Neuroradiology, Department
of Radiology, UF Health Jacksonville,
University of Florida, College of Medicine,
Jacksonville, Florida, USA

MICHAEL S. RUTENBERG, MD, PhD
Department of Radiation Oncology, Mayo
Clinic, Jacksonville, Florida, USA

GAURAV SAIGAL, MD
Professor of Radiology, Department of
Radiology, University of Miami Miller School of
Medicine, Jackson Memorial Hospital, Miami,
Florida, USA

SUKHWINDER JOHNNY S. SANDHU, MD
Division Chair, Department of Radiology,
Mayo Clinic, Jacksonville, Florida,
USA

EMILIO P. SUPSUPIN JR, MD
Associate Professor, Radiology/
Neuroradiology, Associate Program Director,
Radiology Residency Program, University of
Florida College of Medicine, Jacksonville,
Florida, USA; Volunteer Faculty and Staff
Neuroradiologist, University of Texas
Health–Houston, McGovern Medical School,
Department of Diagnostic and Interventional
Imaging, Houston, Texas, USA

FEHIME EYMEN UCISIK, MD
Neuro Oncology Fellow, Department of
Neuroradiology, Division of Diagnostic
Radiology, The University of Texas MD
Anderson Cancer Center, Houston, Texas,
USA

ASHLEIGH WEYH, MD, DMD, MPH
Department of Oral and Maxillofacial Surgery,
University of Florida, College of Medicine,
Jacksonville, Florida, USA

Contents

Marcus J. Lacey and Margaret N. Chapman

Rhinosinusitis is a commonly encountered disease. Imaging is not typically required in acute uncomplicated rhinosinusitis; however, it is integral in the evaluation of patients who present with prolonged or atypical symptoms or when acute intracranial complications or alternate diagnoses are suspected. Knowledge of the paranasal sinus anatomy is important to understand patterns of sinonasal opacification. Bacterial, viral, and fungal pathogens are responsible culprits and, with duration of symptoms, serve to categorize infectious sinonasal disease. Several systemic inflammatory and vasculitic processes have a predilection for the sinonasal region. Imaging, along with laboratory and histopathologic analysis, assist in arriving at these diagnoses.

Natalya Nagornaya, Gaurav Saigal, and Rita Bhatia

Sinonasal tumors are rare, diverse, complex lesions with overlapping demographic and clinical features. Malignant tumors are more common, with a grave prognosis, and require biopsy for accurate diagnosis. This article briefly reviews the classification of sinonasal tumors and provides imaging examples and imaging characteristics of each clinically important nasal and paranasal mass lesions. Although there are no true pathognomonic imaging features, it is important for the radiologist to have a broad knowledge of the various CT and MR imaging findings that can help narrow the differential diagnosis and aid in early diagnosis and mapping of tumor for treatment planning.

Kuang-Chun Jim Hsieh, Kwasi Addae-Mensah, Yahia Alrohaibani, Ashley Goad, and Kim Learned

Perineural tumor spread (PNS) is a well-recognized entity in head and neck cancers and represents a mode of metastasis along nerves. The trigeminal and facial nerves are most affected by PNS, and their connections are reviewed. MRI is the most sensitive modality for detecting PNS, and their anatomy and interconnections are reviewed. MRI is the most sensitive modality for detecting PNS, and imaging features of PNS and important imaging checkpoints are reviewed. Optimal imaging protocol and techniques are summarized as well as other entities that can mimic PNS.

Emilio P. Supsupin Jr., Noelani S. Gonzales, and James Matthew Debnam

 Video content accompanies this article at http://www.oralmaxsurgery.theclinics.com.

The skull base (SB) is the osseous foundation of the cranial vault. It contains many openings that allow communication between the extracranial and intracranial structures. This communication is crucial in normal physiologic processes yet may also arrow spread of disease. This article provides a comprehensive review of SB anatomy including important landmarks and anatomic variants relevant to SB surgery. We also illustrate the diverse pathologies affecting the SB.

Elliott Friedman, Yu Cai, and Bo Chen

Infectious and inflammatory disorders are the commonest pathologies to affect the major salivary glands however frequently overlap in clinical presentation. Imaging plays an important role in diagnosis, usually initially performed by CT or ultrasound. MRI, with its superior soft-tissue characterization compared with CT, provides a better evaluation of tumors and tumor-like conditions. Imaging features may suggest that a mass is more likely to be benign versus malignant, however, biopsy is often needed to establish a definitive histopathologic diagnosis. Imaging plays a key role in the staging of neoplastic disease.

Percutaneous image-guided biopsy has largely replaced open surgical biopsies for many head and neck (H&N) lesions, being very safe and minimally invasive. Although the radiologist plays the primary role in these cases, it requires a multidisciplinary approach. Depending upon numerous factors, these biopsies can be either fine-needle aspiration or core needle biopsy, using ultrasound for superficial lesions and computed tomography for deep neck lesions. The most crucial part of H&N biopsies is planning a trajectory to avoid injury to critical anatomic structures. This article outlines the standard biopsy approaches and key anatomical considerations for H&N procedures.

Proton therapy (PT) is a form of highly conformal external-beam radiotherapy used to mitigate acute and late effects following radiotherapy. Indications for treatment include both benign and malignant skull-base and central nervous system pathologies. Studies have demonstrated that PT shows promising results in minimizing neurocognitive decline and reducing second malignancies with low rates of central nervous system necrosis. Future directions and advances in biologic optimization may provide additional benefits beyond the physical properties of particle dosimetry.

Head and neck and base of skull malignancies are challenging for surgical and radiotherapy treatment due to the density of sensitive tissues. Carbon ion radiotherapy (CIRT) is a form of heavy particle therapy that uses accelerated carbon ions to treat malignancies that may be radioresistant or in challenging anatomic locations. CIRT has an increased biological effectiveness (ie, increased cell killing) at the end of the range of the carbon beam (ie, within the target tissue) but not in the entrance dose. This increased biological effectiveness can overcome the effects of radioresistant tumors, tissue hypoxia, and the need for radiotherapy fractionation.

ORAL AND MAXILLOFACIAL SURGERY CLINICS OF NORTH AMERICA

SERIES OF RELATED INTEREST

Atlas of the Oral and Maxillofacial Surgery Clinics
www.oralmaxsurgeryatlas.theclinics.com

Dental Clinics
www.dental.theclinics.com

THE CLINICS ARE NOW AVAILABLE ONLINE!
Access your subscription at:
www.theclinics.com

Preface

Imaging of Common Oral Cavity, Sinonasal, and Skull Base Pathology

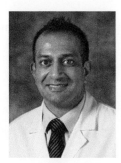

Dinesh Rao, MD
Editor

The management of head and neck and skull base pathologic conditions has evolved over the past several decades. Improvements in surgical technique have allowed surgeons to offer more and better options for the treatment of infectious and inflammatory diseases, trauma, malignancy, and the functional restoration of normal anatomy. The development of nonsurgical treatment options, such as conformal proton radiotherapy for malignancy, has resulted in improved local disease control and longer disease-free survival with less morbidity.

Imaging has played a central role in the diagnosis of disease and pretreatment planning, guiding both surgical and nonsurgical treatments. Over the past 20 years, CT, MRI, and PET imaging techniques have been refined to provide greater anatomic detail and improved lesion localization, which has led to more targeted treatment options for a variety of pathologic conditions. These imaging modalities are routinely used in the setting of presurgical planning, in evaluating for postoperative complications, and in posttreatment disease surveillance. In addition, ultrasound is frequently used as a screening modality and for routine biopsies. Imaging of head and neck disease is often central in multidisciplinary management decision making and is commonly reviewed by physicians and surgeons to guide optimal treatment.

The head and neck encompass many anatomic spaces and organ systems. Surgical management of oral and maxillofacial pathologic conditions intersects with nonsurgical specialties, all of which rely on imaging. This issue focuses on three anatomic areas, which are commonly encountered by oral and maxillofacial surgeons: the oral cavity, the sinonasal complex, and the skull base.

The articles contained in this issue serve as a complement to the surgeon's experience from an imaging standpoint. The included articles are ordered systematically according to each anatomic area and range from the simple to the complex. There is enough repetition within and between each of the articles to serve as a resource for anyone seeking an imaging-based perspective of the anatomy and pathologic conditions that occurs within and between these three regions. Whether you are beginning your journey or a seasoned master, we hope you will find the material contained herein to be helpful.

Dinesh Rao, MD
Department of Radiology
UF Health Jacksonville
655 West 8th Street
Jacksonville, FL 32209, USA

E-mail address:
dinesh.rao@jax.ufl.edu

Oral Maxillofacial Surg Clin N Am 35 (2023) xi
https://doi.org/10.1016/j.coms.2023.03.003

Infections of the Oral Cavity and Suprahyoid Neck

Jeet Patel, MD[a],*, Volodymyr Maymeskul, MD[a], John Kim, MD[b]

KEYWORDS

- Dental infection • Odontogenic abscess • Oral cavity • Tonsillitis • Sialadenitis

KEY POINTS

- Contrast-enhanced computed tomography with multiplanar reformatted images is the best imaging modality to evaluate complex acute infections of the oral and maxillofacial region and suprahyoid neck.
- A rim-enhancing fluid collection in the setting of infection is evidence of an organized abscess.
- The anatomic spaces involved by an abscess must be precisely reported to guide optimal treatment.
- Bone window reconstructed images aid in the detection of osseous sources of infection such as from the teeth and the temporomandibular joint, and in the detection of complications such as osteomyelitis.

INTRODUCTION

Acute infections of the oral and maxillofacial anatomy and suprahyoid neck range from simple superficial conditions that can be treated as an outpatient with oral medication to complex multispatial processes that require surgical intervention, intravenous antibiotics, and inpatient admission. This article will provide the reader with an imaging overview of the range of infections in this anatomic region that may be encountered by oral and maxillofacial surgeons, emergency physicians, and primary care providers.

APPROACH TO IMAGING

In general, diagnostic imaging is not indicated for the workup of superficial infections that can be diagnosed by history and physical examination. However, imaging is indicated when there is concern for deep space infection or for the detection of complications that can alter management. Computed tomography (CT) with intravenous contrast is the gold standard imaging modality in these situations because it tends to be readily available in the emergency department and hospital setting, and provides the ability to evaluate both soft tissues and fine osseous detail.[1] CT of the face or neck should be protocoled to fully include the primary area of concern and adjacent anatomical spaces where involvement needs to be excluded. Multiplanar reformatted images and reconstructed bone window images should be made.

When images are reviewed, there should be emphasis on providing clarity to the clinical problem by identifying the likely cause or site of origin of an infection, conveying the extent of an infection, and identifying key complications that might change management.

On CT, findings that support the presence of infection are nonspecific but associated with inflammation including edema manifesting as

a Department of Radiology, University of Florida College of Medicine – Jacksonville, 655 West 8th Street C90, Clinical Center 2nd Floor, Jacksonville, FL 32209, USA; b Department of Radiology, University of Michigan, 1500 East Medical Center Drive B2A205, Ann Arbor, MI 48109, USA
* Corresponding author. Department of Radiology, University of Florida College of Medicine – Jacksonville, 655 West 8th Street C90, Clinical Center 2nd Floor, Jacksonville, FL 32209.
E-mail address: jeet.patel@jax.ufl.edu

Oral Maxillofacial Surg Clin N Am 35 (2023) 283–296
https://doi.org/10.1016/j.coms.2023.01.001
1042-3699/23/© 2023 Elsevier Inc. All rights reserved.

stranding in fat, thickening of the involved and adjacent soft tissues, and potentially overlying skin thickening; in addition, reactive lymph node enlargement may be present in the regional lymphatic drainage pathway. It should be noted that such findings can also be present because of other causes of edema and soft tissue injury, such as trauma, sequela of radiation therapy, generalized edema from volume overload, and angioedema.

The primary role of intravenous contrast in the workup is to identify an abscess as a complication of an infection that might require drainage. An organized abscess will typically demonstrate a rim-enhancing wall with internal cavitary change. Gas can occasionally also be present in an abscess. In addition, contrast may be helpful to identify subtle inflammation by demonstrating reactive enhancement of inflamed tissue. Furthermore, if contrast has been administered, regional vessels must be evaluated to rule out important vascular complications such as venous thrombophlebitis.

CT image reconstruction in bone window is compulsory because this facilitates the detection of the site of origin in odontogenic infections, detection of osteomyelitis, and detection of radiopaque obstructive sialoliths in the setting of salivary gland infections. Bone window images can also aid in the detection of foreign bodies.

ODONTOGENIC INFECTIONS

Most maxillofacial infections have an odontogenic cause. The pathogenesis of dental infections often begins with dental caries and periapical periodontal disease, which are common chronic conditions. On CT, dental caries can be identified by the presence of erosion of the enamel and/or dentin of the tooth, and periapical disease consists of widening of the periodontal ligament secondary to inflammation and is manifested by periapical lucency on imaging.[2,3] Both these findings are detectable on dental radiography but can also be readily seen on reconstructed bone window CT images (**Fig. 1**). CT can also demonstrate further advanced pathology from periapical lucency including erosion and dehiscence of overlying alveolar process cortical bone encasing the root of a tooth. Each of these findings can be chronic and are not on their own diagnostic for infection but rather evidence of dental disease that may serve as the source of an infection. Therefore, to diagnose a localized acute dental infection on cross-sectional imaging, there must be visible surrounding extension of the inflammation with findings such as adjacent soft tissue thickening or subcutaneous fat stranding from cellulitis.[4] A more advanced localized infection may also result in the formation of an abscess in the adjacent subperiosteal space or in adjacent soft tissues. It should be noted that advanced infections with abscess can also form as a complication of dental procedures such as dental extractions. On confirming the presence of inflammation compatible with an acute infection, the bone window should then be used to identify neighboring dehiscence or erosion in adjacent alveolar cortical bone to help identify the offending tooth.

Many localized infections can be diagnosed with physical examination and treated without obtaining imaging. Panoramic dental radiography is helpful for determining the extent of underlying dental disease and for treatment planning. However, CT with intravenous contrast should be obtained if there is any concern for a deep space infection.[5] In the remainder of this section, a brief overview of pertinent oral cavity and adjacent spatial anatomy (floor of the mouth/sublingual, submandibular, masticator, canine, buccal, and mental spaces) is provided along with some representative cases to demonstrate the extent and type of infections that may be seen on CT examination.

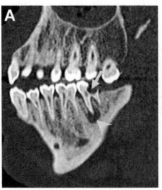
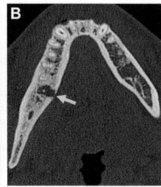

Fig. 1. Dental decay and periodontal disease. Sagittal bone window CT image (*A*) demonstrates dental caries (*arrow*) with erosion of the enamel and dentin of the second mandibular molar and periapical lucency (*arrowhead*) along the root of this tooth; the adjacent first molar serves as a normal comparison. Axial bone window image (*B*) demonstrates additional lingual alveolar cortical erosion (*arrow*) associated with the periapical lucency.

The floor of the mouth is bounded superiorly by the mucosa beneath the tongue, inferiorly by the hammock-like mylohyoid muscle, anteriorly by the posterior surface of the symphyseal mandible, and laterally by the mylohyoid muscle because it curves upward on either side to attach to the bodies of the mandible at the mylohyoid line (**Fig. 2**). Within the floor of the mouth, there are bilateral sublingual spaces divided by the genioglossus and geniohyoid muscles. An odontogenic infection can spread into the sublingual space if it breaches the lingual mandibular cortex above the mylohyoid line (**Fig. 3**); below the mylohyoid line such a breach would lead to direct extension into the submandibular space (**Fig. 4**),[6] which is inferior to the mandible and mylohyoid muscle and anterior and superior to the hyoid bone. There is a posterior edge of the mylohyoid over which the sublingual space communicates with the submandibular space, and it is by this route that an infection in the sublingual space generally spreads into the submandibular space. Clinical suspicion for spread of infection into the sublingual and submandibular spaces is an indication for CT with contrast. A precise description of the involved spaces must be reported because it can affect operative management; in particular, an intraoral approach for drainage might be used for an abscess confined to the sublingual space but an extraoral approach might be used for an abscess in the submandibular space.[7] Furthermore, infection in these spaces can lead to airway compromise from mass effect on the tongue and oral airway. Ludwig angina is a rare clinical situation where a patient presents with acute progressive airway compromise, dysphagia, and firm neck swelling secondary to cellulitis or abscess involving the bilateral sublingual and submandibular spaces, which is usually caused by a dental infection and requires urgent surgical intervention (see **Fig. 3**).[2,7]

The masticator space consists of the muscles of mastication, which surround the ramus, posterior body, and angle of the mandible. These muscles consist of the medial pterygoid and lateral pterygoid muscles medially, and the masseter and temporalis muscles laterally (**Fig. 5**). The temporalis also extends far superiorly along the head because it originates along the calvarium. Masticator space infections tend to arise from the molar teeth (**Fig. 6**), and the broad extent of the space can permit the far spread of an infection if not controlled.[4] Trismus can be a symptom of masticator space involvement.[8]

The canine space extends from the superior lip to the inferior periorbital level and is located between thin muscles of facial expression, which are not well resolved on cross-sectional imaging (**Fig. 7**). Through this space, infections of anterior maxillary teeth can extend to the periorbital tissues.[8] Periorbital/preseptal inflammatory swelling can be an indication for CT in order to exclude postseptal and retrobulbar spread of cellulitis, which can require intravenous antibiotics. This is also a pathway for the intracranial complication of cavernous sinus thrombosis through valveless veins in the orbits.

Typically, an infection breaching through the buccal aspects of the maxillary and mandibular alveolar ridges will do so within the confines of the margin of attachment of the buccinator muscle that originates from both the mandibular and maxillary alveolar processes (**Fig. 8**); as such it will remain a localized vestibular space infection (**Fig. 9**). However, although uncommon, if an

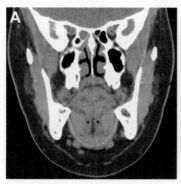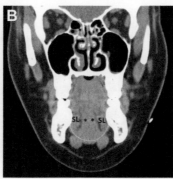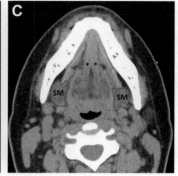

Fig. 2. Sublingual space anatomy. Coronal CT images (*A*, *B*) show the mylohyoid muscle (*white dotted line*) with hammock-like configuration forming the inferior boundary of the floor of the mouth and attaching at the mylohyoid line of the bodies of the mandible, and the sublingual spaces (*orange*) divided by the genioglossus muscles (*asterisk*). The sublingual spaces contain the sublingual glands (SL). Axial image (*C*) demonstrates the posterior edge of the lateral aspects of the mylohyoid (*white dotted line*) abutting the SM, and the sublingual space communicates with the submandibular space along this posterior edge of the mylohyoid.

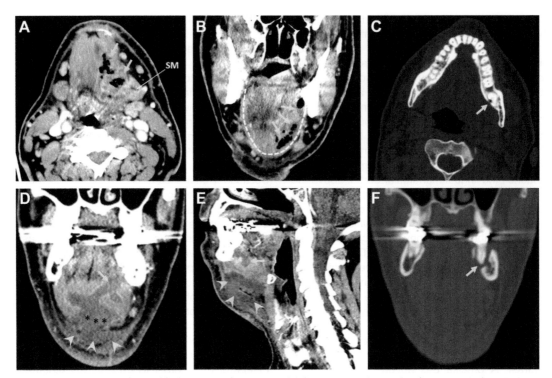

Fig. 3. Sublingual and submandibular space abscess. Axial (*A*) contrast-enhanced soft tissue window CT image demonstrates a gas and fluid-containing abscess (*arrows*) in the left submandibular space at the level of the left SM, and coronal image (*B*) demonstrates the abscess originates in the contiguous sublingual space (*arrows*) bounded by the mylohyoid muscle (*white dashed line*). Axial bone window image (*C*) demonstrates periapical lucency at the third mandibular molar with overlying erosion of the lingual alveolar cortex (*arrow*) as the source of the infection. In a different patient, coronal and sagittal (*D, E*) soft tissue window images demonstrate an abscess in the left sublingual space (*arrows*), which crosses into the right sublingual space and inferiorly through a gap (*asterisks*) in the mylohyoid likely from a mylohyoid boutonniere and into the submandibular/submental space with cellulitis in this area (*arrowheads*); this bilateral involvement and related mass effect may be seen in Ludwig angina, a clinical diagnosis. Coronal bone window image (*F*) demonstrates periapical lucency (*arrow*) at a left mandibular molar with overlying erosion of the lingual cortex as the source of the infection.

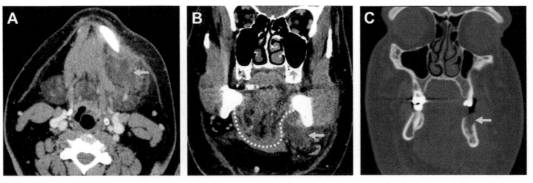

Fig. 4. Direct submandibular abscess. Axial (*A*) and coronal (*B*) contrast-enhanced soft tissue window CT images demonstrate an abscess in the left submandibular space (*arrows*) causing mass effect on and medially displacing the left wall of the mylohyoid muscle (*white dashed line*) without communication of the abscess with the sublingual space. Coronal bone window image (*C*) demonstrates a recent extraction cavity (*arrow*) of a left mandibular molar, from which the infection arose as a postoperative complication.

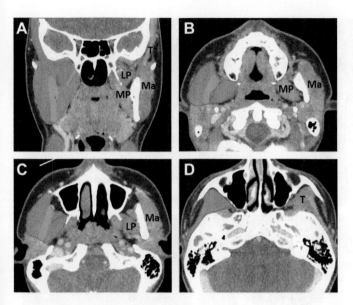

Fig. 5. Masticator space anatomy. Coronal (A) and axial (B–D) CT images demonstrate the masticator space musculature (right masticator space shaded in orange), which includes the medial pterygoid (MP), lateral pterygoid (LP), masseter (Ma), and temporalis (T). Note that the coronal image does not show the full cranial extent of the temporalis.

osseous breach related to periodontal disease occurs beyond the margin of the origin of the buccinator muscle, then a dental infection can spread into the buccal space located lateral to the buccinator muscle.[9]

Finally, the mental space is a potential space anterior to the symphyseal part of the mandible, and dental infections may spread into this space through cortical breaches in the facial alveolar processes of the anterior mandibular teeth (Fig. 10).

Other Osseous Infections

More advanced infection in the bone itself can occur in the form of osteomyelitis of the maxilla or mandible. Osteomyelitis is defined as infection of the cancellous bone and marrow. Findings suggestive of acute osteomyelitis on CT include periosteal reaction along the cortex (Fig. 11),

aggressive bone erosion (Fig. 12B), and adjacent soft tissue inflammation.[10,11] Causes for this include advanced dental disease from caries and periodontal disease, violation of the soft tissues and bone from trauma and fracture, or complications of surgery such as infection along fixation hardware or prostheses. Underlying medical conditions that might predispose a patient to developing osteomyelitis include conditions associated with chronic microvascular disease such as diabetes mellitus, immunocompromising disease, or underlying bone pathologic condition such as osteopetrosis or Paget disease.[4,11] If a patient has had prior radiation therapy in the area, then osteoradionecrosis is a leading differential diagnosis, which can also result in superimposed osteomyelitis. Malignancy such as squamous cell carcinoma invading the bone, osseous metastasis, or other aggressive neoplasms such as

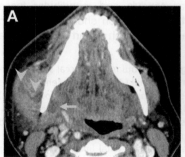 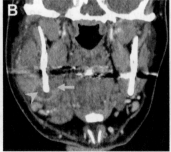 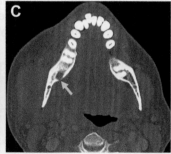

Fig. 6. Masticator space abscess. Axial (A) and coronal (B) contrast-enhanced soft tissue window CT images demonstrate a rim-enhancing abscess in the right medial pterygoid muscle (arrows), which extends under the inferior edge of the mandible and into the right masseter muscle (arrowheads). Axial bone window image (C) demonstrates a recent right third mandibular molar extraction cavity with adjacent erosion of the lingual alveolar cortex (arrow) as the source of the infection.

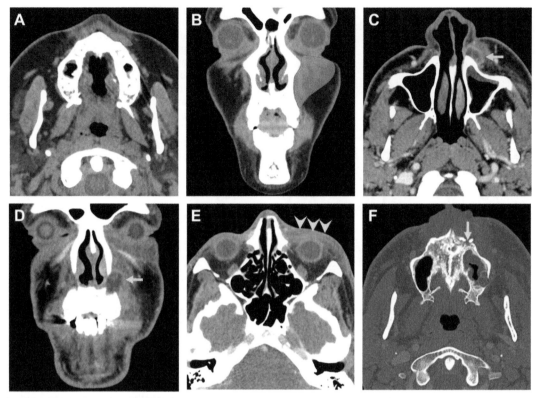

Fig. 7. Canine space anatomy and abscess. Axial (*A*) and coronal (*B*) CT images demonstrate the canine space (*orange*) extending from the soft tissues overlying the maxillary canine and extending superiorly to the inferior periorbital level. In a different patient, axial (*C*) and coronal (*D*) contrast-enhanced soft tissue window images show a rim-enhancing abscess (*arrows*) in the left canine space with a more superior axial image (*E*) showing cellulitis spread to the left periorbital tissues (*arrowheads*); axial bone window image (*F*) demonstrates dental caries and periapical lucency at the left maxillary canine with overlying erosion of the facial alveolar cortex (*arrow*) as the source of the infection.

myeloma must also be considered, especially in the absence of clinical signs of infection and/or if there is an adjacent mass-like soft tissue lesion.

The temporomandibular joint is unique because it is the only synovial joint in the extracranial head and neck, and as such, it can be affected by osteoarthritis, inflammatory arthropathies, and septic arthritis. In early septic arthritis, there may be few signs of an infection. CT may demonstrate increased density of joint fluid and synovial enhancement but these are nonspecific findings that may be present with any inflammatory synovial joint condition. In later stages of infection, CT may demonstrate aggressive lytic erosion from osteomyelitis in the bone of the joint including the mandibular condyle and mandibular fossa (**Fig. 12**). Particular attention should be paid to the mandibular fossa, which is part of the middle

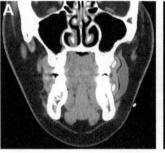
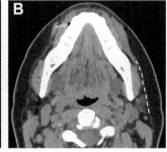

Fig. 8. Vestibular and buccal space anatomy. Coronal (*A*) CT image demonstrates the vestibular spaces (*yellow ovals*) adjacent and lateral to the alveolar processes of the maxilla and mandible and confined laterally by the buccinator muscle (*blue*), and axial image (*B*) shows air (*arrow*) in the inferior right vestibular space. The buccal space (*orange*) is lateral to the buccinator muscle and deep to the platysma muscle (*white dashed line*).

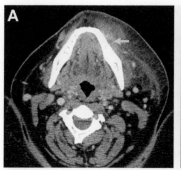 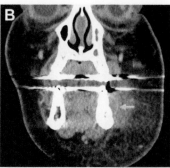 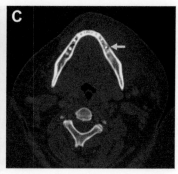

Fig. 9. Vestibular space abscess. Axial (*A*) and coronal (*B*) contrast-enhanced soft tissue window CT images demonstrate a rim-enhancing abscess (*arrows*) immediately adjacent to the buccal aspect of the alveolar process of the left body of the mandible, with the buccinator muscle superficial to the abscess. Axial bone window image (*C*) demonstrates adjacent left second premolar periapical lucency and buccal alveolar cortex erosion (*arrow*) as the source of the infection.

skull base, because full breach through this bone could enable the spread of infection into the intracranial compartment and resulting complications can include meningitis, extra-axial abscess, or cerebral abscess. Additionally, enhanced cross-sectional imaging can reveal a peripherally enhancing collection of the distended inflamed synovium containing pus and surrounding cellulitis in adjacent spaces.[12] The adjacent external auditory canal may also demonstrate inflammatory soft tissue thickening.

SKIN

The skin is the largest organ tissue in the face and neck, and indeed the whole body. One of the prime functions of the skin is to protect the body from infection, and so a breach of the skin can serve as a portal for infection. For example, a deep cut, abrasion, insect bite, or foreign body might all serve as sources of infection. In addition, dermal appendages such as hair follicles, sebaceous glands, and sweat glands can serve as a nidus for bacterial infection if they become plugged and inflamed, and this can give rise to cellulitis or local abscess formation.[13] An infection of the skin should be readily visible on physical examination but imaging can be obtained to assess for a drainable abscess and its deep extent.[14] If the infection is originating from the skin, the epicenter of the inflammation should be superficial and oriented toward the dermis rather than

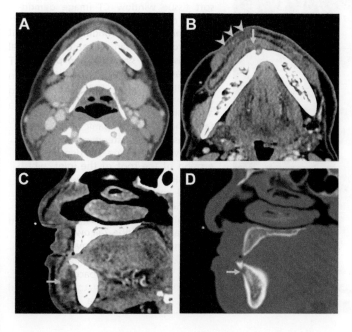

Fig. 10. Mental space anatomy and abscess. Axial CT image (*A*) demonstrates the mental space (*orange*), a potential space immediately anterior to the mandible. In a different patient, axial (*B*) and sagittal (*C*) contrast-enhanced soft tissue window images show a rim-enhancing abscess (*arrows*) in the mental space with surrounding cellulitis (*arrowheads*), and sagittal bone window image (*D*) demonstrates dental caries and periapical lucency at the right mandibular lateral incisor with overlying erosion of the facial alveolar cortex (*arrow*) as the source of the infection.

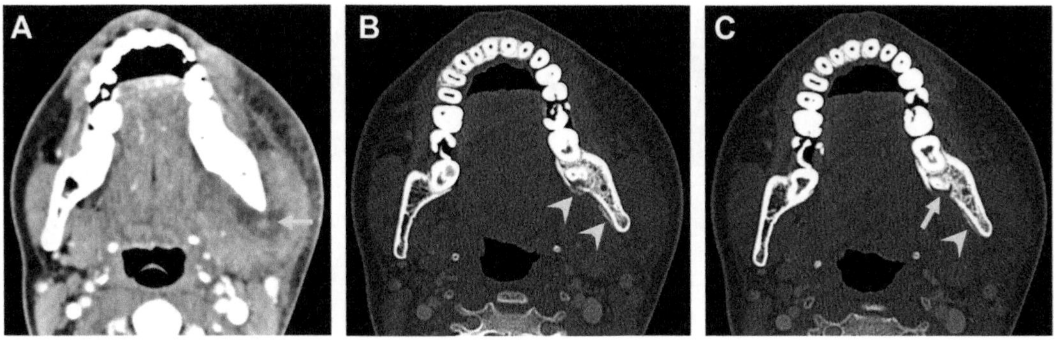

Fig. 11. Mandibular osteomyelitis. Axial (*A*) contrast-enhanced soft tissue window CT image demonstrates odontogenic left masticator space abscess (*arrow*). Axial bone window images (*B, C*) demonstrate periosteal reaction (*arrowheads*) concerning for osteomyelitis along the left mandibular angle and ramus, and periapical lucency and lingual alveolar cortical erosion (*arrow*) as the site of origin of the infection.

emanating from deeper structures. An organized abscess can be diagnosed when there is a fluid collection with peripheral enhancement in the subcutaneous tissue in close proximity to the skin surface (**Fig. 13**). The images should also be carefully reviewed to detect a radiopaque or radiolucent foreign body.

In the lower face, the imager should be careful not to misdiagnose a superficial cutaneous infection as an odontogenic infection extending superficially. On imaging, inflammation that is centered in the superficial subcutaneous tissues and the absence of conspicuous soft tissue thickening immediately adjacent to the buccal or facial aspect of the teeth can help exclude an odontogenic cause. Moreover, the lack of oral physical examination findings can aid in excluding an odontogenic source of infection.

Aggressive infections of the facial skin can lead to postseptal orbital cellulitis and intracranial spread of infection with complications such as cavernous sinus thrombosis. For this reason, the imager must carefully assess the visualized orbits and intracranial compartment as part of their checklist and the patency of vessels if contrast has been administered.

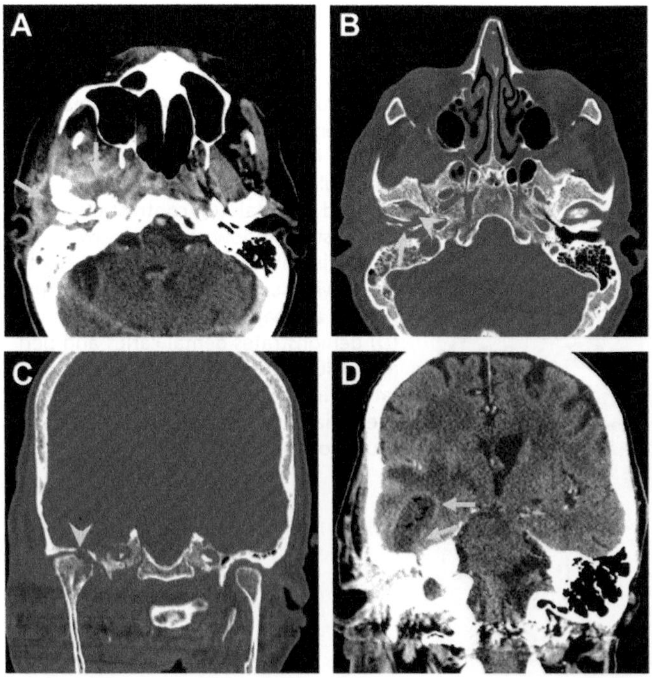

Fig. 12. Temporomandibular joint septic arthritis. Axial (*A*) contrast-enhanced soft tissue window CT image demonstrates a peripherally enhancing collection (*arrows*) surrounding the right temporomandibular joint compatible with distended synovium and pus from septic arthritis extending medially into the parapharyngeal space, and axial bone window image (*B*) demonstrates aggressive erosion of the condylar head (*arrowhead*) and tympanic plate (*arrow*) from associated osteomyelitis. Coronal bone window image (*C*) demonstrates erosion of the roof of the joint, which is the skull base floor (*arrowhead*), and coronal soft tissue image (*D*) demonstrates complication of an intracranial cerebral abscess containing gas in the right temporal lobe (*arrows*) with surrounding vasogenic edema and mass effect.

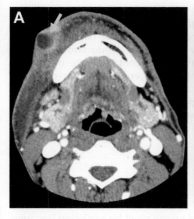
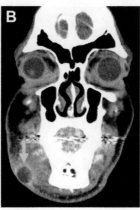

Fig. 13. Subcutaneous abscess of dermal origin. Axial (A) and coronal (B) contrast-enhanced soft tissue window CT images demonstrate a superficial rim-enhancing abscess (arrows) at the level of the mandible immediately deep to the skin surface and with peripheralized regional inflammation in keeping with a dermal source of the infection.

LYMPH NODES

Lymphadenitis is the inflammation of a lymph node secondary to infection. This may be diagnosed with physical examination revealing tenderness and swelling of lymph nodes without the need of imaging. Cross-sectional imaging may be obtained if there is concern to rule out an abscess or other mass lesion. Uncomplicated lymphadenitis will typically demonstrate an enlarged lymph node with inflammatory stranding or haziness in the surrounding adjacent fat. The preservation of a normal fatty hilum in the lymph node can be a reassuring feature of a benign process although this is not completely definitive for benignity.[15,16] Therefore, it is often recommended to obtain clinical follow-up to ensure the resolution of the lymph node enlargement.

On contrast-enhanced imaging, an area of hypoenhancement or nonenhancement representing cavitary change in an inflamed, enlarged lymph node is a sign of suppurative lymphadenitis with abscess formation (Fig. 14). Suppurative lymphadenitis most commonly occurs in the pediatric and young adult population.[15] An important

differential consideration for this is metastatic necrotic lymphadenopathy and, especially in the adult population, this differential diagnosis needs to be excluded.[15,16] Moreover, a careful search should be performed of anatomy drained through the involved lymph node to seek out a neoplastic lesion that may be the cause of this differential possibility; in the pharynx, this may be difficult when there is nonspecific tonsillar hypertrophy that limits the evaluation for detecting a mucosal lesion, and for this reason, visual inspection of the pharynx and larynx should be performed.

OROPHARYNGEAL AND RETROPHARYNGEAL SPACES

Acute pharyngitis involving the oropharyngeal space and, in particular, the palatine tonsils is very common, with viral causes being more common that bacterial. The palatine tonsils are located between the anterior and posterior tonsillar pillars, formed by the palatoglossus and palatopharyngeus muscles, respectively. Tonsillar inflammation can be diagnosed by history and physical examination. CT with contrast can play a role by assessing

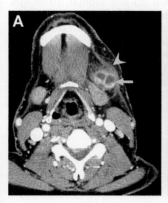
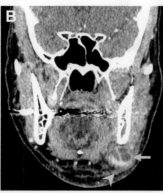

Fig. 14. Suppurative lymphadenitis. Axial (A) and coronal (B) contrast-enhanced soft tissue window CT images demonstrate an enlarged left level 1B lymph node (arrows) containing a multiloculated rim-enhancing abscess compatible with suppurative lymphadenitis, and with overlying inflammatory fat stranding and thickening of the platysma muscle (arrowheads).

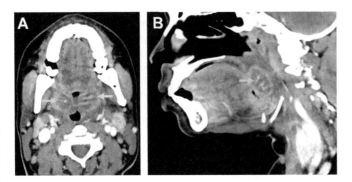

Fig. 15. Palatine tonsillitis. Axial (*A*) and sagittal (*B*) contrast-enhanced soft tissue window CT images demonstrate bilaterally enlarged and edematous palatine tonsils that contact each other and contain a "tiger stripe," striated pattern of enhancement (*arrows*) consistent with tonsillitis, and without any organized rim-enhancing abscess.

for complications such as a drainable tonsillar abscess or deep space extension of the infection. Tonsillitis will demonstrate nonspecific hypertrophy of the tonsillar tissues, usually bilaterally, which might be symmetric or asymmetric. A "tiger stripe" striated pattern of enhancement can be seen in the palatine tonsils when there is nonsuppurative tonsillitis (**Fig. 15**).[17] The presence of a rim-enhancing fluid collection is diagnostic for a tonsillar abscess (**Fig. 16**A, B). On imaging, extension of an abscess into other spaces must be excluded because that could change management. For example, lateral extension of a palatine tonsillar abscess into the parapharyngeal space might necessitate lateral extraoral approach for surgical drainage, whereas a drainable abscess confined to the tonsillar fossa can be drained by intraoral approach.[7] Extension of the infection into the

retropharyngeal space must be excluded because it might necessitate a change to the surgical approach and drain placement (**Fig. 16**C, D). Finally, CT with contrast also helps diagnose septic thrombophlebitis, which along with tonsillitis and septic emboli, makes up a constellation of findings seen in Lemierre syndrome.[18]

The retropharyngeal space is a potential space between the posterior wall of the oropharynx and prevertebral musculature, and it extends from the skull base into the mediastinum. Therefore, the retropharyngeal space can provide a conduit for the spread of infection from the head and neck to the mediastinum. In children, the most common cause of retropharyngeal infection is spread of pharyngitis, tonsillitis or sinusitis related to an upper respiratory tract infection via lymphatic drainage into retropharyngeal

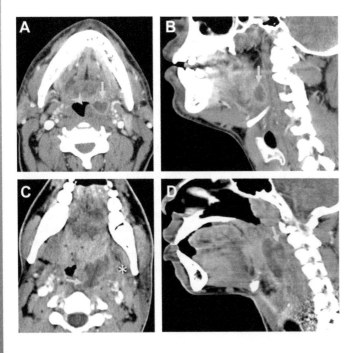

Fig. 16. Palatine tonsillar abscess. Axial (*A*) and sagittal (*B*) contrast-enhanced soft tissue window CT images demonstrate a rim-enhancing fluid collection in the left palatine tonsil (*arrows*) in a patient with acute sore throat and fever consistent with tonsillar abscess, which causes narrowing of the oropharyngeal airway (*arrowhead*). In a different patient, axial (*C*) and sagittal (*D*) images demonstrate a left palatine tonsillar abscess with frank posterior extension of the abscess fluid collection into the retropharyngeal space (*arrows*). The abscess does not extend into the left parapharyngeal space (*asterisk*) (image *C*).

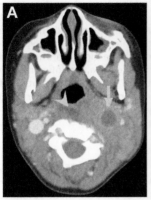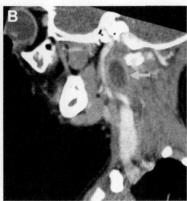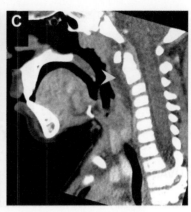

Fig. 17. Retropharyngeal suppurative adenitis. Axial (*A*) and sagittal (*B, C*) contrast-enhanced soft tissue window CT images of a 2-year old male patient with neck pain and swelling demonstrate a lateralized rim-enhancing fluid collection in the retropharyngeal space consistent with retropharyngeal suppurative adenitis/lymph node abscess (*arrows*), and also a retropharyngeal effusion (*arrowheads*) extending inferiorly without an enhancing wall to suggest abscess extension.

space lymph nodes.[19] Retropharyngeal space lymph nodes can be found on CT located just medial to the cervical internal carotid arteries. Retropharyngeal lymphadenitis can be further complicated by suppurative lymphadenitis with abscess formation (**Fig. 17**).[20] This presents a risk for extension of the infection into the broader retropharyngeal space if it ruptures. A key distinguishing finding that an abscess in the retropharyngeal space is originating from a lymph node is that it is lateralized in position in keeping with the nodal anatomic position. In older patients, an injury to or violation of the posterior pharyngeal wall is a more common cause for retropharyngeal abscess (**Fig. 18**).[19] If retropharyngeal infection must be excluded, it is appropriate to obtain a CT of the neck that extends inferiorly through the superior mediastinum so that the whole retropharyngeal space is covered. Edema without a rim-enhancing fluid collection can be seen within the retropharyngeal space in other settings as well including, for example, secondary to trauma in the cervical spine or neck, from postoperative changes after a recent anterior approach cervical spine surgery, or as sequela of radiation therapy.

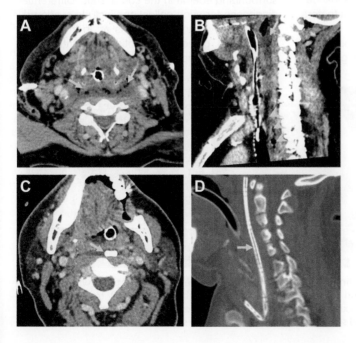

Fig. 18. Retropharyngeal abscess. Axial (*A*) and sagittal (*B*) contrast-enhanced soft tissue window images of a 50-year-old man who ingested antifreeze with complication of esophageal perforation and retropharyngeal abscess (*arrows*) containing gas and fluid extending to the mediastinum (*arrowheads*). Follow-up exam axial (*C*) and sagittal (*D*) images show a retropharyngeal drain (*arrows*) placed as part of treatment.

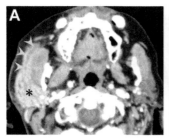
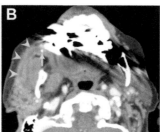

Fig. 19. Parotitis from obstructive calculus. Axial (*A, B*) contrast-enhanced soft tissue window images demonstrate asymmetric enlargement and hyperenhancement of the right parotid gland (*asterisk*) from edema and inflammation consistent with parotitis, and dilation of the right main parotid duct (*arrowheads*) secondary to an obstructive calculus (*arrow*) near its orifice.

SALIVARY GLANDS

The major salivary glands include the parotid, submandibular, and sublingual glands. CT provides excellent depiction of the soft tissue and contours of the parotid glands and submandibular glands (SMs); the sublingual glands are not as well resolved amid adjacent soft tissues of the floor of the month. The parotid duct (Stensen duct) extends anteriorly from the parotid gland, courses lateral to the masseter muscle and through the buccal space fat, and penetrates through the buccinator muscle of the cheek with its orifice at a papilla lateral to the second maxillary molar.[21] The submandibular duct (Wharton duct) extends anteriorly from the SM and courses through the sublingual space before draining via papillae into the oral cavity just lateral to the frenulum of the tongue.[22]

The key findings of salivary gland inflammation—referred to as sialadenitis (or also parotitis in the case of the parotid glands)—on imaging are enlargement of the gland and hyperenhancement of the tissue. There is a variety of risk factors for salivary gland infections but from an imaging perspective, a process causing obstruction or stasis of the secretory output of the salivary glands is

pathologic condition to exclude (**Figs. 19** and **20**). Ductal obstruction will manifest as ductal dilatation proximal to the site of obstruction or stricture. The main submandibular duct is normally not conspicuous on cross-sectional imaging, and the main parotid duct may be delineated but normally no fluid dilatation is visible within the duct. CT is the best modality for detecting radiopaque sialoliths and the expected course of the duct in question should be carefully evaluated to exclude a calculus. A submandibular calculus might be located in the sublingual space because the submandibular duct courses through the sublingual space. Approximately 80% to 90% of salivary duct calculi occur in the SM.[23] Nevertheless, it must be noted that 15% to 20% of sialoliths are not radiopaque and therefore not detectable on CT or radiography.[24]

As the salivary gland infection progresses, phlegmonous change and abscess may develop. An organized abscess would appear as a fluid collection with a peripherally enhancing wall and surrounding edema in the soft tissues. Differential diagnoses for such collections include cystic primary salivary gland neoplasms or, in the case of the parotid gland, a necrotic metastatic intraparotid lymph node; any presence of nodular

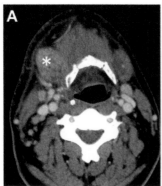
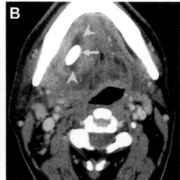
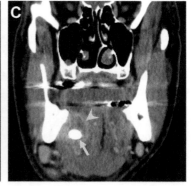

Fig. 20. Submandibular sialadenitis and sublingual abscess. Axial (*A*) contrast-enhanced soft tissue window image demonstrates asymmetric enlargement and hyperenhancement of the right SM (*asterisk*) from edema and inflammation consistent with sialadenitis. Axial (*B*) and coronal (*C*) images demonstrate an obstructive submandibular duct sialolith in the right sublingual space (*arrows*) with surrounding submandibular duct dilatation and abscess (*arrowheads*).

enhancing tissue associated with the lesion and/or a cystic lesion without expected proportionate surrounding inflammation should also raise suspicion for neoplastic disease.

Fluoroscopic sialography using iodinated contrast media can detect radiolucent calculi and other causes of filling defects in the ducts such as mucous plugs, and can also detect ductal strictures.[24] However, sialography is contraindicated in the setting of acute salivary gland infection due to the risk of contrast extravasating into inflamed glandular tissue and causing pain or damaging the glandular tissue.[24,25]

SUMMARY

CT is the best modality to evaluate patients with deep space and complex infections of the oral cavity and suprahyoid neck. To guide definitive treatment, surgeons and radiologists must have a comprehensive knowledge of anatomy and a thorough search pattern to detect the source of an infection, delineate its extent, and identify key complications that can change management.

CLINICS CARE POINTS

- Contrast-enhanced CT is indicated when a deep space infection is suspected and/or when a complication such as an abscess needs to be excluded.

- Bone window reconstructed images should be carefully reviewed to identify osseous sources of infection, osseous complications such as osteomyelitis, foreign bodies, and obstructive calculi in salivary gland ducts.

- An abscess extending into the submandibular space (from the sublingual space) or into the parapharyngeal space (from the palatine tonsil) might require an external approach to drainage rather than an intraoral approach.

- The absence of surrounding inflammation (eg, inflammatory fat stranding, adjacent reactive soft tissue thickening, and overlying skin thickening) or absence of clinical signs and symptoms of infection should raise suspicion for neoplastic disease as a differential consideration.

DECLARATION OF INTERESTS

The authors have no commercial or financial conflicts of interest.

REFERENCES

1. Shuaib W, Hashm M, Vijayasarathi A, et al. The use of facial CT for the evaluation of a suspected simple dentoalveolar abscess in the emergency department. Clin Med Res 2015;13:112–6.
2. Scheinfeld MH, Shifteh K, Avery LL, et al. Teeth: What radiologists should know. Radiographics 2012;32:1927–44.
3. Chapman MN, Nadgir R, Akman AS, et al. Periapical lucency around the tooth: Radiologic evaluation and differential diagnosis. Radiographics 2013;33:E15–32.
4. Patel J, Le RT, Haymes D, et al. Imaging of dental infections. Emerg Radiol 2022;29:197–205.
5. Ogle OE. Odontogenic infections. Dent Clin North Am 2017;61:235–52.
6. Ariji Y, Gotoh M, Kimura Y, et al. Odontogenic infection pathway to the submandibular space: imaging assessment. Int J Oral Maxillofac Surg 2002;31:165–9.
7. Osborn TM, Assael LA, Bell RB. Deep space neck infection: principles of surgical management. Oral Maxillofacial Surg Clin N Am 2008;20:465–73.
8. Lypka M, Hammoudeh J. Dentoalveolar infections. Oral Maxillofacial Surg Clin N Am 2011;23:415–24.
9. Schenck TL, Koban KC, Schlattau A. Updated anatomy of the buccal space and its implications for plastic, reconstructive and aesthetic procedures. J Plast Reconstr Aesthet Surg 2018;71:162–70.
10. Steinklein J, Nguyen V. Dental anatomy and pathology encountered on routine CT of the head and neck. AJR Am J Roentgenol 2013;201:W843–53.
11. Goupil MT, Banki M, Ferneini EM. Osteomyelitis and osteonecrosis of the jaws. In: Hupp JR, Ferneini EM, editors. Head, neck, and orofacial infections: an interdisciplinary approach. St. Louis: Elsevier; 2016. p. 222–31.
12. Gayle EA, Young SM, McKenna SJ, et al. Septic arthritis of the temporomandibular joint: case reports and review of the literature. J Emerg Med 2013;45:674–8.
13. Stulberg DL, Penrod MA, Blatny RA. Common bacterial skin infections. Am Fam Physician 2002;66:119–24.
14. Blankenship RB, Baker T. Imaging modalities in wounds and superficial skin infections. Emerg Med Clin North Am 2007;25:223–4.
15. Eisenmenger LB, Wiggins RH 3rd. Imaging of head and neck lymph nodes. Radiol Clin North Am 2015;53:115–32.
16. Hoang JK, Vanka J, Ludwig BJ, et al. Evaluation of cervical lymph nodes in head and neck cancer with CT and MRI: Tips, traps, and a systematic approach. AJR Am J Roentgenol 2013;200:W17–25.
17. Koontz NA, Seltman TA, Kralik SF, et al. Classic signs in head and neck imaging. Clin Radiol 2016;71:1211–22.

18. Bae YA, Lee IJ, Kim HB. Lemierre syndrome: a case report. J Korean Radiol Soc 2006;54:7–10.

19. Wald ER. Retropharyngeal infections in children. In: Post TW, editor. UpToDate. Waltham (MA): UpToDate; 2022.

20. Chong VFH, Fan YF. Radiology of the retropharyngeal space: pictorial review. Clin Radiol 2000;55: 740–8.

21. Kochhar A, Larian B, Azizzadeh B. Facial nerve and parotid gland anatomy. Otolaryngol Clin North Am 2016;49:273–84.

22. du Toit DF, Nortjé. Salivary glands: applied anatomy and clinical correlates. SADJ 2004;59:65–6, 69–71, 73-74.

23. Abdel Razek AAK, Mukherji S. Imaging of sialadenitis. NeuroRadiol J 2017;30:205–15.

24. Schlieve T, Kolokythas A, Miloro M. Salivary gland infections. In: Hupp JR, Ferneini EM, editors. Head, neck, and orofacial infections: an interdisciplinary approach. St. Louis: Elsevier; 2016. p. 232–47.

25. Reddy SS, Rakesh N, Raghev N, et al. Sialography: report of 3 cases. Indian J Dent Res 2009;20: 499–502.

Imaging of Maxillofacial Trauma

Miguel Fabrega, MD

KEYWORDS

- Nasoseptal • Orbital blowout • Naso-orbito-ethmoidal • Zygomaticomaxillary • LeFort
- Occlusion-bearing maxillary fragment • Markowitz-manson • Facial buttresses

KEY POINTS

- Radiology reports should focus on describing regional injury patterns and discussing factors most pertinent to surgical management.
- LeFort II and III injuries can be thought of as combinations of LeFort 1, zygomaticomaxillary complex, naso-orbito-ethmoidal, internal orbital, and nasoseptal injuries.
- Optimal fixation points for midface injuries coincide with the intersection of fracture pattern lines and regional facial buttresses.

INTRODUCTION

Maxillofacial trauma is commonly encountered in emergency departments. Computed tomography (CT) is the primary diagnostic imaging modality. Interpretation is aided by knowledge of the complex three-dimensional (3D) relationships of anatomy. In particular, understanding the relationship of the major facial buttresses to the zygomaticomaxillary complex (ZMC), naso-orbito-ethmoidal (NOE), and LeFort complex injuries allows for more complete understanding of principles of reduction and fixation. Comprehension of injury patterns allows the radiologist and surgeon to focus on the most clinically relevant features of each region. Using a subunit centered approach, the classic higher order complex pattern injuries can be understood in a manner that facilitates optimal treatment.

Epidemiology

The epidemiology of facial fractures varies depending on population and time period studied. An analysis of data from the Global Burden of Disease Study estimated more than 7 million new facial fractures worldwide during the year of 2017.[1] An earlier review of the US National Trauma Data Bank demonstrated more than 400,000 facial fracture-related ER visits in the United States alone during a single calendar year.[2] The most common injury mechanisms include interpersonal violence, motor vehicle collisions, falls, sports injuries, work accidents, and other mechanisms. A male predilection is often observed. The nasal bones and mandible are the most commonly fractured structures.[1-9]

Nasoseptal Injuries

Nasoseptal injuries are among the most common injuries of the face due to the anterior projection of the nose and its fragility.[10] Knowledge of anatomy aids diagnoses and injury characterization. The bony bridge of the nose consists of paired nasal bones. Lateral to the nasal bones are the frontal processes of the maxilla, interposed between the nasal bones and medial orbital rims. Together these structures form the nasal pyramid, which articulates with the nasal process of the frontal bone at the frontomaxillary and frontonasal sutures (**Fig. 1**A). At the midline, the vertically oriented bony septum is formed by 2 bones, the perpendicular plate of the ethmoid and the vomer. These anchor the nose to the skull base and lower maxilla, respectively. The cartilaginous portion of the nasal septum is located anteriorly below the

Department of Diagnostic and Interventional Imaging, McGovern Medical School at UTHealth Houston, University of Texas at Houston, MSB 2.130B, 6431 Fannin Street, Houston, TX 77030, USA
E-mail address: Miguel.G.Fabrega@uth.tmc.edu

Oral Maxillofacial Surg Clin N Am 35 (2023) 297–309
https://doi.org/10.1016/j.coms.2023.02.001
1042-3699/23/© 2023 Elsevier Inc. All rights reserved.

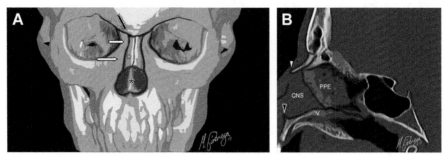

Fig. 1. Nasoseptal anatomy. (*A*) The frontal skull and anatomy of the bony nasal skeleton. The nasal pyramid consists of the nasal bones (*white asterisk*), and the frontal process of the maxilla (*white arrow*). Superiorly, the nasal pyramid articulates with the nasal process of the frontal bone (*black arrow*). The bony nasal septum (*black asterisk*) can be seen within the nasal aperture. (*B*) Sagittal illustration of midline nasoseptal anatomy. The bony nasal septum consists of the perpendicular plate of the ethmoid superiorly (PPE) and the vomer inferiorly (V). The nasal bones protrude anteriorly from the superior aspect of the nasal aperture (*white arrowhead*). The anterior nasal spine (*black arrowhead*) protrudes anteriorly from the midline inferior nasal aperture. All 4 bony structures support the cartilaginous nasal septum (CNS).

nasal bones and interposed between the vomer and perpendicular plate of the ethmoid. The anterior nasal spine protrudes from the inferior midline nasal aperture and anchors the base of the cartilaginous septum (**Fig. 1**A, B). Lateral cartilaginous plates support the lateral soft tissues of the nose and nostrils.[10,11]

Nasoseptal fractures are commonly diagnosed using CT (**Fig. 2**). Immediate management considerations center around managing epistaxis. The septal nasal cartilage is even more fragile than the bony structures but cartilaginous injuries are usually not detected by CT. As such, any bony injury requires assessment by speculum

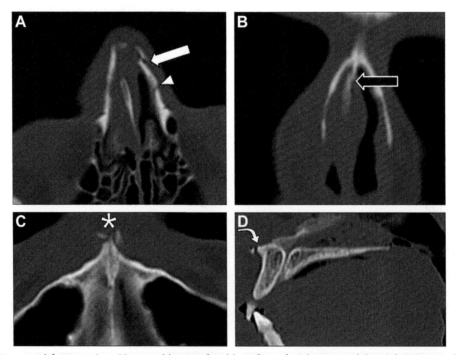

Fig. 2. Nasoseptal fractures in a 23-year-old man after blunt force facial trauma. (*A*) Axial CT image shows displaced nasal bone fracture (*white arrow*) and a nondisplaced fracture of the frontal process of the maxilla (*white arrowhead*). (*B*) Coronal CT reformat demonstrating a mildly displaced fracture of the perpendicular plate of the ethmoid (*black arrow*). (*C*) Axial CT image with fractures of the anterior nasal spine (*white asterisk*). (*D*) Sagittal CT reformat shows a fractured anterior nasal spine (*curved white arrow*).

examination to exclude a septal hematoma. Septal hematomas must be drained acutely because they may result in osteonecrosis, malunion, or abscess.[10,11] Restoring esthetics and normal ventilation can usually be accomplished by closed reduction. This can be performed in the early outpatient setting once soft tissue swelling subsides but before fractures begin to set. In some cases, septorhinoplasty may be necessary to restore form and function.[10] CT evaluation should focus on fracture detection and describing details that may aid reduction planning. Nasal pyramid deviation, angulation, and/or impaction can be described. Reduction of bony septal fractures with acute bowing, telescoping, L-shaped angulation, or stair stepping may require forceps.[11]

Orbital Injuries

CT evaluation of the orbits is imperative to diagnosis of traumatic bony and soft tissue injuries. The orbital walls are often injured by transmission of forces through the orbital rim resulting in "blowout" fractures that increase orbital volume and displace the walls of the orbit outward.[12] Blowout fractures are most common at the orbital floor and medial orbital wall. Classically, blow-out fractures involve the internal orbital walls only, known as "pure" fractures. Involvement of the orbital rim known as "impure" fractures are usually features of other more complex midface injuries (ZMC, NOE, LeFort II, and so forth).[11] Orbital fractures are often managed conservatively with nose-blowing precautions to prevent air from entering the orbit.13 Surgical repair may be indicated for large bony fragments, severe fragment displacement, or significant comminution.[11]

The intraorbital fat and extraocular muscles may herniate through fracture defects (**Fig. 3**)

resulting in enophthalmos or muscle entrapment.[12] Large volumes of herniated soft tissue or clinical evidence of entrapment are also surgical indications. Retrobulbar hematomas can occur (**Fig. 4**) and should be communicated emergently because they may lead to orbital compartment syndrome requiring decompression via lateral canthotomy.[11,13,14] Multiple types of globe injury may be identifiable by CT including lens dislocations, traumatic cataracts, acute corneal rupture, foreign body retention, retinal detachment, vitreous hemorrhage, and globe rupture (**Figs. 5** and **6**).

Naso-Orbito-Ethmoidal Injuries

NOE fractures are complex injuries of the midface that involve the nasal pyramid, the medial orbital walls, and the ethmoid air cells. These injuries involve 2 major facial buttresses and separate a portion of the inferior medial orbit from the remainder of the skull.[11,14,15] The injury pattern includes a fracture across the lateral nasal pyramid from the nasal aperture to the medial orbital rim at the level of frontomaxillary suture, fractures extending between the medial and inferior orbital rims along the medial orbital wall and orbital floor, and a fracture across the anterior maxilla from the inferior orbital rim into the inferior nasal aperture (**Fig. 7**).[11] Two major facial buttresses are involved. The medial maxillary vertical buttress (nasomaxillary buttress) and the upper transverse maxillary buttress (inferior orbital rim) are each traversed twice.[11,14,15] The points of intersection of the fractures and buttresses involve thick bone and are thus ideal fixation points for surgical reduction. As such, the most common sites of plate fixation are the frontomaxillary suture, the inferior orbital rim, and nasomaxillary buttress. If there is nasal

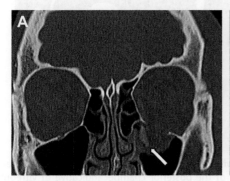
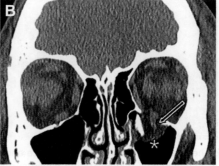

Fig. 3. Left orbital floor blowout fracture in a 25-year-old woman after facial trauma with extraocular muscle herniation. (*A*) Bone window coronal reformat CT image demonstrates an acute fracture fragment (*white arrow*) of the left orbital floor displaced inferiorly into the left maxillary sinus. (*B*) Soft tissue window coronal CT shows a moderate amount of intraorbital fat (*asterisk*) protruding through the orbital floor defect into the maxillary antrum. The left inferior rectus (*black arrow*) also protrudes into the defect with distortion of the muscle belly contour.

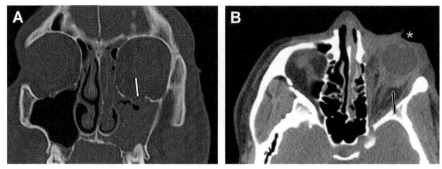

Fig. 4. Left orbital floor blowout fracture in a 33-year-old man after trauma with associated retrobulbar hematoma. (*A*) Coronal CT reformats and bone windows demonstrating a comminuted fracture of the left orbital floor (*white arrow*) with slight depression. (*B*) Axial noncontrast CT in soft tissue windows with a moderate-sized intraconal retrobulbar hematoma (*black arrow*) along the posterior globe at the optic nerve insertion. The patient is status canthotomy with a soft tissue defect seen anteriorly (*asterisk*) and mild anterior globe prolapse after intervention.

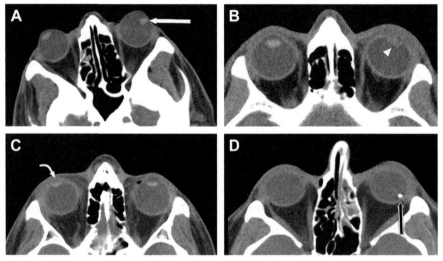

Fig. 5. Various acute injuries to the globes demonstrated on Axial CTs for multiple different trauma patients. (*A*) Lateral displacement of the left ocular lens (*white arrow*) from acute traumatic dislocation in a 58-year-old man. (*B*) Decreased attenuation of the left ocular lens (*white arrowhead*) from an acute traumatic cataract in a 45-year-old man. (*C*) Decreased volume of the right anterior chamber (*curved arrow*) from acute corneal rupture in a 23-year-old man. (*D*) Intraocular foreign body (*black arrow*) with a metallic BB seen in the left globe of a 28-year-old-man.

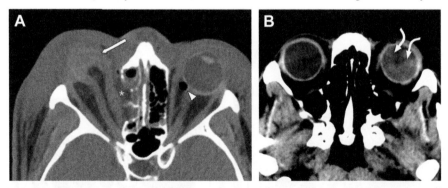

Fig. 6. Globe hemorrhage. (*A*) Right globe rupture and vitreous hemorrhage in a 55-year-old man after trauma. Axial soft tissue window CT demonstrating hyperdensity of the posterior chamber indicative of vitreous hemorrhage, along with marked volume loss and contour deformity of the right globe (*white arrow*) indicative of traumatic globe rupture. Acute fracture of the right medial orbital wall is also seen (*white asterisk*). Intraorbital emphysema (*white arrowhead*) is noted on the left secondary to blowout fracture outside the field of view. (*B*) Left globe retinal detachment in a 46-year-old woman with acute vision loss. Biconvex hyperdense hemorrhagic collections are seen along the medial and lateral globe contour converging posteriorly at the optic disc (*curved white arrows*).

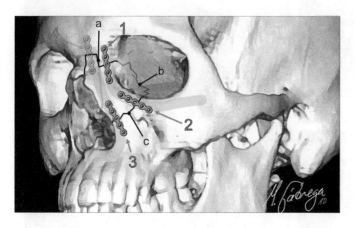

Fig. 7. The NOE fracture pattern, associated facial buttresses, and optimal surgical fixation points. The black lines demonstrate the fractures defining the perimeter of the NOE injuries. A fracture across the lateral nasal pyramid extends from the nasal aperture across the frontal process of the maxilla at the fronto-maxillary suture and into the medial orbital rim above the medial canthal insertion (a). A fracture traverses the inferior medial corner of the orbit descending across the medial orbital wall and exiting through the orbital floor across the inferior orbital rim (b). A fracture traverses the anterior maxillary wall from the inferior orbital rim to the inferior piriform aperture (c). The medial maxillary vertical buttress (*thick light blue line*) and the upper transverse maxillary buttress (*thick light green line*) are each traversed twice by the fracture pattern. The points of intersection of the fractures and buttresses coincide with thick bone and are ideal fixation points, depicted in the illustration as fixation plates across the frontomaxillary suture (1), the inferior orbital rim (2), and the medial maxillary vertical buttress (3). If there is nasal bone involvement, fixation across the frontonasal suture is sometimes performed (4).

bone involvement, fixation across the frontonasal suture is sometimes performed (see **Fig. 7**).[11]

The medial canthal tendon insertion is located at the medial orbital rim above the lacrimal fossa. Injury to this tendon or lateral displacement of a canthal tendon bearing bony fragment results in telecanthus or hypertelorism.[14] As such, describing the degree of comminution of the NOE region is necessary. Potential surgical approaches are determined by the Markowitz-Manson classification (**Fig. 8**). Although the integrity of the tendon cannot be assessed by CT, the degree of comminution is a useful adjunct.[11,14] If the medial canthal bearing fragment is not large enough for fixation, or if the tendon is severed as determined by the surgeon, wire fixation of the tendon (canthopexy) to hardware or to stable contralateral bony structures may be needed.[11] NOE fractures are readily identified on cross-sectional CT images, although 3D reconstruction may be needed to definitively identify the fracture pattern and better assesses the

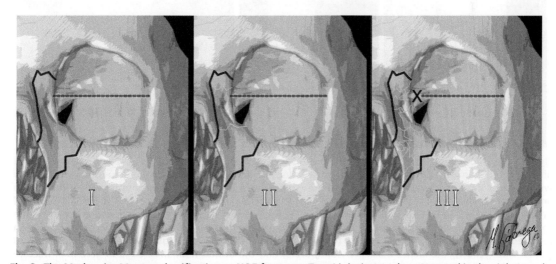

Fig. 8. The Markowitz-Manson classification or NOE fractures. Type I injuries are demonstrated in the right panel, with a single large central NOE fragment. The middle panel demonstrates type II injuries, with moderate comminution but a large medial-canthal ligament-bearing fragment. The medial canthal ligament plane is depicted by the dotted line. Type III injuries are demonstrated in the right panel where there is severe comminution of the NOE region and the medial canthal ligament is disrupted (X).

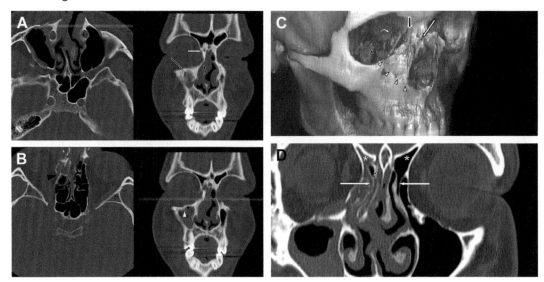

Fig. 9. NOE fracture in a 25-year-old man after trauma. (*A*) Axial and coronal CT images with green localization reference line demonstrating fractures through the right inferior orbital rim (*black arrow*) into the piriform aperture. More superiorly, a fracture line is seen through the frontomaxillary suture (*white arrow*), and there is comminution of the intervening frontal process fragment (*curved black arrow*). (*B*) Axial and coronal CT images with green localization line, demonstrate marked comminution of the right medial orbital wall (*black arrowhead*) and a minimally displaced fracture of the right orbital floor (*white arrowhead*). (*C*) 3D CT reconstruction more easily demonstrates the characteristic fractures of an NOE fracture, with fracture lines from the piriform aperture to the inferior orbital rim across the anterior maxilla (*white arrowheads*), comminuted fractures of the orbital floor (*curved black arrow*) and medial orbital wall (*white curved arrow*), fracture through the frontal process of the maxilla (*black arrow*) and into the nasal aperture (*white arrow*). Moderate comminution and a large fragment at the medial canthal ligament insertion (*asterisk*) are better seen on 3D reformats, with depression of the fragment into the ethmoid air cells. (*D*) Coronal CT reformat demonstrating the frontal sinuses (*asterisks*) and frontal recesses (*white arrows*), obstructed on the right and patent on the left. Slight bony disruption of the recess is noted on the right (*curved black arrow*).

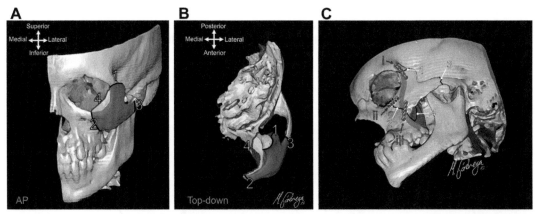

Fig. 10. The ZMC subunit anatomy, associated buttresses, and optimal fixation points. (*A*) Left half of the skull and zygomatic region. The zygoma is in blue. Black lines simulate the characteristic fractures of a ZMC injury with fractures through the lateral orbital rim at the zygomaticofrontal suture (1), the anterior wall of the maxilla and inferior orbital rim (2), the zygomatic arch (3), and the inferior lateral orbit (4) through the partially obscured orbital floor (*green*) and lateral orbital wall (*yellow*). (*B*) A top–down view of the ZMC region after removing the top of the skull and superior orbit at the level of the zygomaticofrontal suture. The medial orbit has also been removed at inferior orbital rim. This exposes the deep attachments of the ZMC region, which consist of the lateral orbital wall (*yellow*), the lateral maxillary wall (*purple*) and the orbital floor (free edge in *green*). A fracture through these structures (4) would free the zygoma as a floating piece. (*C*) A semirecumbent lateral view of the left skull. The characteristic fractures of a ZMC injury (1–4) traverse the upper transverse maxillary buttress (*broad light green line*) and the lateral maxillary vertical buttress (*broad pink line*). Points of intersection coincide with thick bone and are optimal sites for fixation, demonstrated here as fixation plates at the zygomaticofrontal suture (i), the inferior orbital rim (ii), and the lateral maxillary vertical buttress (iii).

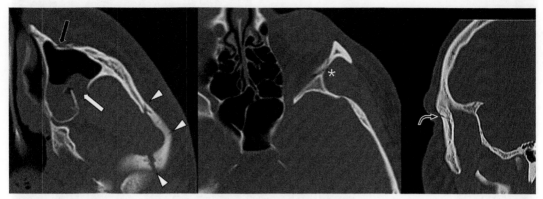

Fig. 11. ZMC fracture in a 22-year-old man after blunt trauma to the face. Characteristic fractures of the anterior wall of the maxilla (*black arrow*), the posterior lateral wall of the maxillary sinus (*white arrow*), the zygomatic arch (*white arrowheads*), and the lateral orbital wall (*asterisk*) are shown, with diastasis of the zygomaticofrontal suture (*curved black arrow*) to complete the pattern.

degree of comminution for surgical planning (**Fig. 9**A–C).[11] The radiologist should try to identify and draw attention to obstruction of the frontal recess (**Fig. 9**D) and the presence and degree of comminution of the posterior table of the frontal sinus. These 2 features are used by the surgeon to determine the need for frontal sinus obliteration or cranialization.[11,14]

Zygomaticomaxillary Complex Fractures

ZMC fractures are multibuttress injuries that separate the zygoma from the remainder of the skull. The ZMC injury pattern includes fractures of the anterior and posterolateral maxillary walls, the orbital floor, the inferior orbital rim, the lateral orbital wall, and the lateral orbital rim.[11,14] The older term "tripod fracture" has been abandoned

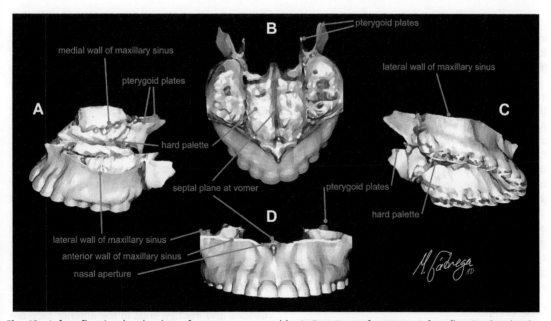

Fig. 12. A free-floating hard palette fragment as caused by LeFort I type fractures. A free-floating hard palate fragment is shown disarticulated from the remainder of the midface. This fragment results from an axial dissection plane through the pterygoid plates and walls of the maxillary sinuses, above the hard palette but below the orbits, and extending into the nasal aperture. The resulting free-floating fragment is shown with the various free edges labeled in detail in the diagram. Right facing and oblique (A), top down (B), left facing and oblique (C), and frontal (D) views are shown.

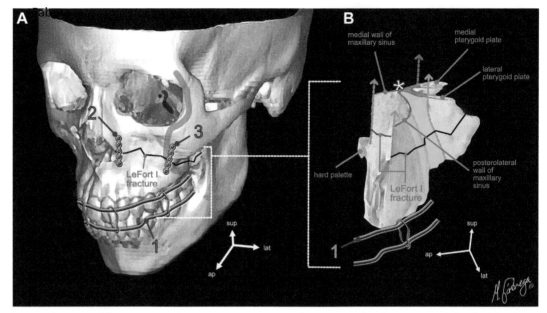

Fig. 13. The optimal fixation sites of LeFort Type I injuries with respect to facial buttresses. (*A*) Left oblique view of the skull depicted demonstrating a LeFort I type fracture pattern (*jagged black line*) traversing multiple facial buttresses including the medial maxillary vertical buttress (*broad light blue line*), the lateral maxillary vertical buttress (*broad pink line*), and the partially concealed posterior maxillary vertical buttress (*broad bright green*) at the pterygoid plates. Optimal maxillomandibular fixation is achieved by arch bars and wires (1), while the points where the fracture lines traverse the medial (2) and lateral (3) maxillary vertical buttresses are ideal locations for plate fixation to the upper midface. (*B*) Magnified cut-out view of the inferior lateral corner of the maxilla at the posterior maxillary vertical buttress (*green*), which is traversed by a LeFort I fracture (*jagged black line*). The confluence of the maxillary walls and pterygoid plates functions as an "I beam" (bony cross section at *white asterisk*) providing a vertical attachment (*dotted green arrows*) for the posterior aspect of the maxilla to the central skull base. When severed, the resulting "floating palette" requires maxillomandibular fixation using arch bars and wires (1) to restore and/or maintain proper occlusion.

in favor of the term "tetrapod fracture" to account for the deep attachments of the ZMC subunit (**Fig. 10**A, B).[14]

Fracture lines traverse 2 major facial buttresses including the upper transverse maxillary buttresses and the lateral maxillary vertical buttress. Again, the points of intersection of buttresses and fractures provide optimal sites for hardware fixation. The 3 most common fixation sites are the inferior orbital rim, the zygomaticofrontal suture, and the zygomaticomaxillary buttress (**Fig. 10**C).[11,14,15]

ZMC fracture assessment on CT should focus on confirmation of the injury pattern (**Fig. 11**) while describing any displacement and/or rotation of the zygomatic body because the most important surgical goal is the preservation of normal orbital volumes.[11,14]

LeFort I Injuries

LeFort I fractures are multibuttress injuries of the midface that separate the hard palette containing segment of the maxilla from the remainder of the face. The resulting fragment has been referred to as the occlusion-bearing maxillary

segment.[11] The injury pattern involves an axially oriented fracture plane through the pterygoid plates and the walls of the maxillary sinuses into the nasal aperture. The fracture plane is above the hard palate and inferior to the orbits. This results in a "floating-palette" fragment (**Fig. 12**).[11,12,14,16]

Three vertical facial buttresses are involved. These include the medial maxillary vertical buttress at the nasal aperture, the lateral maxillary vertical buttress at the zygoma, and the posterior maxillary vertical buttress at the pterygoid plates.[11,14,15] Severance from the vertical attachments allows for free movement of the occlusion-bearing maxillary fragment, which may result in malocclusion.[11,14] Restoration of normal bite is the most important surgical goal and is usually achieved by maxillomandibular fixation via arch bars and wires. The 2 intersections of buttresses and fracture lines in the anterior face are optimal sites for plate fixation (**Fig. 13**).[11] CT evaluation should focus on confirmation of injury pattern (**Fig. 14**) and comment on possible impediments to reduction and fixation, such as impacted or incomplete fractures.[11]

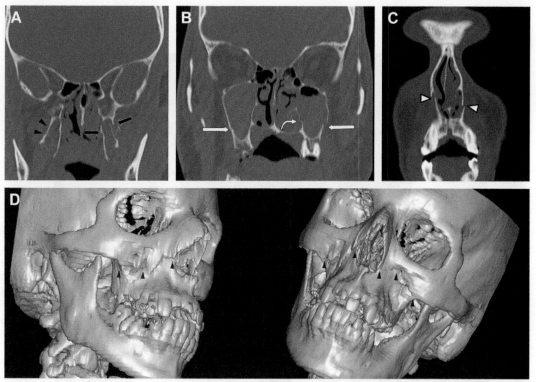

Fig. 14. LeFort I type fracture pattern in a 42-year-old man after blunt trauma to the face. (*A*), (*B*), and (*C*) coronal CT images of the face demonstrating fractures through the left pterygoid plates (*black arrows*), the bilateral lateral maxillary walls (*white arrows*), the medial wall of the left maxillary sinus (*curved white arrow*). and through the anterior maxilla into the nasal aperture (*white arrowheads*). Pattern is characteristic of LeFort I injuries, although the right pterygoid plates (*black arrowhead*) seem intact, which suggests an incomplete injury on the right. (*D*) 3D CT reconstruction demonstrates the typical appearance of bilateral LeFort I fractures with fractures traversing the walls of the maxillary sinuses into the nasal aperture (*blue arrowheads*).

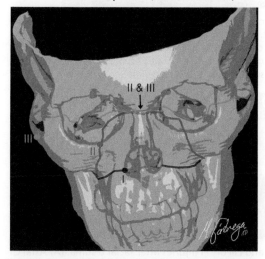

Fig. 15. Symmetric bilateral LeFort injuries, including their shared and unique characteristics. Fracture lines for each injury pattern are drawn. Among the 3 injury types, LeFort I fractures (*blue line*) are unique in that they spare the orbits and enter the inferior nasal aperture (*blue dot*). LeFort II (*pink line*) and LeFort III (*green line*) fractures both have interorbital components and often cross across the midline at the level of the frontonasal/frontomaxillary; however, the involvement of the inferior orbital rim (*pink dot*) is unique to LeFort II injuries, whereas the involvement of the zygomatic arch (*green dot*) is unique to LeFort III injuries. All LeFort injuries traverse the pterygoid plates posteriorly, not shown here.

LeFort II and III Injuries

Similar to LeFort I injuries, LeFort II and III injuries sever the vertical posterior maxillary buttress at the pterygoid plates and separate portions of the midface from the remainder of the skull. Both traverse the midline face with interorbital components.[11,12,14]

LeFort II injuries extend through the inferior orbital rim and result in a free-floating pyramidal fragment, a "floating maxilla," with the nasoseptal region at its apex and the occlusion-bearing maxillary segment as its base. LeFort III injuries extend through the lateral orbital walls, lateral orbital rims, and the zygomatic arch with complete dissociation of the midface from the remainder of the skull, resulting in a "floating face" (**Fig. 15**).[11,12,14,16]

To aid in differentiation, it has been suggested one focus on the unique features of each injury, such as extension into the nasal aperture below the orbits (LeFort I), fractures through the inferior orbital rim (LeFort II), and fractures through the zygomatic arches (LeFort III) (**Fig. 15**).[16]

LeFort II and III injuries can be regarded as combinations of nasoseptal, NOE, ZMC, and LeFort I

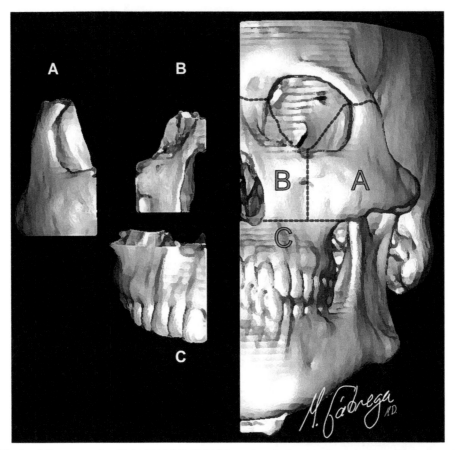

Fig. 16. The 3 midface subunits. Right ZMC (*A*), NOE (*B*), and occlusion-bearing maxillary (*C*) fragments are depicted as disarticulated free-floating fragments. On the left, these subunits are outlined in their native positions within the skull. Each LeFort injuries can be thought of as combination of these subunits, with LeFort I injuries corresponding to segment C, LeFort II fractures consisting of segments (*B*+ *C*), and LeFort III injuries consisting of segments (*A*+ *B*+ *C*). Any combination of conjoined or separate subunits is possible.

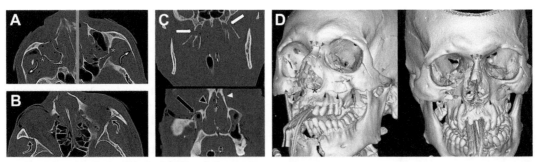

Fig. 17. A 36-year-old man with bilateral LeFort I, LeFort II, and LeFort III injuries after facial trauma. (*A*) Axial CT demonstrating fractures of the bilateral zygomatic arches (*curved arrows*) and posterolateral walls of the maxillary sinuses (*asterisks*). (*B*) Axial CT with bilateral fractures of the lateral orbital walls (*curved black arrows*). (*C*) Displaced bilateral pterygoid plate fractures (*white arrows*), with fractures through the medial orbital walls on the right (*black arrowhead*) and left (*white arrowhead*). A trans-septal injury is noted at the midline (*black asterisk*). Pattern is in keeping with bilateral LeFort type III injuries. Fracture through the inferior orbital rim (*black arrow*) supports a right LeFort II injury as well. (*D*) 3D CT reconstructions better demonstrating some of the fracture characteristics not well seen on standard axial and conormal images. LeFort I (*blue arrowheads*), LeFort II, (*pink arrowheads*), and LeFort III (*green arrowheads*) fracture patterns can be demonstrated bilaterally, Fractures through the inferior nasal aperture (*blue asterisk*), inferior orbital rim (*pink asterisk*), and zygomatic arch (*green asterisk*) represent the unique features of injury. These injuries could also be described as separate NOE, ZMC, and LeFort I injuries bilaterally, with intervening nasoseptal injuries.

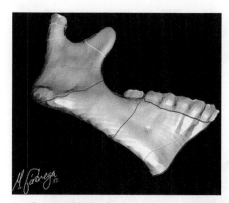

Fig. 18. The mandibular fracture nomenclature. A disarticulated right mandibular half is depicted with numerous color-coded fracture lines. Mandibular fractures are classified by their anatomic location. Symphyseal (*dark blue line*), parasymphyseal (*light blue line*), body (*pink line*), angle (*red line*), ramus (*orange*), coronoid (*white*), subcondylar (*yellow*), condylar (*bright green*), and alveolar ridge fractures (*black line*) are shown.

subunits (**Fig. 16**), with the management of the higher order injuries identical to the management of individual subunits already discussed.[11] Any combination of unilateral or bilateral LeFort I, II, and/or III injuries are possible.[14,16] CT evaluation should focus on the detection of the fracture patterns and reporting of clinically relevant information for each subunit as discussed in earlier sections (**Fig. 17**).[11]

Mandible fractures

After the nasoseptal region, the mandible is the second most common site of facial fracture.[12] Mandibular fractures are described by their anatomic location (**Fig. 18**).[12,17] Because the mandible is an arch, fractures often occur at 2 locations or may be associated with temporomandibular joint dislocation. About half the time, only one fracture is detected.[12,18]

CT evaluation should focus on the detection of fractures (**Fig. 19**A) and dislocations if present. Degree of fracture comminution should be described.[12] Displaced alveolar ridge fragments containing teeth may be present (**Fig. 19**B). Fractures extending into periapical lucencies should be reported because this increases the risk of subsequent hardware or soft tissue infection (**Fig. 20**).

SUMMARY

Maxillofacial injuries are common and complex. CT is the primary imaging tool used for diagnosis. Understanding 3D anatomy, patterns of injury, and the concept of functional subunits aids communication between radiologist, emergency physicians, and surgeons. Complex facial skeleton injuries can be understood and described by referring to individual nasoseptal, internal orbital, NOE, ZMC, LeFort, and mandibular injuries. This helps ensure production of radiology reports that go beyond simply listing fractured bones, while drawing attention to clinically relevant details and

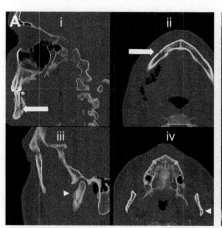
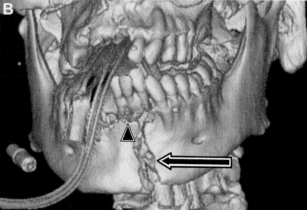

Fig. 19. Mandibular fractures in 2 different patients after trauma. (*A*) Bilateral mandibular fractures on multiple CT images in a 28-year-old man with jaw pain after trauma. The top 2 panels (i and ii) demonstrate an injury on the patient's right side, with a minimally displaced parasymphyseal fracture (*white arrows*), whereas the bottom 2 panels (iii and iv) demonstrate a subcondylar fracture (*white arrowheads*) on the patient's left side. (*B*) 3D CT reconstruction of the jaw in a 36-year-old male trauma victim (same patient as in **Fig. 17**) with a displaced left parasymphyseal fracture (*black arrow*) contiguous with a transverse alveolar ridge fracture (*black arrowhead*), separating multiple central mandibular teeth from the jaw.

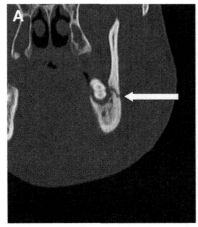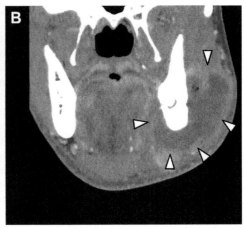

Fig. 20. A 42-year-old man 2 weeks after trauma with untreated mandibular fracture, complicated by left facial abscess. (*A*) Coronal CT image on bone windows with a left mandibular angle fracture (*white arrow*) extending into the periapical lucency of a mandibular molar. (*B*) Coronal CT image with soft-tissue windows demonstrating a large submandibular and submasseteric abscess (*white arrowheads*).

downplaying others that do not affect management.

CLINICS CARE POINTS

- When any nasoseptal fracture is detected on imaging, a speculum examination is needed to exclude septal hematoma.

- When evaluating orbital trauma on CT, assess the soft tissues for signs of entrapment and to exclude retrobulbar hematoma.

- When evaluating NOE fractures, assess the degree of comminution at the medial canthal insertion and look for signs of frontal recess obstruction.

- When analyzing higher order injuries, focus on the individual nasoseptal, orbital, NOE, ZMC, and maxillary occlusion-bearing subunits.

- When evaluating mandibular fractures, comment on the involvement of periodontal disease.

CONFLICT OF INTEREST

The author has no conflicts of interest to disclose.

REFERENCES

1. Lalloo R, Lucchesi LR, Bisignano C, et al. Epidemiology of facial fractures: incidence, prevalence and years lived with disability estimates from the Global Burden of Disease 2017 study. Inj Prev 2020; 26(Suppl 2):i27–35.

2. Allareddy V, Allareddy V, Nalliah RP. Epidemiology of facial fracture injuries. J Oral Maxillofac Surg 2011; 69(10):2613–8.

3. Gassner R, Tuli T, Hächl O, et al. Cranio-maxillofacial trauma: a 10 year review of 9543 cases with 21 067 injuries. J Cranio-Maxillofacial Surg 2003;31(1):51–61.

4. Afrooz PN, Bykowski MR, James IB, et al. The epidemiology of mandibular fractures in the United States, part 1: a review of 13,142 cases from the US National Trauma Data Bank. J Oral Maxillofac Surg 2015;73(12):2361–6.

5. Lee KH. Interpersonal violence and facial fractures. J Oral Maxillofac Surg 2009;67(9):1878–83.

6. Haug RH, Prather J, Indresano AT. An epidemiologic survey of facial fractures and concomitant injuries. J Oral Maxillofac Surg 1990;48(9):926–32. Available at: https://www.joms.org/article/0278-2391(90)90004-L/pdf.

7. Gaddipati R, Ramisetti S, Vura N, et al. Analysis of 1,545 fractures of facial region—a retrospective study. Craniomaxillofacial Trauma Reconstr 2015; 8(4):307–14.

8. Erdmann D, Follmar KE, DeBruijn M, et al. A retrospective analysis of facial fracture etiologies. Ann Plast Surg 2008;60(4):398–403.

9. Kucik CJ, Clenney TL, Phelan J. Management of acute nasal fractures. Am Fam Physician 2004; 70(7):1315–20. Available at: https://www.aafp.org/pubs/afp/issues/2004/1001/p1315.html.

10. Chan J, Most SP. Diagnosis and management of nasal fractures. Operat Tech Otolaryngol Head Neck Surg 2008;19(4):263–6.

11. Dreizin D, Nam AJ, Diaconu SC, et al. Multidetector CT of midfacial fractures: classification systems,

principles of reduction, and common complications. Radiographics 2018;38(1):248–74.

12. Gómez Roselló E, Quiles Granado AM, Artajona Garcia M, et al. Facial fractures: classification and highlights for a useful report. Insights into Imaging 2020;11(1):1–15.

13. Døving M., Lindal F.P., Mjøen E., et al., Orbital fractures. Tidsskrift for Den norske legeforening, Available at: https://tidsskriftet.no/en/2022/04/clinical-review/orbital-fractures, 2022. Accessed December 11, 2022.

14. Hopper RA, Salemy S, Sze RW. Diagnosis of Midface Fractures with CT: what the surgeon needs to know. Radiographics 2006;26(3):783–93. https://doi.org/10.1148/rg.263045710.

15. Gentry LR, Manor WF, Turski PA, et al. High-resolution CT analysis of facial struts in trauma: 1. Normal

anatomy. Am J Roentgenol 1983;140(3):523–32. Available at: https://www.ajronline.org/doi/epdf/10.2214/ajr.140.3.523.

16. Rhea JT, Novelline RA. How to simplify the CT diagnosis of Le Fort fractures. Am J Roentgenol 2005;184(5):1700–5. Available at: https://www.ajronline.org/doi/full/10.2214/ajr.184.5.01841700.

17. Cornelius CP, Audigté L, Kunz C, et al. The comprehensive AOCMF classification system: mandible fractures-level 2 tutorial. Craniomaxillofacial Trauma Reconstr 2014;7(1_suppl):15–30. Available at: https://www.ncbi.nlm.nih.gov/pmc/articles/PMC4251718/pdf/10-1055-s-0034-1389557.pdf.

18. Fraioli RE, Branstetter BF 4th, Deleyiannis FW. Facial fractures: beyond Le Fort. Otolaryngol Clin 2008; 41(1):51–76.

Malignant and Nonmalignant Lesions of the Oral Cavity

Jeanie Choi, MD[a],*, Derek Huell, BS[b], Fehime Eymen Ucisik, MD[a],
Kim Learned, MD[a]

KEYWORDS

• Oral cavity • Benign • Malignant • Imaging

KEY POINTS

- The oral cavity is a complex anatomic space bordered by but separate from the oropharynx.
- Knowledge of oral cavity subsites is important to form an accurate differential diagnosis of the many pathologies, both benign and malignant that may occur.
- There is a wide spectrum of benign pathologies including congenital and vascular lesions with characteristic imaging appearances.
- The most common oral cavity malignancy is squamous cell carcinoma.

INTRODUCTION

The oral cavity is the entry way to the aerodigestive tract and is a complex anatomic site serving multiple essential functions. The components of the oral cavity, bounded anteriorly by the lips, posteriorly by the oropharynx, laterally by the buccoalveolar regions, superiorly by the hard palate, and inferiorly by the floor of mouth, can give rise to a multitude of lesions, spanning benign and malignant etiologies. Although the oral cavity is readily accessible for physical examination, imaging plays a critical role in delineating oral cavity lesions. Here we will highlight a practical approach to the imaging assessment of oral cavity lesions and review the major differential diagnoses of both benign and malignant lesions.

ANATOMY
Gingivobuccal Region

The oral vestibule lies between the cheeks, lips, and teeth (**Fig. 1**). The mucosa of the lips and cheeks serves as the external boundary of the oral vestibule whereas the teeth and gingiva serve as the internal boundary.[1] The buccal mucosa covers the inner cheeks and reflects superiorly over the maxilla and inferiorly over the mandible. The buccal and gingival mucosae meet at the GBS.

Deep to the mucosal covering of the cheek lies the buccinator muscle covered by the buccal fat pad. The parotid gland (Stensen's) duct courses through the buccal fat pad and pierces the buccinator muscle exiting at the level of the second maxillary molar.

The retromolar trigone is a triangular region just posterior to the mandibular third molar and is close to the pterygomandibular raphe.[2] This fibrous band extends from the hamulus of the medial pterygoid to the mandibular mylohyoid ridge and forms a boundary between the oral cavity and oropharynx, attaching to the buccinator muscle anteriorly and superior pharyngeal constrictor muscle posteriorly.[3] Although not well seen on imaging, the pterygomandibular raphe can serve as a conduit for the spread of tumor between the oral cavity and oropharynx.

Oral Tongue

The oral cavity proper is bounded superiorly by the hard palate, inferiorly by the floor of mouth, and

---

[a] Department of Neuroradiology, Division of Diagnostic Radiology, The University of Texas MD Anderson Cancer Center, 1400 Pressler Street Unit 1482, Houston, TX 77030, USA; [b] New York University Grossman School of Medicine, 550 1st Avenue, New York, NY 10016, USA
* Corresponding author.
E-mail address: jchoi1@mdanderson.org

Oral Maxillofacial Surg Clin N Am 35 (2023) 311–325
https://doi.org/10.1016/j.coms.2023.02.008
1042-3699/23/Published by Elsevier Inc.

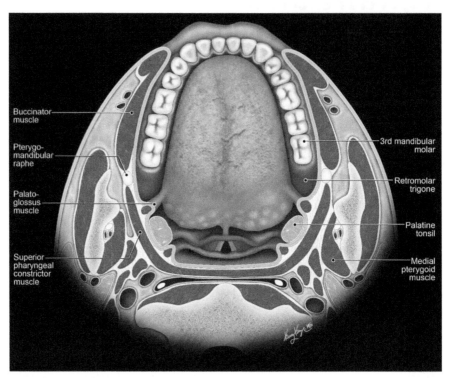

Buccinator muscle

Pterygo-mandibular raphe

Palato-glossus muscle

Superior pharyngeal constrictor muscle

3rd mandibular molar

Retromolar trigone

Palatine tonsil

Medial pterygoid muscle

Fig. 1. Diagram of the oral cavity. (*Courtesy of* Kelly Kage, MFA, CMI, Houston, TX.)

anteriorly by the teeth with the oral tongue as its largest anatomic structure (see **Fig. 1**; **Figs. 2** and **3**). The anterior two-thirds of the tongue is considered the oral tongue and is delineated from the base of the tongue by the circumvallate papillae. The posterior one-third of the tongue is the tongue base, which is a subsite of the oropharynx. The intrinsic muscles of the oral tongue include the inferior and superior longitudinal lingual muscles, which curl the tongue upward and downward, respectively, and the transverse and vertical lingual muscles, responsible for elongating and flattening the tongue, respectively.[4] The extrinsic muscles of the tongue include the genioglossus, styloglossus, hyoglossus, and palatoglossus muscles. The extrinsic muscles have bony attachments whereas the intrinsic muscles do not. The genioglossus, styloglossus, and hyoglossus muscles are innervated by the hypoglossal nerve; the palatoglossus is innervated by the pharyngeal branch of the vagus nerve.[4] The genioglossus divided by the lingual septum is responsible for protruding the tongue, whereas the hyoglossus muscle retracts the tongue. The styloglossus controls the rising of the sides of the tongue to form a channel for swallowing. The palatoglossus is responsible for elevating the posterior tongue and contributes to the initiation of swallowing.[4]

Floor of Mouth

The floor of the mouth is bounded inferiorly by the sling-shaped mylohyoid muscle (see **Figs. 2** and **3**). The mylohyoid muscles originate along the length of the mylohyoid ridge of the mandible and extend to the last molar teeth posteriorly. A gap exists between the posterior border of the mylohyoid muscle and the hyoglossus, where the submandibular gland extends around the mylohyoid muscle. The anterior bellies of the digastric muscle run inferiorly along the mylohyoid muscle in an anterior-posterior direction providing additional support for the floor of the mouth.

Sublingual and Submandibular Space

The sublingual space, containing the sublingual glands, lies beneath the tongue and is bounded inferiorly by the mylohyoid muscle, anteriorly by the mandible, and medially by the genioglossus geniohyoid muscle complex (see **Figs. 2** and **3**). The hyoglossus, styloglossus, and palatoglossus muscles run along the sublingual space. Posteriorly, the sublingual space communicates with the submandibular space with the deep lobe of the submandibular gland wrapping around the posterior border of the mylohyoid muscle and extending into the sublingual space. The submandibular gland (Wharton's) duct, lingual nerve, artery, and

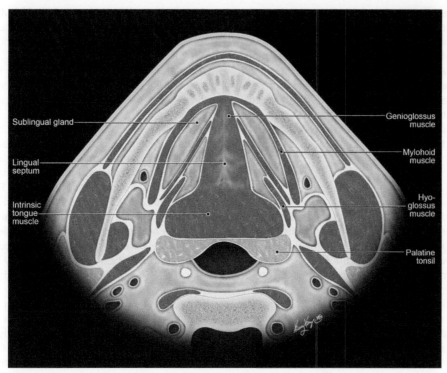

Fig. 2. Diagram of the oral cavity. (*Courtesy of* Kelly Kage, MFA, CMI, Houston, TX.)

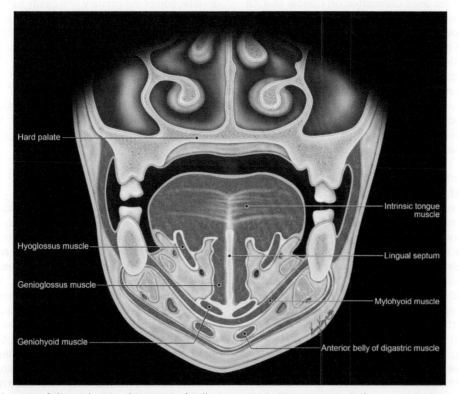

Fig. 3. Diagram of the oral cavity. (*Courtesy of* Kelly Kage, MFA, CMI, Houston, TX.)

vein course through the sublingual space as do the glossopharyngeal nerve and hypoglossal nerve.

The sublingual and submandibular spaces are separated by the mylohyoid muscle. The submandibular space is bordered inferiorly by the hyoid bone, superiorly by the mylohyoid muscle, anteriorly and laterally by the mandible, and medially by the anterior bellies of the digastric muscles. Within the submandibular space lies the superficial portion of the mandibular gland, facial artery, and vein.

IMAGING MODALITIES

Panorex radiographs image the entire complement of teeth and allow evaluation of the alveolar bone around the teeth.[5] X-ray imaging of the mandible via panorex is helpful in assessing any bony asymmetry and secondary bony effects of soft tissue lesions.

Computed tomography (CT) and MRI are the mainstays of imaging the oral cavity. CT offers precise evaluation of cortical bone which is essential in staging oral cavity cancers and is readily available. Contrast-enhanced CT (CECT) has been shown to have the highest specificity in detecting bone erosion,[6] an upstaging feature in oral cavity cancer. Invasion of extrinsic tongue musculature has been replaced as a T4 upstaging feature in the American Joint Committee on Cancer (AJCC) 8th edition by depth of invasion (DOI).[7] DOI is not synonymous with the measurement of tumor thickness on cross-sectional imaging and is determined histologically.

Techniques to improve CT image quality in the face of dental amalgam artifacts include a second pass CT with angled gantry and metal reduction reconstruction algorithms.[8] A puffed cheek technique can be employed to improve the detection of mucosal lesions along the buccal and gingival surfaces.[9]

MRI offers superior soft tissue resolution compared with CT. Delineation of typical signal characteristics such as fat signal within benign dermoid cysts and the depiction of tumor infiltration, perineural spread, and marrow involvement are some of the advantages of MRI. MRI is also better able to delineate anatomic structures such as the extrinsic muscles of the tongue when compared with CT. Disadvantages of MRI include longer imaging time with increased motion artifact and pulsation artifact from vascular structures in the head and neck.[10] The lack of beam-hardening artifact due to metal is an advantage of MRI over CT, and metal suppression MRI techniques may aid in further decreasing metallic susceptibility artifact.[11]

Dynamic contrast-enhanced (DCE)-MRI is a technique that evaluates the microvascular features of tumors. As in perfusion imaging of the brain, DCE-MRI of head and neck tumors, including oral cavity tumors, can provide information about the presence of abnormal leaky vessels and resulting permeability between the intravascular and extravascular environments.[12] There is also evidence DCE-MRI may be a useful noninvasive method of helping to predict human papilloma virus (HPV) and epidermal growth factor receptor (EGFR) status before treatment in oropharyngeal and oral cavity tumors with implications for prognosis and expected response to therapy.[13]

Ultrasound is useful in evaluating nodal disease in the neck and for guidance for fine needle aspiration. Intraoral ultrasound can provide accurate estimates of tumor thickness in oral cavity cancers pre-operatively and intraoperatively and can aid in improving margin resection.[14]

Fluorodeoxyglucose (FDG) PET-CT plays an important role in the initial staging of oral cavity cancers. Oral cavity cancers are currently staged using the AJCC 8th edition.[15] FDG PET-CT plays an important role in the delineation of the extent of primary tumor which can sometimes be obscured by dental amalgam artifacts on CT and motion artifacts on MRI.[16] Compared with CT or MRI alone, FDG PET-CT has reported sensitivities for detection of the primary oral cavity tumor of up to 98%.[17] Nodal involvement is one of the most important prognostic indicators at initial diagnosis, and FDG PET-CT has demonstrated a sensitivity of 83%, specificity of 85%, and superior negative predictive value of 93% compared with CT and MRI alone.[17] In addition, FDG PET-CT images the entire body, detecting distant metastatic disease and possible additional primary tumors, both of which alter prognosis and management.

NONMALIGNANT PATHOLOGY
Cystic Lesions

Of the spectrum of nonmalignant lesions that develop in the oral cavity, congenital lesions make up a major category. The most commonly encountered lesions include epidermoid and dermoid cysts, vascular malformations, and anomalies.

Epidermoid cysts result from inclusion of ectodermal elements during neural tube closure. Acquired epidermoid cysts are rare and may result from surgery or penetrating trauma. On CT, epidermoid cysts demonstrate low attenuation similar to cerebrospinal fluid (CSF) and may contain internal calcifications. Lesions are typically low signal on T1-weighted images but rare "white"

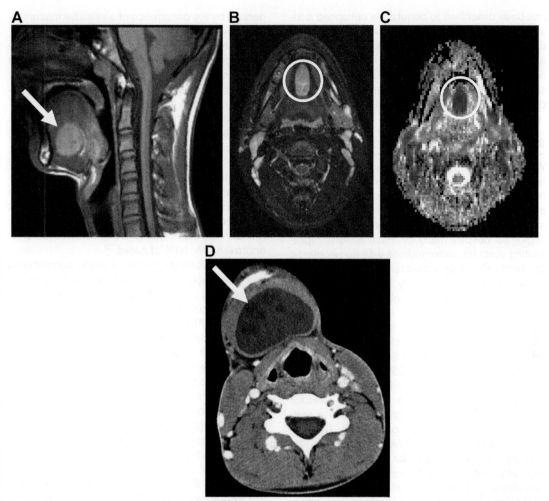

Fig. 4. Epidermoid and dermoid cysts. Sagittal T1-weighted image (*A*) shows a relatively hyperintense mass in the floor of mouth (*arrow*). Axial T2 image (*B*) shows the mass demonstrating T2 hyperintensity and restricted diffusion on ADC map (*C*) of epidermoid cyst (*circles*). Axial post-contrast CT (*D*) shows the characteristic sack of marbles appearance (*arrow*) of dermoid cyst.

epidermoid cysts demonstrate T1 hyperintense signal due to increased proteinaceous content (**Fig. 4**).[18] MRI demonstrates T2 hyperintense signal within the lesion but incomplete nulling of signal on fluid-attenuated inversion recovery (FLAIR) resulting in increased signal within the lesion as compared with CSF. Epidermoid cysts classically demonstrate internal restricted diffusion and show no enhancement.

Dermoid cysts are derived from totipotent stem cells that form the ectodermal germ layer. Dermoid cysts may contain any ectodermal elements including cutaneous appendages such as hair, sebaceous glands, and teeth.[19] This is in contrast to epidermoid cysts, which do not contain sebaceous glands, sweat glands, and hair follicles. On imaging, the different ectodermal elements within dermoid cysts help make the diagnosis. CT may show hyperdense teeth and fat attenuation within the lesion, and MRI will show fat signal intensity within the lesions or a characteristic sack of marbles appearance of fat globules with no enhancement (see **Fig. 4**).

Ranulas represent mucous retention cysts of the sublingual glands or minor salivary glands in the floor of mouth and may result from trauma to the gland or from obstruction. Ranulas confined to the floor of mouth are termed simple ranulas whereas those extending inferior to the floor of mouth are termed plunging or diving (**Fig. 5**).

On MRI, ranulas will demonstrate fluid signal and may show thin peripheral enhancement. If infected, they may show a thickened peripherally enhancing wall. A tapered narrowed "tail sign" has been described to denote the collapsed sublingual space component of the lesion.[20] Differentiating ranula from dermoid cysts can be made by assessing for the absence of fat within the lesion on CT or MRI, and differentiation from epidermoid cysts can be made by the absence of restricted diffusion within the lesion on MRI.

Vascular anomalies

When designating vascular and lymphatic anomalies, there has been extensive controversy in nomenclature that has caused marked complexity in their classification. Previously, many vascular lesions have been referred to as hemangiomas and angiomas despite many of these lesions representing vascular malformations with no neoplastic potential. Creating consistency and clarity in nomenclature is increasingly important in clinical care as many vascular anomalies require multidisciplinary care, necessitating mutual understanding. The initial classification system proposed in 1982 by Mulliken and Glowacki has been formally refined into the International Society for the Study of Vascular Anomalies (ISSVA) classifications, which was most recently revised in 2018.[21] The ISSVA classification system separates vascular anomalies into two primary groups: vascular malformations and vascular tumors (**Fig. 6**). This diagram illustrates the ISSVA designations for vascular anomalies. Vascular anomalies are first separated into vascular tumors and vascular malformations. Thereafter, vascular tumors are divided into benign, locally aggressive/borderline, and malignant groups. Vascular malformations are separated into simple, combined, of major vessels, and associated with other anomaly groups.

Vascular Malformations

Vascular malformations are classified into four subtypes: simple malformations, combined malformations, malformations of major named vessels, and malformations associated with other anomalies. Simple malformations can be separated into capillary, lymphatic, venous, and arteriovenous malformations. High-flow malformations include arteriovenous malformations and fistulas and slow-flow malformations include venous, venolymphatic and lymphatic malformations (**Figs. 7** and **8**).[21] Combined vascular malformations are defined as lesions with multiple vascular malformations present. Malformations of major named vessels are composed of deformities of significant blood vessels that are anatomically differentiated with names. Lastly, vascular malformations associated with other anomalies are

defined by the occurrence of a vascular malformation amid other confounding symptoms.[21]

Venolymphatic and lymphatic malformations are slow-flow lesions and are often trans-spatial in the head and neck. Lymphatic malformations can be defined morphologically as macrocystic, microcystic, or combined. Macrocystic lymphatic malformations are composed of one to three large (>1 cm) lesions whereas microcystic lymphatic malformations are composed of many smaller (<1 cm) lesions clustered together. Combined lymphatic malformations are composed of macrocystic and microcystic lesions present in the same area. Lymphatic malformations can be found throughout the body but are most commonly found in the head and neck, which accounts for approximately 50% of cases.[22]

These lesions demonstrate cystic components that may show different signal characteristics on T1-weighted and T2-weighted MRI depending on the presence of internal hemorrhage and fluid-fluid levels (**Fig. 9**). Venolymphatic malformations consist of lymphatic malformations with slow-flow venous vessels and possible phleboliths within the venous component. They may demonstrate heterogeneous enhancement.

Several treatment options exist for lymphatic malformations including surgery and sclerotherapy. Although surgical resection has been the most longstanding treatment, a high recurrence rate necessitated clinicians pivot toward a new procedure.[23] Complete resection is difficult due to the proximity of lymphatic malformations to critical structures in the head and neck. Particularly for lymphatic malformations of the oral cavity, surgical resection alone has proven to be highly difficult. Instead, a multifaceted approach involves sclerotherapy and surgery given the often trans-spatial nature of these lesions.[22] There is also research showing the potential benefits of molecular drugs to eliminate lymphatic malformations. Drugs are currently being designed to inhibit mTOR, a catalytic subunit of two protein complexes that contributes to cell proliferation in lymphatic malformations.[24]

Vascular tumors

Vascular tumors have rapidly multiplying vascular endothelial cells whereas vascular malformations exhibit dilation of vessels but lack proliferating endothelial cells. Vascular tumors are separated into three subtypes: malignant, locally aggressive/borderline, and benign tumors. Benign vascular tumors, also known as hemangiomas, are the result of errors in vascular development.[25] Over 60% of all cases occur in the head and neck.[25] Hemangiomas occur at a greater rate in

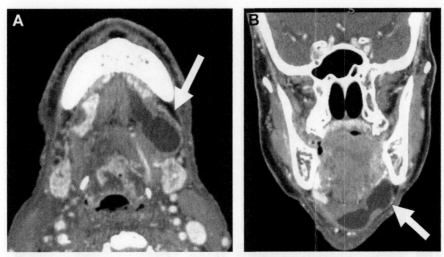

Fig. 5. Diving/plunging ranula. Axial (*A*) and coronal (*B*) post-contrast CT images show a well-circumscribed low-attenuation collection along the left floor of mouth (*arrows*) extending through the mylohyoid muscle.

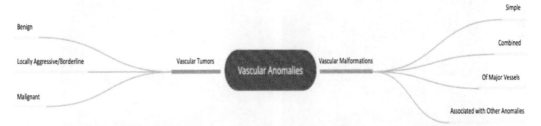

Fig. 6. This diagram illustrates the ISSVA designations for vascular anomalies. Vascular anomalies are first separated into vascular tumors and vascular malformations. Thereafter, vascular tumors are divided into benign, locally aggressive/borderline, and malignant groups. Vascular malformations are separated into simple, combined, of major vessels, and associated with other anomaly groups.

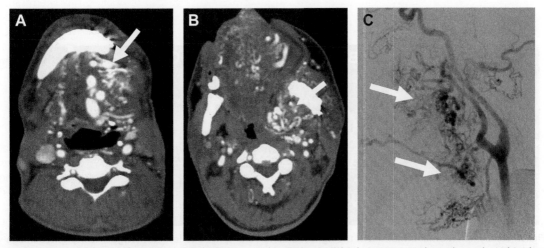

Fig. 7. Arteriovenous malformation. Axial CTA images (*A, B*) show multiple tortuous enlarged vessels within the oral tongue (*A, arrow*) and left masticator space (*B, arrow*). Digital subtraction angiography (*C*) shows multiple enlarged tortuous external carotid artery branches supplying the arteriovenous malformation (*arrows*).

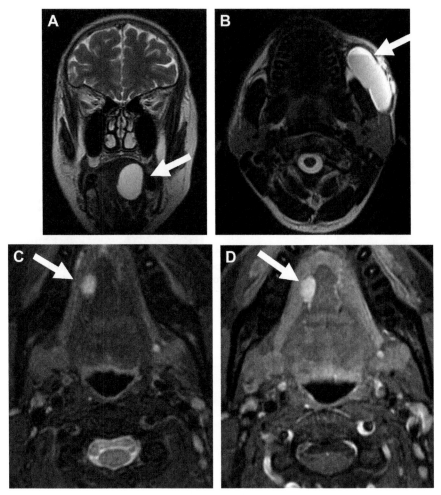

Fig. 8. Slow-flow vascular malformation. Macrocystic lymphatic malformation: coronal (*A*) and axial (*B*) T2-weighted images show well-circumscribed lesions in the oral tongue (*A, arrow*) and left buccal fat pad with fluid-fluid level (*B, arrow*). Venous malformation: axial T2 (*C, arrow*) and T1 post-contrast images (*D, arrow*) show T2 hyperintense, avidly enhancing lesions along the right oral tongue.

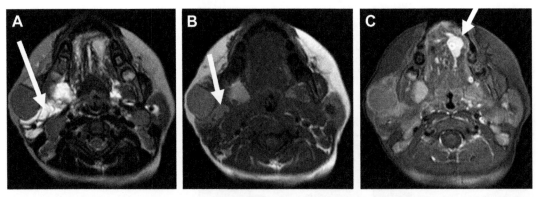

Fig. 9. Venolymphatic malformations in the right submandibular space and left oral tongue. T2-weighted image (*A*) shows hyperintense cystic right submandibular space lesion with fluid-fluid levels (*arrow*) and T1 hyperintense fluid within the cysts (*B, arrow*). T1 post-contrast image (*C*) shows avid enhancement within the left oral tongue lesion (*arrow*).

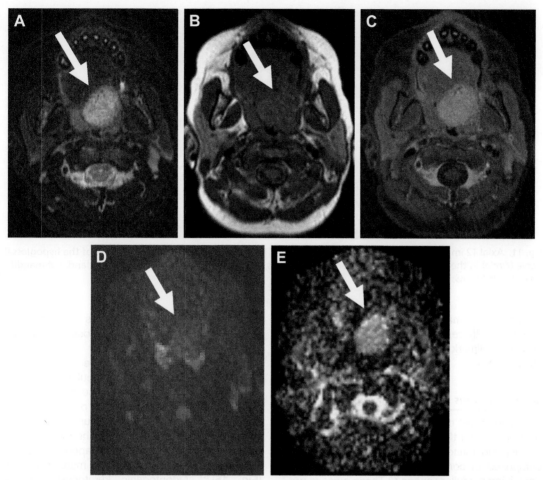

Fig. 10. Posterior tongue congenital hemangioma. T2-weighted image (*A*) shows a hyperintense ovoid mass in the posterior left tongue (*arrow*) and T1-weighted image (*B*) shows hypointense signal within the lesion (*arrow*). Post-contrast T1-weighted image (*C*) shows homogeneous enhancement (*arrow*) and DWI sequence (*D*) and ADC map (*E*) show no restricted diffusion within the mass (*arrows*).

Caucasians, women, and premature infants.[26] They are categorized as either infantile or congenital hemangiomas. Infantile hemangiomas develop in the first few months of life, proliferate for the first year, and then typically undergo slow involution over several years.[26] Congenital hemangiomas are present at birth, show no proliferation, and may or may not involute.[25] MRI depicts the full extent of these lesions and their relation to adjacent structures. These lesions are typically well-circumscribed and demonstrate avid enhancement (**Fig. 10**).

Benign tumors

Peripheral Nerve Sheath Tumors
Peripheral nerve sheath tumors including neurofibromas and schwannomas are common in the head and neck but relatively rare in the oral cavity.

It is approximated that perineural spread of tumors (PNSTs) account for 0.5% of biopsied lesions in the oral cavity.[27]

Neurofibromas are the most common benign PNST of the oral cavity, representing approximately 32% of all cases.[27] Neurofibromas are caused primarily by the proliferation of Schwann cells, but their composition may also include perineural cells, endoneural fibroblasts, axons, and inflammatory features. In the oral cavity, the tongue, buccal mucosa, and posterior mandible are the most frequent locations for neurofibromas to arise.[27] Schwannomas account for 20% of PNSTs found in the oral cavity.[27] Schwannomas are derived from Schwann cells and have a more homogeneous composition than neurofibromas.

On MRI, peripheral nerve sheath tumors are typically well circumscribed with T2 hyperintensity (**Fig. 11**) and show variable enhancement.

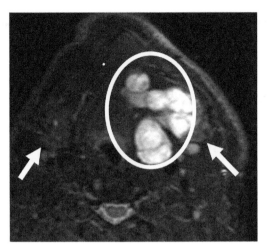

Fig. 11. Axial T2 image with fat saturation shows tubular T2 hyperintense nerve sheath tumor of the hypoglossal nerve (*circle*) in the sublingual and submandibular spaces, displacing the left submandibular gland. Submandibular glands (*arrows*).

Schwannomas may show internal cystic change. When in or adjacent to bone, smooth bony remodeling is a hallmark imaging feature of benign nerve sheath tumors.

Osseous lesions

Tori is the most common benign osseous lesion occurring along the cortical surfaces of both the maxilla and mandible (**Fig. 12**). Tori is primarily composed of compacted bone without marrow containing medullary space.[28] These masses present bilaterally in 90% of cases, and their cause has not been explicitly defined with some studies hypothesizing a genetic component.[28] Most tori are asymptomatic, and those smaller in size do not necessitate treatment. If they are suspected to interfere with dental implants or with eating and drinking, large tori may be removed.[28]

Fibro-osseous lesions stem from proliferations of spindle cells with interwoven bone.[29] Although previous classification of subtypes was unclear, the World Health Organization reviewed groupings in 2017 and formalized three subtypes: fibrous dysplasia, cemento-ossifying fibroma, and cemento-osseous dysplasia.

Fibrous dysplasia lesions are expansile and classically described as having a "ground glass" matrix on CT (**Fig. 13**). Heterogeneous enhancement on MRI can sometimes be misleading for a more aggressive lesion. Cemento-ossifying fibromas and fibrous dysplasia share a similar radiographic appearance, but cemento-ossifying fibromas tend to have more well-defined borders and tend to occur more often in the mandible versus the maxilla in fibrous dysplasia (**Fig. 14**).[30]

Cemento-osseous dysplasia is distinguished from other subtypes as it is associated with the apex of the tooth.

Benign odontogenic cysts are common and include dentigerous cysts, radicular cysts, and odontogenic keratocyst. These lesions are frequently diagnosed on panorex or CT. Dentigerous cysts are associated with an unerupted tooth, and radicular cysts are found at the root of a previously inflamed tooth. Both will appear as lucent lesions with well-circumscribed margins on CT (**Fig. 15**).[31] Odontogenic keratocyst appears most commonly as a smoothly bordered unilocular cystic lesion and can share overlapping imaging features with ameloblastoma (see **Fig. 15**).[32]

Ameloblastoma is the most common odontogenic tumor and shows a tendency for local recurrence.[32] More common in the mandible versus the maxilla, ameloblastoma demonstrates a unilocular or multilocular expansile appearance with mixed internal densities on CT (see **Fig. 15**).[32]

Malignant Pathology

Squamous cell carcinoma
Greater than 90% of oral cavity cancers are SCC with the remainder including lymphoma, salivary gland neoplasms, and sarcomas.[33] Up to 33% of oral cavity SCC will originate from the oral tongue, making it the most common site in the oral cavity.[34] Major risk factors for oral cavity SCC include tobacco, alcohol, and HPV infection with betel nut chewing playing a significant role in certain parts of South East Asia and the Pacific regions.[35]

The majority of oral tongue SCC originate from the lateral surface or undersurface of the tongue

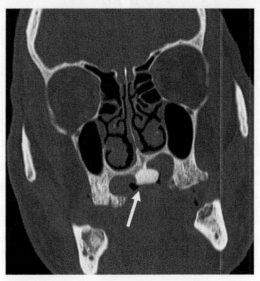

Fig. 12. Torus palatinus in the midline hard palate (*arrow*).

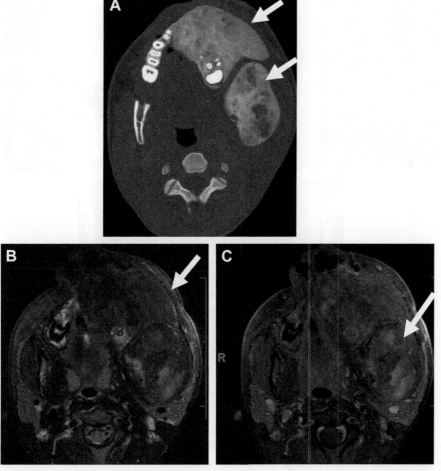

Fig. 13. Fibrous dysplasia. Axial CT (*A*) shows expansile ground glass matrix lesion of the left maxilla and mandible (*arrows*). T2-weighted image (*B*) and post-contrast T1 with fat saturation image (*C*) show hypointense T2 signal (*arrow*) and heterogeneous enhancement within the lesion (*arrow*).

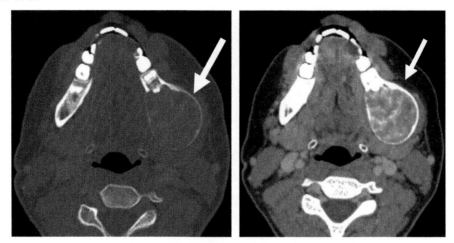

Fig. 14. Cemento-ossifying fibroma. Axial CT images show well-defined expansile lesions (*arrows*) in the left angle of the mandible with a mixture of calcification and soft tissue matrix and without cortical breach.

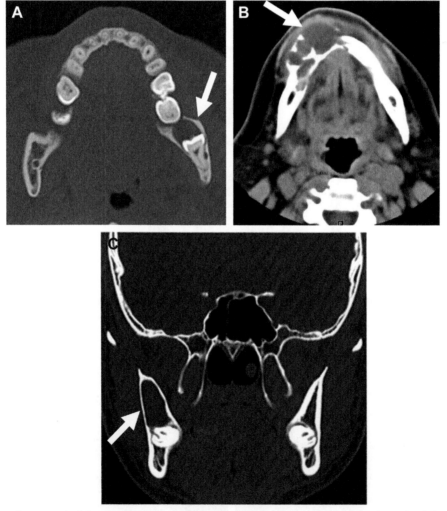

Fig. 15. Dentigerous cyst, (*A*) Axial CT image shows a well-defined lucent lesion in the left angle of the mandible associated with the crown of an impacted molar (*arrow*). Ameloblastoma, (*B*) Axial CT image shows multilocular expansile lytic lesion in the right mandibular symphysis and parasymphyseal region with focal soft tissue (*arrow*). Odontogenic keratocyst (*arrow*), (*C*) Coronal CT shows well-defined lucent lesion in the right mandible.

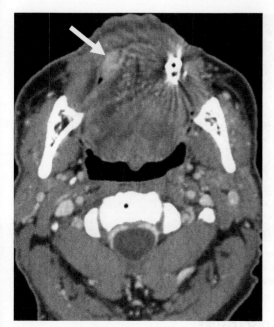

Fig. 16. Oral tongue SCC. Axial CT image shows an enhancing tumor along the right lateral oral tongue (*arrow*).

(**Fig. 16**).[2] The most recent AJCC 8th edition included DOI as a new feature in assigning T status. DOI is not synonymous with tumor thickness. DOI is defined in the AJCC 8th edition as measured from the adjacent normal mucosa basement membrane to the deepest margin of tumor invasion.[36] Although the depth of invasion is determined histologically, some say it can be estimated by measuring the margins of enhancement of the tumor on coronal T1-enhanced images.[34] Imaging

features such as involvement of adjacent structures including cortical bone erosion and encasement of the internal carotid artery are critical to mention as they are T4 upstaging features.[34] The hyoglossus muscle is closely approximated to the neurovascular bundle, and involvement depicted by MRI can be highly suggestive of neurovascular invasion.[34]

Salivary gland neoplasms
Minor salivary gland rests are scattered throughout the aerodigestive tract with the majority located in the oral cavity. Minor salivary gland malignancies arising from these rests most often occur in the palate with the junction of the hard and soft palate being a common location. Other sites in the oral cavity for minor salivary gland tumors include the buccal space, lips, tongue and retromolar trigone (**Fig. 17**).[37] Adenoid cystic and mucoepidermoid carcinoma are the most common salivary gland malignancies with acinic cell carcinoma and adenocarcinoma rounding out the top epithelial salivary gland malignancies.[38]

Imaging features of salivary gland benign and malignant neoplasms have overlapping features, but the role of imaging is to evaluate the full extent of spread. Recognizing features of minor salivary gland malignant tumor spread such as bone destruction and foraminal widening are imperative in describing the full extent of spread. CT may demonstrate bony involvement and erosion associated with palate tumors, but MRI is superior in tracing the perineural extent of tumor spread (**Fig. 18**). Oral cavity minor salivary gland malignant tumors have been shown to have an overall worse prognosis compared with minor salivary

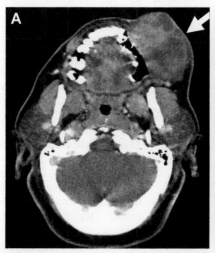
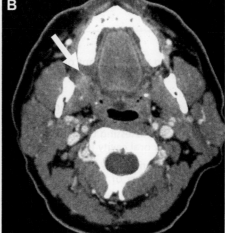

Fig. 17. Minor salivary gland ACC. (*A*) Axial CT shows a large bulky tumor of the left buccal space (*arrow*). (*B*) Axial CT shows an ill-defined enhancing tumor involving the right retromolar trigone (*arrow*).

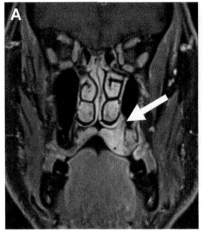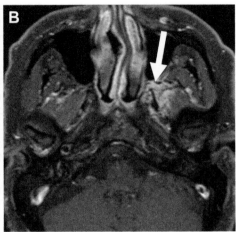

Fig. 18. ACC of the hard palate. Coronal post-contrast T1 image (*A*) shows enhancing tumor of the left hard palate growing through the enlarged left greater palatine foramen (*arrow*). Axial post-contrast T1 image (*B*) shows perineural tumor in the expanded left pterygopalatine foramen (*arrow*).

gland tumors elsewhere in the aerodigestive tract, however, several factors including the stage at diagnosis, surgical margins, presence of perineural and lymphovascular invasion, also influence prognosis.[39]

SUMMARY

The oral cavity is a complex anatomic region from which many pathologies, both nonmalignant and malignant can arise. Knowledge of imaging patterns as well as key anatomic relationships of the structures in the oral cavity is essential to forming an accurate and succinct differential diagnosis for lesions found in this region.

CLINICS CARE POINTS

- Many malignant and nonmalignant oral cavity lesions have characteristic imaging patterns.
- CT with its superior bone delineation and MRI with its superior soft tissue characterization are complementary in assessing typical imaging features of many oral cavity lesions.
- Squamous cell carcinoma is by far the most common malignant tumor of the oral cavity.
- The majority of minor salivary gland malignant tumors occur in the oral cavity and knowledge of potential patterns of spread is essential in evaluating the full extent of the tumor on imaging.

DISCLOSURE

Authors have no disclosures.

REFERENCES

1. Laine FJ, Smoker WRK. Oral cavity: Anatomy and pathology. Semin Ultrasound CT MRI 1995;16(6): 527–45.
2. Aiken AH. Pitfalls in the Staging of Cancer of Oral Cavity Cancer. Neuroimaging Clin 2013;23(1): 27–45.
3. Meesa IR, Srinivasan A. Imaging of the Oral Cavity. Radiol Clin 2015;53(1):99–114.
4. Dotiwala AK, Samra NS. Anatomy, Head and Neck, Tongue. In: StatPearls. StatPearls Publishing. 2022. Available at: http://www.ncbi.nlm.nih.gov/books/ NBK507782/. Accessed November 19, 2022.
5. Agostinelli C, Agostinelli A, Berardini M, et al. Radiological Evaluation of the Dimensions of Lower Molar Alveoli. Implant Dent 2018;27(3):271–5.
6. Goerres GW, Schmid DT, Schuknecht B, et al. Bone Invasion in Patients with Oral Cavity Cancer: Comparison of Conventional CT with PET/CT and SPECT/CT. Radiology 2005;237(1):281–7.
7. Glastonbury CM. Critical Changes in the Staging of Head and Neck Cancer. Radiol Imaging Cancer 2020;2(1):e190022.
8. Diehn FE, Michalak GJ, DeLone DR, et al. CT Dental Artifact: Comparison of an Iterative Metal Artifact Reduction Technique with Weighted Filtered Back-Projection. Acta Radiol Open 2017;6(11). 2058460117743279.
9. Weissman JL, Carrau RL. Puffed-cheek" CT Improves Evaluation of the Oral Cavity. AJNR Am J Neuroradiol 2001;22(4):741–4.

10. Chi JM, Hagiwara M. Update on MRI for Oral Cavity. Top Magn Reson Imag 2021;30(2):85–96.

11. Hagiwara M, Nusbaum A, Schmidt BL. MR Assessment of Oral Cavity Carcinomas. Magn Reson Imag Clin N Am 2012;20(3):473–94.

12. Sideras P, Singh G. MRI Dynamic Contrast Imaging of Oral Cavity and Oropharyngeal Tumors. Top Magn Reson Imag 2021;30(2):97–104.

13. Choi YS, Park M, Kwon HJ, et al. Human Papillomavirus and Epidermal Growth Factor Receptor in Oral Cavity and Oropharyngeal Squamous Cell Carcinoma: Correlation With Dynamic Contrast-Enhanced MRI Parameters. Am J Roentgenol 2016;206(2):408–13.

14. Klein Nulent TJW, Noorlag R, Van Cann EM, et al. Intraoral ultrasonography to measure tumor thickness of oral cancer: A systematic review and meta-analysis. Oral Oncol 2018;77:29–36.

15. Amin MB, Greene FL, Edge SB, et al. The Eighth Edition AJCC Cancer Staging Manual: Continuing to build a bridge from a population-based to a more "personalized" approach to cancer staging. CA Cancer J Clin 2017;67(2):93–9.

16. Pasha MA, Marcus C, Fakhry C, et al. FDG PET/CT for Management and Assessing Outcomes of Squamous Cell Cancer of the Oral Cavity. Am J Roentgenol 2015;205(2):W150–61.

17. Linz C, Brands RC, Herterich T, et al. Accuracy of 18-F Fluorodeoxyglucose Positron Emission Tomographic/Computed Tomographic Imaging in Primary Staging of Squamous Cell Carcinoma of the Oral Cavity. JAMA Netw Open 2021;4(4):e217083.

18. Mishra SS, Panigrahi S, Dhir MK, et al. Intrinsic brainstem white epidermoid cyst: An unusual case report. J Pediatr Neurosci 2014;9(1):52–4.

19. Edwards RM, Chapman T, Horn DL, et al. Imaging of pediatric floor of mouth lesions. Pediatr Radiol 2013; 43(5):523–35.

20. Jain P. Plunging Ranulas and Prevalence of the "Tail Sign" in 126 Consecutive Cases. J Ultrasound Med 2020;39(2):273–8.

21. Kunimoto K, Yamamoto Y, Jinnin M. ISSVA Classification of Vascular Anomalies and Molecular Biology. Int J Mol Sci 2022;23(4):2358.

22. Kulungowski AM, Patel M. Lymphatic malformations. Semin Pediatr Surg 2020;29(5):150971.

23. Perkins JA, Manning SC, Tempero RM, et al. Lymphatic malformations: review of current treatment. Otolaryngol Neck Surg Off J Am Acad Otolaryngol-Head Neck Surg. 2010;142(6):795–803 1.

24. Sabatani DM. Twenty-five years of mTOR: Uncovering the link from nutrients to growth. Proc Natl Acad Sci U S A 2017;114(45):11818–25.

25. Johnson EF, Davis DM, Tollefson MM, et al. Vascular Tumors in Infants: Case Report and Review of Clinical, Histopathologic, and Immunohistochemical Characteristics of Infantile Hemangioma, Pyogenic Granuloma, Noninvoluting Congenital Hemangioma, Tufted Angioma, and Kaposiform Hemangioendothelioma. Am J Dermatopathol 2018;40(4):231–9.

26. Drolet BA, Esterly NB, Frieden IJ. Hemangiomas in children. N Engl J Med 1999;341(3):173–81.

27. Franco T, Freitas Filho SA, Muniz LB, et al. Oral peripheral nerve sheath tumors: A clinicopathological and immunohistochemical study of 32 cases in a Brazilian population. J Clin Exp Dent 2017;9(12): 1459–65.

28. Platzek I, Schubert M, Sieron D, et al. Mandibular tori as an incidental finding in MRI. Acta Radiol Short Rep 2014;3(2). 2047981614522790.

29. Edward FM. Fibro-osseous lesions of the maxillofacial bones. Head Neck Pathol 2013;7(1):5–10.

30. Katti G, Khan MM, Chaubey SS, et al. Cemento-ossifying fibroma of the jaw. Case Rep 2016;2016. bcr2015214327.

31. Gohel A, Villa A, Sakai O. Benign Jaw Lesions. Dent Clin North Am 2016;60(1):125–41.

32. Alves DBM, Tuji FM, Alves FA, et al. Evaluation of mandibular odontogenic keratocyst and ameloblastoma by panoramic radiograph and computed tomography. Dentomaxillofacial Radiol 2018;47(7): 20170288.

33. Ettinger KS, Ganry L, Fernandes RP. Oral Cavity Cancer. Oral Maxillofac Surg Clin N Am 2019; 31(1):13–29.

34. Abdel Razek AAK, Mansour M, Kamal E, et al. MR imaging of Oral Cavity and Oropharyngeal Cancer. Magn Reson Imag Clin N Am 2022;30(1):35–51.

35. Chamoli A, Gosavi AS, Shirwadkar UP, et al. Overview of oral cavity squamous cell carcinoma: Risk factors, mechanisms, and diagnostics. Oral Oncol 2021;121:105451.

36. Lydiatt WM, Patel SG, O'Sullivan B, et al. Head and neck cancers—major changes in the American Joint Committee on cancer eighth edition cancer staging manual. CA Cancer J Clin 2017;67(2):122–37.

37. Hiyama T, Kuno H, Sekiya K, et al. Imaging of Malignant Minor Salivary Gland Tumors of the Head and Neck. Radiographics 2021;41(1):175–91.

38. Abdel Razek AAK, Mukherji SK. State-of-the-Art Imaging of Salivary Gland Tumors. Neuroimaging Clin 2018;28(2):303–17.

39. Hay AJ, Migliacci J, Zanoni DK, et al. Minor Salivary Gland tumors of the Head and Neck- Memorial Sloan Kettering experience. Incidence and outcomes by site and histological type. Cancer 2019; 125(19):3354–66.

The Role of Imaging in Mandibular Reconstruction with Microvascular Surgery

Dinesh Rao, MD[a],*, Ashleigh Weyh, MD, DMD, MPH[b],
Anthony Bunnell, MD, DMD[b], Mauricio Hernandez, PhD[a]

KEYWORDS

- Mandibular reconstruction • Squamous cell carcinoma • Facial trauma • Fibular free flap
- Microvascular reconstruction • Virtual surgical planning

KEY POINTS

- Imaging plays a key role in diagnosis, preoperative planning, and disease surveillance.
- Proper surgical decision-making requires accurate imaging protocols and interpretation.
- Virtual surgical planning is used routinely for mandibular resection and reconstruction including autologous harvest site planning.

INTRODUCTION

Imaging plays a critical role in the preoperative assessment of patients undergoing mandibular reconstruction. Segmental mandibular defects can arise from neoplasm, trauma, and less commonly infection and congenital deformities.[1–7] Deformities of the face can result in impaired function, increased psychosocial stress, isolation, and depression.[1] The main goal of mandibular reconstruction is to reestablish mandibular function and to return patients to their pre-disease state.[8] The surgeon's tasks include preserving the normal contours and structure of the lower third of the face while restoring the normal functions of swallowing, mastication, and speech production. Proper dental occlusion and temporomandibular joint (TMJ) function should also be preserved to allow for dental rehabilitation.[1,9] Oral cavity anatomy consists of different types of tissue including skin, bone, mucosa, connective tissue, and muscle. Free tissue transfer allows resected tissue to be replaced with the same tissue types harvested from a distant site of the patient's own body. This "like-with-like" resection and reconstruction strategy has been shown to achieve the goals and objectives of oral cavity reconstruction while preserving structural integrity, function, and aesthetics.[10] Microvascular free tissue transfer is typically reserved for large mandibular defects usually spanning greater than 6 cm, whereas nonvascularized grafts and reconstruction plates can be used for smaller defects.[11,12]

Several classification systems for detailing mandibular defects have been proposed, although none have gained widespread acceptance.[12] The main benefit of adopting a standardized classification system is the ability to develop an algorithmic treatment strategy that encompasses both reconstruction and harvest site surgical planning.[13]

This article serves as an imaging-based review of the different etiologies of mandibular defects, including major proposed defect classification systems. We also review and illustrate reconstruction options including the advantages and morbidity of different flap sources, including

---

The authors have no disclosures.
[a] Department of Radiology, University of Florida, College of Medicine, 655 West 8th Street, Jacksonville, FL 32209, USA; [b] Department of Oral and Maxillofacial Surgery, University of Florida, College of Medicine, 655 West 8th Street, Jacksonville, FL 32209, USA
* Corresponding author.
E-mail address: rao.dinesh@mayo.edu

Oral Maxillofacial Surg Clin N Am 35 (2023) 327–344
https://doi.org/10.1016/j.coms.2023.01.002
1042-3699/23/© 2023 Elsevier Inc. All rights reserved.

options for mandibular condyle reconstruction. Imaging examples related to pathology, management decisions, and complications are provided. Lastly, we describe recent advances in presurgical planning, specifically the utility of imaging in computer-aided virtual surgical planning (VSP).

MANDIBULAR RECONSTRUCTION INDICATIONS

Segmental mandibular defects can be caused by many etiologies, the most common of which is surgical resection related to oral cavity squamous cell carcinoma (SSCA).[10] Tumor can be localized to the mucosal layer of the oral cavity or invade deeper tissue layers including bone, muscle, connective tissues, and overlying skin. Because mucosal lesions are amenable to visual inspection, smaller or lower-grade lesions can be staged primarily by clinical examination and are frequently not evident on imaging. However, the overall extent of a tumor may be underestimated on physical examination due to the depth of invasion of adjacent osseous and soft-tissue structures. Different classification systems have been proposed to take into account the different tissue types that must be resected and reconstructed.[6] SSCA can arise from any mucosal or submucosal surface within the oral cavity. The anatomic subsites of the oral cavity include the lips, floor of mouth, the oral tongue, the buccal mucosa, the upper and lower gingival surfaces, the hard palate, and the retromolar trigone. Approximately 75% of oral cavity SSCA arises from the lower lip, oral tongue, or floor of mouth, and the mandible can be involved secondarily from any subsite by direct extension. The presence of osseous involvement indicates a T4 lesion, and as such, imaging can be used to assess for both cortical and marrow space involvement.[14] Computed tomography (CT), MRI, and/or PET/CT are commonly used for complete assessment and staging. On CT, the most sensitive findings of osseous involvement include cortical erosion adjacent to the musical primary lesion, aggressive periosteal reaction, abnormal marrow space attenuation, and pathologic fractures (**Fig. 1**). CT has a sensitivity of 95% when section thickness of 1 mm and multiplanar reformats are obtained in bone windows.[15] However, these osseous changes are often difficult to discern due to the presence of beam hardening related to dental amalgam and hardware.

MRI is used for staging with relatively high sensitivity (96%) but relatively low specificity (54%).[16] The most common finding of tumor invasion into the mandible is replacement of normal hyperintense fat signal on T1-weighted images by lower

signal intensity and tumor and enhancement within the tumor and bone marrow. T2-weighted and short tau inversion recovery (STIR) images may show intermediate to hyperintense signal depending on the degree of tumor cellularity (**Fig. 2**). False positive findings on MRI can occur due to similar signal changes related to recent tooth extraction, or post-treatment-related changes such as radiation-induced fibrosis and osteoradionecrosis (ORN) (**Fig. 3**).

When invasion of the mandible is present, the preferred treatment is a partial mandibulectomy. The degree of resection depends on the extent of osseous involvement by tumor. In marginal mandibulectomy, the tumor is excised with the adjacent cortex without sacrificing the whole segment. Marginal mandibulectomy can be performed if a lesion abuts the mandible but is freely mobile on examination, or if minimal cortical invasion is present on physical examination and imaging. However, if there is gross cortical and marrow space invasion, or involvement of the inferior alveolar nerve or mental foramen, then a segmental mandibulectomy is required followed by segmental reconstruction.[17] The specific type of mandibular reconstruction performed is based on the surgical margins after tumor resection.

The timing of reconstruction following mandibular resection due to tumor has been historically debated among reconstructive surgeons. In the past, a delayed or staged approach was used with reconstruction after a period of observation to evaluate for the development of recurrent disease. Delayed reconstruction was assumed to be critical for wound bed maturation to allow for graft placement. However, due to the evolution of microsurgical techniques it has become widely accepted that immediate reconstruction can be performed without risk of recurrent disease.[18] Healing of the reconstruction flap is essential because adjuvant radiation therapy must be performed within 6 weeks of surgery to improve patient survival.[19,20] Additionally, most patients prefer immediate reconstruction as it results in higher quality of life as compared with staged reconstruction.[21–25]

The types of defects caused by trauma and ORN are similar to those resulting from tumor ablative surgery; however, each poses unique challenges. Avulsive segmental fractures can occur from gunshot wounds, industrial accidents, and occasionally motor vehicle collisions (**Fig. 4**). Blunt trauma usually does not have enough kinetic injury to cause the kind of segmental defects that necessitate reconstruction. The kinetic energy associated with missile projectiles, such as bullets, dramatically increases the impact on bone and

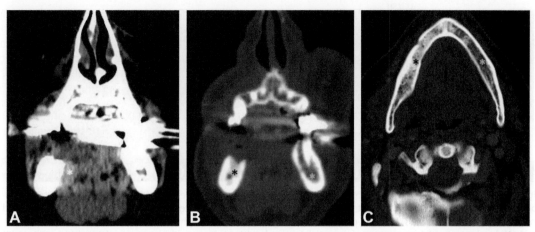

Fig. 1. A 79-year-old man with biopsy-proven right mandibular alveolar ridge SCCA. (*A*) Enhanced coronal CT reconstructed image showing a soft-tissue component of tumor along the lingual mucosa of the right mandible. (*B*) Coronal and (*C*) axial bone window reconstructions show increased attenuation within the marrow space of the mandibular body (*black asterisk*) in comparison to the normal density of the contralateral mandibular body marrow (*blue asterisk*). On examination, the exophytic component of the tumor was fixed to the mandible.

soft tissues and results in devitalization due to vascular compromise.[8] For complex mandibular defects due to trauma, microvascular free flap reconstruction has become the mainstay of treatment.[26]

ORN is a severe complication following radiation therapy for head and neck malignancies. ORN is defined as a condition in which the necrotic bone becomes exposed through a wound in the overlying mucosa or skin.[27] Owing to its tenuous blood supply, ORN is more likely to occur in the mandible than the other bones of the head and neck.[28] The

presence of dental decay, minor trauma, and tooth extraction can increase the chances of developing ORN.[29] ORN-related mandibular necrosis results from radiation-induced vascular compromise, and therefore carries a less favorable prognosis for reconstruction than from other etiologies.[4] On CT, ORN is characterized by lytic bony destruction, cortical disruption, and a loss of marrow trabeculations (**Fig. 5**). On MRI, ORN is characterized by bone destruction without a soft-tissue mass. The bone may be low or intermediate in signal intensity on T1-weighted-images and

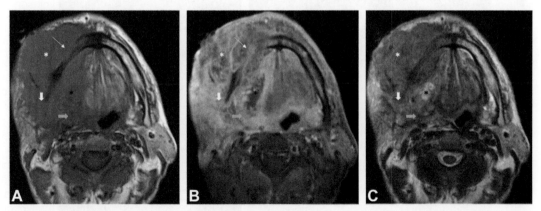

Fig. 2. A 61-year-old man with biopsy-proven anterior floor of mouth SCCA with lingual and buccal mucosa with mandibular invasion and extension anteriorly to the cutaneous surface. The posterior tumor invades the masticator space and the parotid gland (*white block arrows*). The medial portion of the tumor extends along the floor of mouth posteriorly to the base of tongue (*blue block arrows*). (*A*) Axial T1-weighted image show hypointense tumor (*white asterisk*) invading the mandibular cortex. Note the cortical destruction and marrow space invasion by tumor (*thin white arrows*). (*B*) Axial T1-weighted fat-saturated image with gadolinium shows heterogeneous enhancement. The relative hypointense T1 area in the right floor of mouth (*black asterisk*) shows no evidence of enhancement and is hyperintense on the axial T2-weighted image (*C*) indicating tumor necrosis.

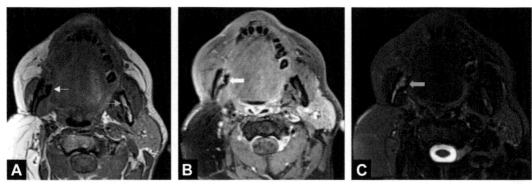

Fig. 3. MRI from a 51-year-old male who underwent resection of the right external auditory canal and parotidectomy for cutaneous SCCA. The patient had ADA tooth 32 removed prior to radiotherapy. (*A*) Axial T1-weighted image demonstrates loss of normal hyperintense fat signal within the right mandibular marrow (*thin white arrow*). Note the normal hyperintense fat signal in the healthy left mandibular ramus (*thin blue arrow*). (*B*) Enhanced Axial T1-weighted image with fat-saturation demonstrates enhancement of the marrow space (*thick white arrow*) due to the recent tooth extraction. (*C*) Axial STIR image demonstrates hyperintense signal within the marrow, reflective of reactive edema-like signal from the recent traumatic extraction. These signal changes can easily be mistaken for tumor.

hyperintense on T2 or STIR. Adjacent soft tissues may show hyperintense T2/STIR signal and enhancement[30] (**Figs. 6** and **7**). ORN with or without superimposed osteomyelitis can be difficult to distinguish from tumor recurrence.

Recurrent tumor often occurs at the surgical resection margins. The margin between the resection site, also known as the recipient bed, and the flap is the most common site of local disease recurrence[31] (**Fig. 8**). The presence of a solid or cystic soft-tissue mass is strongly associated with tumor recurrence[32] (**Fig. 9**). Other

complications along the margins of a flap include dehiscence and fistula formation. Soft-tissue infections can also occur with nonspecific imaging features including soft-tissue swelling and stranding. Distinguishing recurrent tumor for infection or post-treatment changes from tumor recurrence may be difficult on imaging alone, and therefore surgical debridement or biopsy may be necessary[31] (**Fig. 10**). Early stages of ORN are treated conservatively with antibiotics, daily chlorhexidine rinses, and occasionally hyperbaric oxygen therapy. However, more advanced stages of ORN

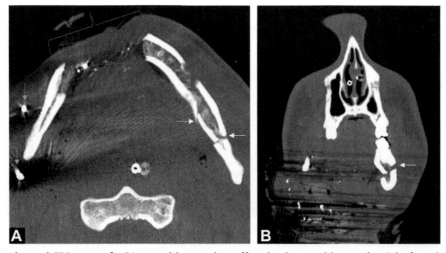

Fig. 4. Unenhanced CT images of a 21-year-old man who suffered a shotgun blast to the right face. (*A*) Axial image shows a large segmental defect of the right anterior mandible (*red bracket*). A nondisplaced fracture of the left mandibular body was present due to blunt force (*white arrows*). Metallic debris from the buckshot was present throughout the lower face (*blue arrows*). (*B*) Coronal image show the large segmental defect (*red bracket*) with overlying severe soft-tissue injury of the skin, submental and submandibular spaces, and floor of mouth. Note the fracture of the left mandible (*white arrow*).

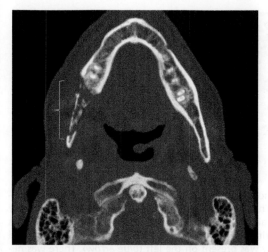

Fig. 5. Axial CT image of a 63-year-old woman show a lytic lesion in the posterior mandibular body extending to the angle. The dot-dash and fragmented appearance without a soft-tissue mass is characteristic of osteoradionecrosis. The patient had oropharyngeal squamous cell carcinoma treated with chemotherapy and radiation therapy 5 years prior.

often require surgical intervention including mandibular resection with microvascular reconstruction.

Similar to ORN, the mandible is the most commonly affected bone for medicine-related osteonecrosis of the jaw (MRONJ). MRONJ is related to the systemic uptake of pharmaceuticals, most commonly bisphosphonate medications. However, it has also been associated with immunosuppressive and antiangiogenic drugs such as Avastin.[5,33,34] MRONJ is primarily diagnosed on CT. Imaging findings are nonspecific, and this entity can be radiographically indistinguishable from ORN. A wide spectrum of findings has been reported in MRONJ including bone sclerosis, erosion of cortical bone, periosteal reaction, disruption of trabecular bone, and pathologic fractures.[35] The presence of a bony sequestrum and adjacent soft-tissue swelling are found in approximately 50% of patients[36] (**Fig. 11**). In contrast to ORN of the mandible, treatment of MRONJ is primarily palliative with fastidious dental hygiene with mouthwashes and antimicrobials. Surgery is generally avoided because it can aggravate the degree of necrosis.[34]

MANDIBULAR DEFECT CLASSIFICATION

When the mandible is invaded by tumor, segmental resection is the first and most important step in the treatment process.[37] Mandibular and other oral cavity defects resulting from tumor resection determine the type of reconstruction that can be offered. The goal of a classification is to aid in the development of a reconstructive treatment strategy. An ideal classification system would be logical and simple, with defects falling into categories that are reflective of increasing complexity and difficulty of achieving the objectives of surgical reconstruction.[37] Although there is no established standard, classification systems are helpful as they can highlight the size and

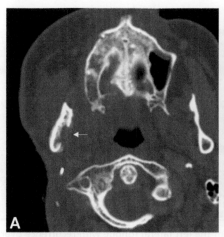
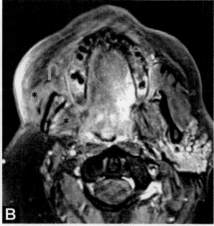

Fig. 6. A 49-year-old man who underwent parotidectomy, resection of the right EAC, and mastoidectomy for cutaneous SCCA followed by reconstruction and flap failure. (*A*) Axial enhanced CT of the neck in bone window show periosteal reaction, mixed cortical thickening, and erosion with disruption of the normal trabecular pattern (*white arrow*) suggestive of ORN. An MRI was obtained (*B*) 1 year after ALT flap reconstruction show enhancement of the mandibular angle marrow space (*red asterisk*), the adjacent masticator space musculature (*black asterisk*), and the adjacent left facial soft tissues and buccal space (*curved blue arrow*). The enhancement of normal soft tissues without a mass lesion can be seen adjacent to an area of ORN.

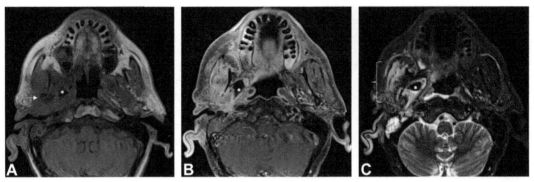

Fig. 7. 55-year-old male with a history of multiple recurrences of benign mixed tumor who had undergone multiple resections in the superficial and deep parotid lobes. The patient had malignant transformation with tumor located in the parapharyngeal space, underwent gross total surgical resection followed by radiotherapy 5 years prior. (*A*) Axial T1 MRI demonstrating loss of normal hyperintense fat signal within the mandibular condyle and ramus (*white arrow*). The normal healthy condylar marrow was present on the left (*blue arrow*). There was necrosis of the masticator, parapharyngeal, and overlying mucosal soft tissues with fistula formation with the oropharynx (*white asterisks*). (*B*) Enhanced Axial T1 fat saturated image demonstrating enhancement of the soft tissues surrounding the necrotic bone (*red bracket*). On Axial STIR (*C*), these tissues demonstrate hyperintense signal (*white bracket*).

location of the defects, as well as the associated functional and esthetic deficits. The primary difficulties in mandibular reconstruction arise from the anatomic complexity of the mandibular arch, the relation to the opposing maxillary dentition, as well as its articulation with the temporal bone. The mandible can be divided into three major sections: the horizontal body, the vertical ramus, and the anterior (central) segment. The horizontal or lateral body extends from the mandibular angle to the canine teeth. Lateral resections that spare the ramus or central mandible portend good

functional and esthetic outcomes[19,38]. The symphyseal or anterior portion of the mandible is located between the canine teeth, including the incisors, and serves as the attachment of the paired geniohyoid and digastric muscles, which are important for mouth opening. Anterior symphyseal defects present greater challenges in successful reconstruction related to the functional objectives of swallowing, mastication, speech, and breathing. Tumor involving the anterior segment of the mandible may necessitate resection of either the anterior floor of mouth or lower lip, which can

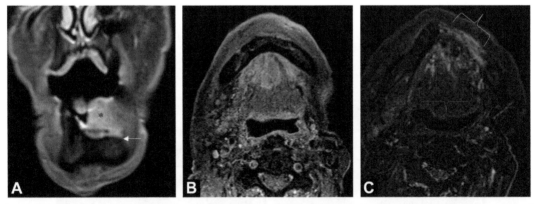

Fig. 8. MRI of a 78-year-old man with a history of SCCA of the left lateral tongue with recurrence over a decade later. Patient underwent composite resection of the left posterior tongue, floor of mouth, and marginal mandibulectomy. (*A*) Enhanced coronal T1-weighted image with fat saturation show the left symphyseal marginal mandibulectomy defect (*white arrow*) and recurrent tumor along the superior margin (*red asterisk*). (*B*) Enhanced axial T1-weighted image with fat saturation show recurrent enhancing tumor along the posterior margin of the mandible invading the floor of mouth (*red bracket*). (*C*) Axial STIR image 5 mm superior to (*B*) show the recurrent tumor along the superior margin of the mandibulectomy defect (*blue bracket*) and the posterior extent of tumor along the floor of mouth (*red bracket*).

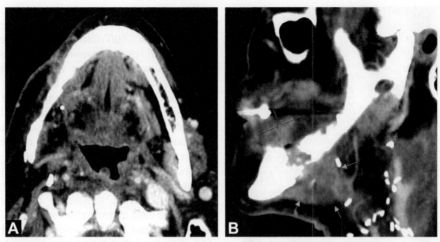

Fig. 9. Enhanced CT images of a 61-year-old woman with history of right oral cavity SCCA, underwent marginal mandibulectomy and nodal dissection followed by chemotherapy and radiotherapy several years prior. The patient developed ORN in the native mandible. (*A*) Axial image shows a cystic/necrotic soft-tissue mass along the lingual and buccal cortical surfaces of the mandible (*red asterisks*). (*B*) Sagittal obliqued reconstructed image shows a fragmented left mandibular body (*red bracket*) and necrotic soft-tissue mass inferior to the mandible worrisome for recurrent tumor (outlined by *blue arrows*).

cause problems with speech, swallowing, incompetent oral cavity closure, and esthetics. Vertical segments extend from the mandibular angle to the ramus including the condyle and coronoid process. Condylar resection poses unique problems, as stability of the TMJ is necessary for proper dental occlusion, oral intake and speech.

Pavlov published the first mandibular defect classification in 1974.[39] In this classification system, mandibular defects were placed into three different classes depending on the number of remaining mandibular arch fragments (1, 2, or 3) after resection. This classification recognized the functional problems posed by resection of the

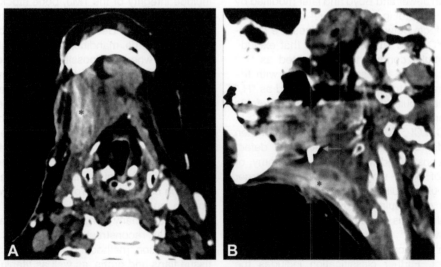

Fig. 10. Enhanced CT images of an 81-year-old woman with history of right lateral tongue SCCA who underwent right hemiglossectomy and selective node dissection, chemotherapy, and radiation 10 years prior. The patient underwent segmental mandibulectomy and reconstruction and developed an orocutaneous fistula with an adjacent area of swelling on clinical examination. (*A*) Axial oblique CT shows an enhancing soft-tissue lesion (*red asterisk*) in the right submental area. (*B*) Enhanced sagittal oblique reconstruction show enhancing mass-like lesion (*red asterisk*) extending posteriorly and inferior to the hyoid bone (*blue arrow*). This was debrided and pathology returned chronic inflammatory changes related to treatment and the fistula.

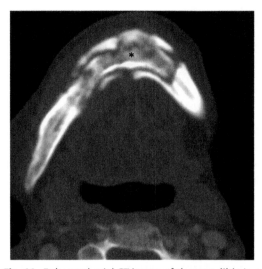

Fig. 11. Enhanced axial CT image of the mandible in a 72-year-old woman with MRONJ. The patient had undergone treatment with bisphosphonates for several years for osteoporosis. Note the sequestered bone fragment in the central mandibular segment (*black asterisk*) with surrounding fragmented and irregular cortex and trabecular bone. A sequestered bone fragment is present in 50% of MRONJ cases.

condyle and the symphysis, and technical difficulties in achieving the goals of reconstruction of these anatomic regions. Since that time, many classification systems have been proposed, of which, the most widely cited is the HCL classification by both Jewer and Boyd and later modified by Boyd.[40,41] According to the Jewer classification, central defects between both canines are designated as "C," and lateral segments that exclude the mandibular condyle are designated as "L." When the condyle is resected together with the lateral mandible, the defect is designated as "H," or hemi-mandibular (**Fig. 12**). Mandibular defects can be combined into eight combinations—C, L, H, LC, HC, LCL, HCL, and HH—which can then be used for surgical planning. A lateral defect can be reconstructed with a single osteotomy, or segment of bone, whereas a central or larger defect would require multiple osteotomies and potentially mandibular condyle reconstruction.[42] Boyd modified this system to include soft-tissue defects, with "t" representing a large tongue defect, "m" a mucosal defect, and "s" an external skin defect. Further classification includes the mucosal and soft-tissue components of the defect with "o", no muscle/skin, "m" muscle only, and "s" skin only.

Urken developed a comprehensive classification of composite oral cavity and mandibular defects, including the presence of neurologic deficits if the inferior alveolar, lingual, hypoglossal, or facial nerves are involved.[43] This system is complex with over 3500 different combinations when nerve structures are involved, and 400 if considering only soft-tissue and bony defects. When classifying the mandible by bone defects: *C*ondyle, *R*amus, *B*ody, *S*ymphysis, and incorporates soft-tissue defect: Mucosa- *L*abial, *B*uccal, *SP* soft palate, *FOM* floor of mouth, as well as *T*ongue, and *C*utaneous. A major criticism of the Urken classification is that it is purely descriptive, and individual cases cannot be stratified into categories based on complexity or the technical difficulty of achieving successful reconstruction.[37] More simplified classification systems have since been proposed based solely on defect location and laterality, while taking into account the need for mandibular ramus and condyle resection, and the viability of ipsilateral vasculature with which the flap can be anastomosed.[37,44] Mandibular defects fall into either lateral or anterior defects within these simplified classification systems.

MANDIBULAR RECONSTRUCTION OPTIONS

An understanding of native mandibular functionality with regard to swallowing, mastication, and speech production is necessary for successful reconstruction of mandibular defects. Proper dental occlusion and TMJ function is necessary for biomechanical function and stability. Factors that influence the biomechanics of the mandible include integrity of the TMJ, bone stock distribution, and the forces associated with postoperative scar contracture. Because the TMJ is difficult to reconstruct, the mandibular condyle should be preserved whenever possible.[42] The contour of the mandible is important to facial symmetry as well as oral and tongue function. The anterior midline portion of the mandible has greater trabecular bone density, as it serves as an attachment of extrinsic and submental muscles.[45] The mandibular symphysis serves as the anchor to the mylohyoid muscle, which supports the proper function of the tongue. Disruption of the mandibular arch can result in problems with swallowing, speech, and articulation.

There are many surgical options available for mandibular reconstruction. The most common reconstruction methods use osseous and soft-tissue flaps and grafts, as well as titanium reconstruction plates used to span smaller segmental defects.[20] Both grafts and flaps are blocks of tissue transferred from the patient. Whereas flaps include tissues with their own blood supply, grafts rely on angiogenesis via blood supply from the recipient bed. Microvascular free flaps are

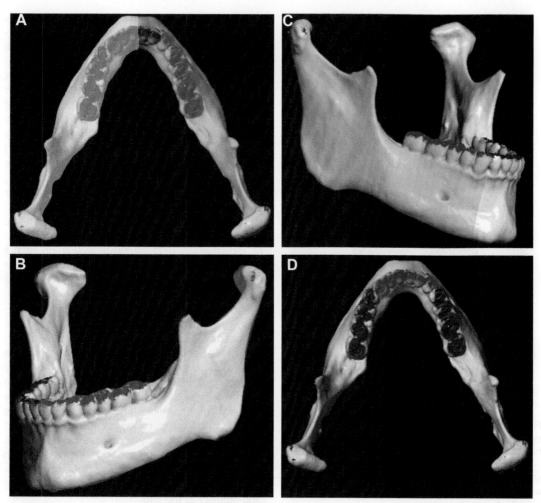

Fig. 12. 3D-reconstructed images of a normal mandible to illustrate the Jewer classification. (*A*) Superior downward 3D image of a normal mandible. The yellow-shaded area of the right mandible corresponds to a theoretic "H" defect involving the mandibular symphysis to the condyle. The blue shaded area corresponds to a theoretic "L" defect involving the base of the ipsilateral canine tooth to the condylar neck sparing the condyle. (*B*) Right lateral oblique 3D image. The shaded yellow portion of the left mandible denotes a theoretic "H" type of defect from the symphysis up to and including the mandibular condyle. (*C*) Right lateral oblique 3D image. The shaded blue portion of the right mandible denotes a lateral or "L" type of defect extending from the canine tooth to the base of the articular process not including the condyle. (*D*) Superior downward view reconstructed 3D image of a normal mandible. The shaded green portion of the mandible corresponds to a central or "C" defect of the central mandibular segment including the incisors and bilateral canine teeth.

harvested to include an artery and vein, which then require microsurgical anastomosis to major vessels of the neck near the defect.[46,47] Flaps and grafts may be from the donor (autograft), from other people or cadavers (allograft), or from man-made materials (alloplastic). For superficial cosmetic portions of reconstruction, the surgeon can choose either full-thickness skin flaps, which contain complete epidermis and dermis or split-thickness grafts with complete epidermis but the varying thickness of the dermis.[48,49]

For more complex restoration procedures, such as those needed for mandibular reconstruction,

flaps are generally superior to grafts because of the larger bulk of tissue needed to fill the resection defect. Because of the blood supply, flaps typically show superior healing with less contracture and better cosmesis. This is especially important when reconstructing a mandible with compromised blood supply, as in cases of osteonecrosis or osteomyelitis.[50,51]

The most common sources of autologous bone free-tissue transfer for mandibular reconstruction are the fibula, the iliac crest, the scapula, and the radius.[52] The fibular free flap (FFF) is the gold standard and workhorse for the reconstruction of

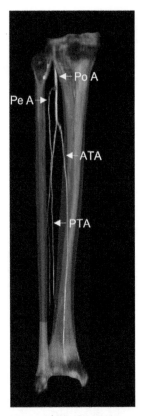

Fig. 13. Reconstructed 3D CT angiogram of a lower extremity. 25 cm of fibular length (*red area*) can be harvested for mandibular reconstruction. At least 7 cm of the distal fibula (*green area*) must be preserved to maintain ankle stability. AT A, anterior tibial artery; Pe A, peroneal artery; PT A, posterior tibial artery; Po A, popliteal artery.

mandibular defects. Reconstructions using the FFF have been shown to have the shortest operation time, the least amount of blood loss, and with low donor site morbidity.[52] The FFF receives arterial blood supply from the peroneal artery and periosteal branches. The rich blood supply to the lower extremity and foot renders the fibula an excellent supply of bone, muscle, and skin if necessary. Signs of previous surgery, trauma, or signs of impaired perfusion should be evaluated clinically and with imaging. Doppler ultrasound, CT, and MR angiography can also be performed to assess for patent three-vessel flow to the lower extremity[53] (**Fig. 13**). The peroneal artery terminates above the ankle joint, with the anterior and posterior tibial arteries supplying the dorsal and plantar surfaces in the foot respectively. In 7% to 12% of patients, atherosclerotic disease-related stenosis of the tibial arteries results in a dominant peroneal artery, making it the main blood supply for the distal leg and foot and therefore unsuitable for flap harvest. Rarely, an arteria peronea magna,

a congenital anomaly in which the peroneal artery is the sole vessel supplying the foot may be present. This is estimated to occur in 0.2% to 0.9% of the population.[54,55]

Evaluation of the anticipated mandibular defect should be performed with the aid of a panoramic radiograph and CT of the mandible. Evaluation of the recipient vessels in the head and neck is also critically important. The ipsilateral facial artery and vein are most commonly anastomosed to the flap vasculature when reconstructing the mandible (**Fig. 14**). The superior thyroid artery, the external jugular vein, and the internal jugular vein, as well as contralateral neck vessels, can also be used as recipient's vessels. In patients who have undergone previous neck dissections or radiotherapy (RT), accurate evaluation of the head and neck vasculature is critical to ascertain the presence or absence of the above-named vessels.[53]

Approximately 25 cm of bone length can be supplied by the fibula, which is longer than any other donor site.[53] The rich blood supply and the uniformity of the bone in width and length allow the fibula to be osteotomized as many times as necessary for reconstruction.[56] Multiple osteotomies can be used to shape the anterior arch, body, angle, or ramus of the mandible (**Fig. 15**). The skin of the lower lateral leg can be incorporated into the flap in cases of malignancy or avulsed tissues due to trauma where wide excision is needed to reach healthy tissues.[42] A portion of soleus or flexor hallucis longus muscle can be used to provide bulk and stability to the flap.[50]

Complications of the FFF include flap loss caused by vessel thrombosis. The incidence of total flap loss is 5% or less in high-volume centers with experienced surgeons, and in cases without prior radiation treatment.[19,56] Morbidity of the donor site is low. If a 7 cm or greater distal fibular segment is preserved, with maintenance of the tibio-fibular interosseous membrane, then ankle joint stability will be preserved.[57] Patients generally return to normal function in 5 to 6 weeks postoperatively.[58] Complications include peroneal muscle weakness, sensory loss, and inability to run.

The scapular free flap (SFF) can be harvested for complex composite defects of large tissue loss. The subscapular artery supplies the circumflex humeral and thoracodorsal arteries which supply blood to the latissimus dorsi and anterior serratus muscles which can be used in large facial reconstructions. The vascular pedicle length is 11 to 14 cm.[58,59] The circumflex scapular artery supplies the lateral aspect of the scapula through periosteal branches, which allows for the harvesting of

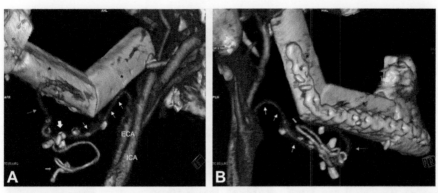

Fig. 14. 3D reconstructed views (*A*: medial view, *B*: lateral view) of a microvascular anastomosis of a fibular free flap in a 46-year-old man for an ameloblastoma. The facial artery (*white arrows*) was anastomosed to the peroneal artery (*blue arrows*) with a microvascular anastomotic coupler (*white block arrow*). The fibular flap was osteotomized into two segments (*black asterisks*) and placed adjacent to the native anterior mandible (*red asterisk*). Tubing related to an intraoperative ultrasound device was captured in the image (*blue block arrows*).

10 to 14 cm of bone for an osteocutaneous reconstruction. The major advantage of this flap is that the subscapular arterial system allows the surgeon to harvest a composite of bone, muscle, and skin for large complex reconstructions. A major disadvantage of this flap is the difficulty in patient positioning. Patients must be placed in a decubitus position to harvest the flap, and then repositioned for mandibular reconstruction. In comparison, the

FFF and iliac crest free flap (ICFF) can be harvested and reconstructed by two separate teams without repositioning which shortens operative time. Another disadvantage of the SFF is the thin bone stock, which makes it unsuitable for dental implants, and the inability to create multiple osteotomies.[60]

The anatomy of the ICFF has been described by Taylor and colleagues.[61] The ICFF can be used for

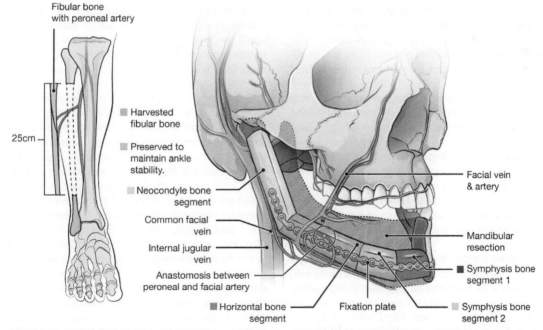

Fig. 15. Artistic rendering show the versatility of the FFF in reconstructing the different segments of the resected mandible. Up to 25 cm of fibula can be harvested and osteotomized into different bone segments to replace the vertical and horizontal segments of the mandible. Several smaller bone segments can be used to reconstruct the central area. (Christopher M. Brown, BFA, MS, Indianapolis, IN.)

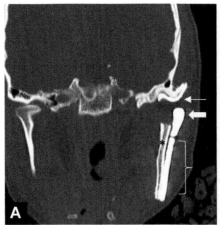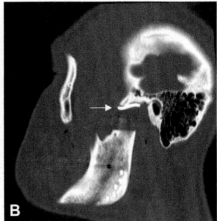

Fig. 16. Unenhanced coronal (*A*) and sagittal (*B*) CT of Left TMJ prosthesis in a 24-year-old woman with malocclusion secondary to craniofacial dysplasia. Black asterisk (*)—native mandible. White bracket—prosthetic TMJ mandibular ramus component. Thick white arrow—prosthetic TMJ condylar head component. Thin white arrow—TMJ glenoid fossa component.

large mandibular defects. The iliac crest provides a large bone stock, muscle, and skin for adequate tissue coverage. Both anterior and hemi-mandible defects can be reconstructed using the anterior superior iliac spine to recreate the mandibular angle.[62,63] The osteocutaneous flap is supplied by the DCIA. The main disadvantage of this flap is its short vascular pedicle, which often necessitates a vein graft to increase the pedicle length to carry out the anastomosis.[53] The ICFF has been shown to have the highest rate of flap loss in comparison to other flaps. Finally, donor site morbidity is also relatively higher in comparison with other flaps, including chronic pain, gait problems, and fractures of the anterior superior iliac spine.[52]

The radial forearm osteocutaneous free flap (RFFF) relies on the patency of the radial artery. The RFFF provides a small amount of bone and a skin paddle that can be used for intraoral lining. Although an advantage of this flap is the long vascular pedicle length, the osteocutaneous variant of this flap is seldom used for mandibular reconstruction due to the lack of sufficient bone height and width. The thickness of the bone graft is inadequate to support multiple osteotomies and bone implants.[60] Additionally, the harvested bone does not provide enough structural strength for mastication.[63] Also, there is high morbidity with high rates of fractures of the remaining radius. Grip, pinch, and range of motion may also be reduced in the affected hand when fractures occur. The most feared complication of RFFF harvest is an ischemic hand. Although Doppler ultrasound can be used to determine patency of the radial artery, the Allen's test remains the most

accurate method for preoperative evaluation of blood flow to the hand.[64]

MANDIBULAR CONDYLE RECONSTRUCTION

Resection of the mandibular condyle may be necessary when defects involve the mandibular ramus. When condylar resection is necessary, options for reconstruction are limited. The anatomy of the TMJ is complex and its function is difficult to recreate. Mandibular resections that involve mandibular condyle disarticulation can result in facial deformities and impaired occlusion, mastication, and speech. Joint ankylosis can occur if reconstruction is not performed which can impair function.

Generally, the condyle is planned for resection if the remaining bone stock would not allow for at least three titanium screws to be placed to stabilize the reconstruction plate that fixates the flap segments to the native mandible. There are several options for condylar replacement. Titanium joint prostheses have been used; however, these are only used on a short-term basis (2 years) because of complications related to hardware failure, dehiscence, and intracranial migration[65] (**Fig. 16**). Another option to maintain TMJ function is to add the resected condyle to the fibular flap[66] (**Fig. 17**). However, this may not allow for adequate surgical margins and risks tumor residual or recurrence. Also, resection of the condyle from the native mandible may result in devascularization that can increase the risk of flap failure and ORN.

Although there is no consensus, using a segment of fibula to reconstruct the mandibular condyle has been shown to provide long-term

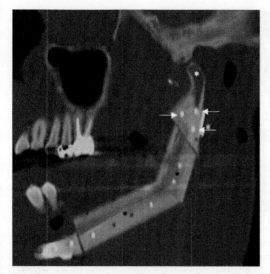

Fig. 17. Oblique sagittal CT image of a 72-year-old man with ORN of the mandibular angle. The patient underwent resection of the mandibular body, angle and ramus. There was enough normal bone below the mandibular condyle (*white asterisk*) to attach the microplate to the fibular flap segments (*black asterisks*) with 3 screws (*white arrows*).

stability in patients requiring condylar resection.[67] In this technique, the glenoid fossa is preserved and the end of the fibula is reshaped into a rounded neocondyle. The articular disc is very important for the function of the TMJ reconstruction and is preserved to articulate with the neocondyle[65] (**Fig. 18**). The fibular flap is fitted into the mandibular segmental flap and held in place by a fitted plate or reconstruction bar. A bar is usually adapted prior to the resection and contoured to the planned reconstructed FFF. The fibular neocondyle must be maintained within the glenoid fossa. After the flap is placed and the vascular anastomosis is completed, the masseter muscle can be sutured to the angle of reconstruction plate to maintain the condylar position and function.

VIRTUAL SURGICAL PLANNING

Prior to the development of preoperative three-dimensional (3D) planning, surgical decisions were based on physical examination findings, preoperative imaging, and intraoperative findings. A successful reconstruction, therefore, relied heavily on the surgeon's experience level and skill.[68] Each step from tumor ablation, flap harvesting, shaping, and placing the neomandible into the defect were performed by hand and based on two-dimensional imaging scans.[69] This resulted in a lack of standardization between surgeons of different skill levels. This further led to heterogeneous outcomes

among surgeons, particularly in complex cases wherein prolonged operative times resulted in complications such as flap failure.[70–72]

Preoperative 3D planning is also known as computer-aided design, computer-aided manufacturing, and VSP. VSP has been evolving since the 1990's and has revolutionized how surgeons perform free tissue transfer to reconstruct mandibular defects. As discussed previously, the complex anatomy and functional relationships of the mandible requires deep understanding and surgical precision to achieve the goals of reconstruction. In comparison to the free-hand approaches of the past, VSP technology allows for improved understanding of each patient and takes the guesswork out of determining resection margins, osteomotizing the flap to create the neomandible, bending fixation plates, and in-setting the free flap.[73] This has led to improved outcomes, and less time spent in the operating room.[74,75]

VSP can be divided into three phases:[76] (1) presurgical planning, (2) modeling, and (3) prototyping, and the surgical phase. During the planning phase, a high-resolution CT scan of the patient's maxillofacial skeleton is sent to the vendor and reconstructed into 3D images. Computed tomographic angiogram (CTA) images of the lower extremity are also obtained to evaluate the fibula harvest site and associated vasculature. The mandibular resection margins and placement of the FFF are planned and marked on the 3D reconstruction images. The FFF is created virtually and superimposed on the virtual mandibular defect. In cases in which the condyle must be resected, a prosthetic or neo-condyle can be incorporated into the 3D plan.[73] The fibula can be virtually osteotomized to precisely recreate the shape of the native mandible. During the modeling phase, stereolithographic components are manufactured. A model of the craniofacial skeleton is made to assist the surgeons and patients. Cutting guides are created that fit onto the mandible that allows the actual resection to match that which was created virtually during the planning phase. Patient-specific reconstruction plates can be pre-bent to match the virtual plate design. Prefabricated cutting guides are used for both the resection and reconstruction phase of the surgery. If applicable, simultaneous placement of dental implants is planned into the cutting guide and included within the design (**Fig. 19**).

One disadvantage of VSP is that the presurgical planning sessions can be time-consuming. Planning sessions with VSP vendors can range from 15 to 60 min and the modeling phase has been reported to take between 8 and 15 days.[73,77,78] Although these times can vary depending on the

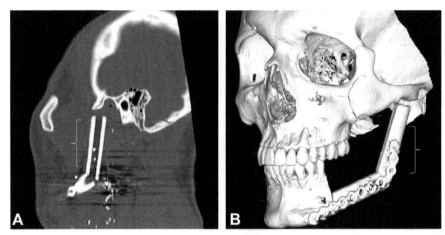

Fig. 18. Sagittal (*A*) and 3D-reconstructed left anterior oblique (*B*) postoperative CT in a 28-year-old man with comminuted mandibular fracture involving the condyle requiring mandibular reconstruction with FFF and TMJ reconstruction with a vertical fibular segment (*white bracket*) articulating with the glenoid fossa (*black asterisk*).

institution and vendor, shorter treatment windows have been associated with lower locoregional recurrence for malignant oral cavity lesions.[79] Another drawback of VSP is that less experienced surgeons may over-rely on the prefabricated cutting guides. If the intraoperative findings no longer mirror the virtual plan because of interval tumor progression or other factors, the surgeon may

have to revert to a traditional free hand approach to achieve adequate resection margins and reconstruction.[80] Finally, VSP is currently unable to account for both the soft-tissue components of tumor resection and soft-tissue reconstruction. Therefore, anticipated defects resulting from soft-tissue resection are made clinically during treatment planning.

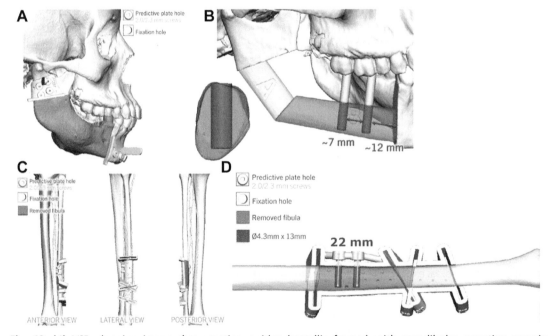

Fig. 19. (*A*) VSP planning image show cutting guides (metallic frames) with mandibular resection margin (mandible in *red*). (*B*) VSP images show metallic cutting guides to assist with fibular osteotomy segments (*dark and light green*). (*C*) Simulation image show the fibular segments (*light and dark green*) inset into the defect after mandibular resection. Endosseous dental implants (*gray and yellow cylinders*) can be planned during the planning phase. (*D*) VSP data show incorporation of the dental implants guides into the fibula cutting guides. This allows for simultaneous dental implant placement at the time of harvest of the fibula-free flap.

SUMMARY

Segmental mandibular defects can occur from several etiologies, including oral cavity SSCA, ORN, trauma, and infection. Mandibular defects must be reconstructed to restore oral cavity function, cosmesis, and to avoid psychosocial morbidity resulting from disease. Many classification systems exist to aid surgeons in decision-making. The basic tenet of all classification systems is to stratify patients according to the difficulties of achieving the goals of reconstruction, particularly when the central mandibular segment and mandibular condyle are involved. The role of imaging in mandibular reconstruction has expanded beyond its traditional role in diagnosis, cancer staging, and disease surveillance. As microvascular surgical techniques have evolved over the past 20 years to allow autologous free tissue transfer for osseous and soft-tissue oral cavity defects, so too has the role of imaging in preoperative 3D computer-assisted planning of both resection and flap harvest sites. These advances are particularly important in complex resections and have shown value in reaching the goals of reconstruction with improved efficiency, decreased operative time, and decreased morbidity.

CLINICS CARE POINTS

- Squamous cell carcinoma arises from the lower lip, oral tongue, and floor of mouth in 75% of oral cavity cancers and can invade the mandible by direct extension.

- New or residual tumor, recent dental extractions, osteoradionecrosis (ORN), and osteomyelitis can have similar appearances on computed tomography and MRI. The presence of a soft-tissue mass increases the probability of residual or recurrent tumor.

- Recurrent tumor most commonly occurs at the surgical resection margins.

- Imaging features of ORN overlap with medicine-related osteonecrosis of the jaw (MRONJ); 50% of MRONJ cases show a sequestrum.

- Anterior and condylar mandibular defects are more difficult to reconstruct than lateral defects.

- The fibular free flap is the gold standard for mandibular reconstruction due to the length and thickness of the bone for reconstruction and the rich blood supply and length of the peroneal artery.

- Virtual surgical planning helps in mandibular segmental resection, reconstruction, and harvest site planning.

REFERENCES

1. Batstone MD. Reconstruction of major defects of the jaws. Aust Dent J 2018;63(Suppl1):S108–13.
2. Paré A, Joly A. Oral cancer: risk factors and management. Presse Medicale Paris Fr 2017;46:320–30.
3. Khatib B, Gelesko S, Amundson M, et al. Updates in management of craniomaxillofacial gunshot wounds and reconstruction of the mandible. Facial Plast Surg Clin North Am 2017;25(4):563–76.
4. Rommel N, Kesting MR, Rohleder NH, et al. Surgical management of severe osteoradionecrosis of the mandibular bone by using double free flap reconstruction. J Cranio-Maxillo-Fac Surg 2018;46(1):148–54.
5. Neto T, Horta R, Balhau R, et al. Resection and microvascular reconstruction of bisphosphonate-related osteonecrosis of the jaw: the role of microvascular reconstruction. Head Neck 2016;38(8):1278–85.
6. Paré A, Joly A, Laure B, et al. A chronic swelling of the mandible in a child. J Stomatol Oral Maxillofac Surg 2018;119(1):81–2.
7. Baur DA, Altay MA, Flores-Hidalgo A, et al. Chronic osteomyelitis of the mandible: diagnosis and management—an institution's experience over 7 years. J Oral Maxillofac Surg 2015;73(4):655–65.
8. Namaki S, Matsumoto M, Ohba H, et al. Masticatory efficiency before and after surgery in oral cancer patients: comparative study of glossectomy, marginal mandibulectomy and segmental mandibulectomy. J Oral Sci 2004;46(2):113–7.
9. Kumar VV, Jacob PC, Ebenezer S, et al. Implant supported dental rehabilitation following segmental mandibular reconstruction-quality of life outcomes of a prospective randomized trial. J Cranio-Maxillo-Fac Surg 2016;44(7):800–10.
10. Butler DP, Dunne JA, Wood SH, et al. A Unifying Algorithm in Microvascular Reconstruction of Oral Cavity Defects Using the Trilaminar Concept. Plast Recontr Surg Glob Open 2019;7:e2267.
11. Foster RD, Anthony JP, Sharma A, et al. Vascularized bone flaps versus nonvascularized bone grafts for mandibular reconstruction: an outcome analysis of primary bony union and endosseous implant success. Head Neck 1999 Jan;21(1):66–71.
12. Nandra B, Fattahi T, Martin T, et al. Free Bone Grafts for Mandibular Reconstruction in Patients Who Have Not Received Radiotherapy: The 6-cm Rule-Myth or Reality? Craniomaxillofac Trauma Reconstr 2017;10(2):117–22.

13. Paré A, Bossard A, Laure B, et al. Reconstruction of segmental mandibular defects: Current procedures and perspectives. Laryngoscope Investig Otolaryngol 2019;4(6):587–96.

14. Trotta BM, Pease CS, Rasamny JJ, et al. Oral cavity and oropharyngeal squamous cell cancer: key imaging findings for staging and treatment planning. Radiographics 2011;31(2):339–54.

15. Brockenbrough JM, Petruzzelli GJ, Lomasney L. DentaScan as an Accurate Method of Predicting Mandibular Invasion in Patients With Squamous Cell Carcinoma of the Oral Cavity. Arch Otolaryngol Head Neck Surg 2003;129(1):113–7.

16. Imaizumi A, Yoshino N, Yamada I, et al. A potential pitfall of MR imaging for assessing mandibular invasion of squamous cell carcinoma in the oral cavity. AJNR Am J Neuroradiol 2006;27(1):114–22.

17. Wein RO, Weber RS. Malignant neoplasms of the oral cavity. In: Cummings CW, Flint PW, Harker LA, et al, editors. Cummings otolaryngology: head and neck surgery. 4th ed. Philadelphia, Pa: Elsevier Mosby; 2005. p. 1591–607.

18. Schusterman MA, Harris SW, Raymond AK, et al. Immediate free flap mandibular reconstruction: significance of adequate surgical margins. Head Neck 1993;15:204.

19. Kakarala K, Shnayder Y, Tsue TT, et al. Mandibular reconstruction. Oral Oncol 2018;77:111–7.

20. Koyfman SA, Ismaila N, Crook D, et al. Management of the neck in squamous cell carcinoma of the oral cavity and oropharynx. ASCO clinical practice guideline. J Oncol Pract 2019;15(5):273–8.

21. Cordeiro PG, Hidalgo DA. Conceptual considerations in mandibular reconstruction. Clin Plast Surg 1995;22:61.

22. Baker A, McMahon J, Parmar S. Immediate reconstruction of continuity defects of the mandible after tumor surgery. J Oral Maxillofac Surg 2001;59:1333.

23. Li X, Zhu K, Liu F, et al. Assessment of quality of life in giant ameloblastoma adolescent patients who have had mandible defects reconstructed with a free fibula flap. World J Surg Oncol 2014;12:201.

24. Netscher DT, Meade RA, Goodman CM, et al. Quality of life and disease specific functional status following microvascular reconstruction for advanced (T3 and T4) oropharyngeal cancers. Plast Reconstr Surg 2000;105:1628.

25. Weymuller EA, Yueh B, Deleyiannis FWB, et al. Quality of life in patients with head and neck cancer. Arch Otolaryngol Head Neck Surg 2000;126:329.

26. Khatib B, Gelesko S, Amundson M, et al. Updates in Management of Craniomaxillofacial Gunshot Wounds and Reconstruction of the Mandible. Oral Maxillofac Surg Clin N Am 2021;33(3):359–72.

27. Schwartz HC, Kagan AR. Osteoradionecrosis of the mandible: scientific basis for clinical staging. Am J Clin Oncol 2002;25(2):168–71.

28. Bras J, de Jonge HK, van Merkesteyn JP. Osteoradionecrosis of the mandible: pathogenesis. Am J Otol 1990;11(4):244–50.

29. Kim JW, Hwang JH, Ahn KM. Fibular flap for mandible reconstruction in osteoradionecrosis of the jaw: selection criteria of fibula flap. Maxillofac Plast Reconstr Surg 2016;38(1):46.

30. Glastonbury CM, Parker EE, Hoang JK. The postradiation neck: evaluating response to treatment and recognizing complications. AJR Am J Roentgenol 2010;195(2):W164–71.

31. McCarty JL, Corey AS, El-Deiry MW, et al. Imaging of Surgical Free Flaps in Head and Neck Reconstruction. AJNR Am J Neuroradiol 2019;40(1):5–13.

32. Alhilali L, Reynolds AR, Fakhran S. Osteoradionecrosis after radiation therapy for head and neck cancer: differentiation from recurrent disease with CT and PET/CT imaging. AJNR Am J Neuroradiol 2014;35(7):1405–11.

33. Estilo CL, Fornier M, Farooki A, et al. Osteonecrosis of the jaw related to bevacizumab. J Clin Oncol 2008;26(24):4037–8. https://doi.org/10.1200/JCO.2007.15.5424.

34. Zebic L, Patel V. Preventing medication-related osteonecrosis of the jaw. BMJ 2019;365:l1733.

35. Cardoso CL, Barros CA, Curra C, et al. Radiographic Findings in Patients with Medication-Related Osteonecrosis of the Jaw. Int J Dent 2017;2017:3190301.

36. Baba A, Goto TK, Ojiri H, et al. CT imaging features of antiresorptive agent-related osteonecrosis of the jaw/medication-related osteonecrosis of the jaw. Dentomaxillofac Radiol 2018;47(4):20170323.

37. Brown JS, Barry C, Ho M, et al. A new classification for mandibular defects after oncological resection. Lancet Oncol 2016;17(1):e23–30. https://doi.org/10.1016/S1470-2045(15)00310-1. Epub 2015 Dec 23.

38. Cordeiro PG, Henderson PW, Matros E. A 20-year experience with 202 segmental mandibulectomy defects: a defect classification system, algorithm for flap selection, and surgical outcomes. Plast Reconstr Surg 2018;141(4):571e–81e.

39. Pavlov BL. Klassifikatsiia defektov nizhnei cheliusti [Classification of mandibular defects]. Stomatologiia (Mosk) 1974;53(5):43–6. Russian.

40. Jewer DD, Boyd JB, Manktelow RT, et al. Orofacial and mandibular reconstruction with the iliac crest free flap: a review of 60 cases and a new method of classification. Plast Reconstr Surg 1989;84:391–405.

41. Boyd JB, Gullane PJ, Rotstein LE, et al. Classification of mandibular defects. Plast Reconstr Surg 1993;92(7):1266–75.

42. Kumar BP, Venkatesh V, Kumar KAJ, et al. Mandibular Reconstruction: Overview. J. Maxillofac. Oral Surg. 2016;15(4):425–41.

43. Urken ML, Weinberg H, Vickery C, et al. Oromandibular reconstruction using microvascular composite free flaps. Arch Otolaryngol Head Neck Surg 1991; 117:733–44.

44. Schultz BD, Sosin M, Nam A, et al. Classification of mandible defects and algorithm for microvascular reconstruction. Plast Reconstr Surg 2015;135(4): 743e–54e.

45. Urken ML. Atlas of Regional and free flaps for head and neck reconstruction. New York: Raven Press; 1995.

46. Conley J, Patow C, editors. Flaps in head & neck surgery. 2nd edition. NewYork: Thieme; 1989.

47. Goldenberg D, Goldstein BJ, editors. 7.3 facial reconstruction. Stuttgart: Thieme; 2011.

48. Weiland AJ, Phillips TW, Randolph MA. Bone grafts: a radiologic, histologic, and biomechanical model comparing autografts, allografts, and free vascularized bone grafts. Plast Reconstr Surg 1984;74: 368–79. CrossRef Medline.

49. Sparks DS, Wagels M, Taylor GI. Bone reconstruction: a history of vascularized bone transfer. Microsurgery 2018;38:7–13. CrossRef Medline.

50. Kuriloff DB, Sullivan MJ. Mandibular re-construction using vascularized bone graft. Otolaryngol Clin North Am 1991;24:1391–418.

51. Kelly AM, Cronin P, Hussain HK, et al. Preoperative MR Angiography in Free Fibular Flap Transfer for Head and Neck Cancer: Clinical Application and Influence on Surgical Decision Making. Am J Roentgenol 2007;188:268–74.

52. Wilkman T, Husso A, Lassus P. Clinical Comparison of Scapular, Fibular, and Iliac Crest Osseal Free Flaps in Maxillofacial Reconstructions. Scand J Surg 2019;108(1):76–82.

53. Fernandes R. Fibula Free Flap in Mandibular Reconstruction. Atlas Oral Maxillofacial Surg Clin N Am 2006;14:143–50.

54. Lohan DG, Tomasian A, Krishnam M, et al. MR angiography of lower extremities at 3 T: presurgical planning of fibular free flap transfer for facial reconstruction. AJR Am J Roentgenol 2008;190(3): 770–6.

55. Lutz BS, Wei FC, Ng SH, et al. Routine donor leg angiography before vascularized free fibula transplantation is not necessary: a prospective study in 120 clinical cases. Plast Reconstr Surg 1999; 103(1):121–7.

56. Frodel JL Jr, Funk GF, Cappis DT, et al. Osseointegrated implants: a comparative study of bone thickness in four vascularized bone flaps. Plast Reconstr Surg 1993;92:449–55.

57. Wol KD, Ervens J, Herzog K, et al. Experience with the osteocutaneous fibula flap: an analysis of 24 consecutive reconstructions of composite mandibular defects. J Cranio-Maxillo-Fac Surg 1996;24: 330–8.

58. Chim H, Salgado CJ, Mardini S, et al. Reconstruction of mandibular defects. Semin Plast Surg 2010; 24(2):188–97.

59. Baker SR, Sullivan MJ. Osteocutaneous free scapular flap for one stage mandibular reconstruction. Arch Otolaryngol Head Neck Surg 1988;114: 267–77.

60. Urken ML, Buchbinder D, Weinberg H, et al. Primary placement of osseointegrated implants in microvascular mandibular reconstruction. Otolaryngol Head Neck Surg 1989;101:58–73.

61. Taylor GI, Townsend P, Corlett R. Superiority of the deep circumflex iliac vessels as the supply for free groin flaps. Clinical work. Plast Reconstr Surg. 1979;64(6):745–59.

62. Urken ML, Buchbinder D, Costantino PD, et al. Oromandibular reconstruction using microvascular composite flaps: report of 210 cases. Arch Otolaryngol Head Neck Surg 1998;124(1):46–55.

63. Manchester WM. Some technical improvements in the reconstruction of the mandible and temporomandibular joint. Plast Reconstr Surg 1972;50(3): 249–56.

64. Jaquet Y, Enepekides DJ, Torgerson C, Higgins KM. Radial forearm free flap donor site morbidity: ulnar-based transposition flap vs split-thickness skin graft. Arch Otolaryngol Head Neck Surg 2012;138(1): 38–43.

65. Wolford LM, Rodrigues DB, McPhillips A. Management of the infected temporomandibular joint total joint prosthesis. J Oral Maxillofac Surg 2010;68:2810.

66. Hidalgo DA. Condyle transplantation in free flap mandible reconstruction. Plast Reconstr Surg 1994;93:770–81.

67. Guyot L, Oliver R, Layoun W, et al. Long term radiologic findings following reconstruction of the condyle with fibular free flaps. J Cranio-Maxillo-Fac Surg 2004;32:98–102.

68. Deek NFAL, Wei FC. Computer-Assisted Surgery for Segmental Mandibular Reconstruction with the Osteoseptocutaneous Fibula Flap: Can We Instigate Ideological and Technological Reforms? Plast Reconstr Surg 2016;137(3):963–70.

69. Li C, Cai Y, Wang W, et al. Combined application of virtual surgery and 3D printing technology in postoperative reconstruction of head and neck cancers. BMC Surg 2019;19:182.

70. Ayoub N, Ghassemi A, Rana M, et al. Evaluation of computer-assisted mandibular reconstruction with vascularized iliac crest bone graft compared to conventional surgery: a randomized prospective clinical trial. Trials 2014;15:114.

71. Zhang L, Liu Z, Li B, et al. Evaluation of computer-assisted mandibular reconstruction with vascularized fibular flap compared to conventional surgery. Oral Surg Oral Med Oral Pathol Oral Radiol 2016; 121(2):139–48.

72. Pucci R, Weyh A, Smotherman C, et al. Accuracy of virtual planned surgery versus conventional free-hand surgery for reconstruction of the mandible with osteocutaneous free flaps. Int J Oral Maxillofac Surg 2020;49(9):1153–61.

73. Weyh AM, Quimby A, Fernandes RP. Three-Dimensional Computer-Assisted Surgical Planning and Manufacturing in Complex Mandibular Reconstruction. Atlas Oral Maxillofac Surg Clin North Am 2020;28(2):145–50.

74. Bell RB. Computer planning and intraoperative navigation in cranio-maxillofacial surgery. Oral Maxillofac Surg Clin North Am 2010;22(1):135–56.

75. Antony AK, Chen WF, Kolokythas A, et al. Use of virtual surgery and stereolithography-guided osteotomy for mandibular reconstruction with the free fibula. Plast Reconstr Surg 2011;128(5):1080–4.

76. Hirsch DL, Garfein ES, Christensen AM, et al. Use of computer-aided design and computer-aided manufacturing to produce orthognathically ideal surgical outcomes: a paradigm shift in head and neck reconstruction. J Oral Maxillofac Surg 2009;67(10):2115–22.

77. Steinbacher DM. Three-Dimensional Analysis and Surgical Planning in Craniomaxillofacial Surgery. J Oral Maxillofac Surg 2015;73(12 Suppl):S40–56.

78. Succo G, Berrone M, Battiston B, et al. Step-by-step surgical technique for mandibular reconstruction with fibular free flap: application of digital technology in virtual surgical planning. Eur Arch Oto-Rhino-Laryngol 2015;272(6):1491–501.

79. Rosenthal DI, Liu L, Lee JH, et al. Importance of the treatment package time in surgery and postoperative radiation therapy for squamous carcinoma of the head and neck. Head Neck 2002;24(2):115–26.

80. Kirke DN, Owen RP, Carrao V, et al. Using 3D computer planning for complex reconstruction of mandibular defects. Cancers Head Neck 2016;1:17.

Normal and Variant Sinonasal Anatomy

Richard D. Beegle, MD[a], John V. Murray Jr, MD[b,*], Sukhwinder Johnny S. Sandhu, MD[b]

KEYWORDS

- Paranasal sinuses • Anatomic variants • Functional endoscopic sinus surgery (FESS)
- Computed tomography (CT)

KEY POINTS

- This article reviews the complex anatomy of the paranasal sinuses and the multiple anatomic variants.
- It is important for the radiologist and surgeon to have knowledge of the anatomy of the paranasal sinuses to help determine the cause of disease and increase success of surgical treatment.
- There are many anatomic variants that can predispose the patient to complications during endoscopic sinus surgery, which are presented in this article.

INTRODUCTION

The nasal cavity is pyramidal-shaped, located midline between the frontal sinuses and the oral cavity, surrounded by the air-filled paranasal sinuses. The nasal cavity receives and conditions air before passage to the more distal respiratory tract.[1] The function of the paranasal sinuses includes immunological defense, decreasing the weight of the head, buffering against facial trauma, and increasing voice resonance.[2] The paranasal sinuses subdivide into air-filled cavities lined by ciliated mucosa, which communicate directly with the nasal cavity.

A thorough understanding of the anatomy of the paranasal sinuses, nasal cavity, and many anatomic variants is essential in achieving successful and safe functional endoscopic sinus surgery (FESS) outcomes. Many anatomic variants are incidental but some can obstruct sinonasal drainage pathways, whereas others present potential for iatrogenic injury during FESS. This article will provide a detailed review of the anatomy and anatomic variants of the nasal cavity and paranasal sinuses.

IMAGING TECHNIQUES

Noncontrast computed tomography (CT) is the primary imaging modality used to evaluate inflammatory mucosal disease of the paranasal sinuses. CT precisely defines anatomy and potential surgical hazards before FESS. Preoperative CT also provides image-guided navigation during FESS. Thin slice high-resolution CT with multiplanar reconstructions in the axial, coronal, and sagittal planes in both bone and soft tissue kernels are useful to define anatomy and mucosal disease. MRI of the sinuses obtained without and with contrast is necessary to evaluate sinonasal masses. MRI can also be helpful in the evaluation of intracranial and soft tissue extension of pathologic condition, skull base encephaloceles, and aggressive infectious processes such as invasive fungal sinusitis.

NASAL CAVITY AND SKULL BASE

The paranasal sinuses drain into the nasal cavities. The nasal cavity contains the superior, middle, and inferior turbinates, which divide the nasal cavity into the superior, middle, and inferior meatus,

[a] AdventHealth Medical Group, 2600 Westhall Lane, 4th Floor, Maitland, FL 32751, USA; [b] Mayo Clinic Florida, 4500 San Pablo Road South, Jacksonville, FL 32224, USA
* Corresponding author. Mayo Clinic Florida, Department of Radiology, 4500 San Pablo Road South, Jacksonville, FL 32224.
E-mail address: Murray.John@mayo.edu

Oral Maxillofacial Surg Clin N Am 35 (2023) 345–357
https://doi.org/10.1016/j.coms.2023.02.002

respectively. Some patients also have a supreme turbinate. The posterior ethmoid air cells and sphenoid sinuses drain through the sphenoethmoidal recess into the superior meatus. The ostiomeatal unit (OMU) is the anatomical complex that drains the frontal sinuses, anterior ethmoidal air cells, and maxillary sinuses into the middle meatus. The OMU comprises the maxillary sinus ostium, ethmoid infundibulum, uncinate process, hiatus semilunaris, middle meatus, ethmoid bulla, and frontal recess (**Fig. 1**). The nasolacrimal duct drains into the inferior meatus, beneath the inferior turbinate. The nasal cavity is divided at the midline by the nasal septum.

Knowledge of the many anatomic variants that occur in the nasal cavities is essential for successful FESS and to reduce the risk of intraoperative complications. A deviated nasal septum is one of the most common variants.[3] Nasal septal deviations can be unilateral or have an S-shaped configuration with deviations along both sides of the midline.[4] A prominent deviated septum can displace the middle turbinate laterally and obstruct the OMU.[5] It may also interfere with surgical access to the middle meatus. Nasal septal spurs, particularly those that contact either the turbinates or lateral wall of the nasal cavity, can lead to obstruction and cause contact point headaches. Pneumatization of the posterior bony nasal septum can narrow the sphenoethmoidal recess and impede access to the sphenoid ostium.[4]

The ethmoid infundibulum is a thin passage, which connects the maxillary ostium to the hiatus semilunaris and is the primary drainage pathway of the maxillary sinuses. The uncinate process is a thin bone that forms the medial wall of the ethmoid infundibulum and is typically resected

during FESS. It attaches anteriorly to the lacrimal bone and posteriorly has a free concave margin. The inferior attachment is to the inferior turbinate insertion of the lateral nasal cavity wall. The superior attachment of the uncinate process can be variable. It may attach to the anterior skull base, middle turbinate, or lamina papyracea. The attachment determines the location of frontal sinus drainage. When the uncinate process attaches to the lamina papyracea, the frontal sinus drains into the middle meatus and creates a blind pouch called the recessus terminalis. If it attaches to the anterior skull base or the middle turbinate, then the frontal sinus drains into the ethmoid infundibulum. An atelectatic uncinate process as occurs in maxillary sinus hypoplasia or acquired atelectasis can efface the infundibulum and increase the risk of orbital penetration during FESS. The uncinate process can be pneumatized, potentially leading to infundibulum narrowing.[4]

The middle turbinate has a complex shape and attaches to the nasal cavity in all 3 planes.[4] Anatomic variants of the middle turbinate include concha bullosa, paradoxical middle turbinate, and pneumatized basal lamella. A concha bullosa, a pneumatized middle turbinate, can occur with nasal septal deviation, narrowing of the nasal air passages, or narrowing of the ethmoid infundibulum (**Fig. 2**). The middle turbinate usually forms a medial convex curvature. A paradoxical lateral convexity can occur and may result in obstruction/narrowing of the middle meatus or ethmoid infundibulum (see **Fig. 2**).[5] The basal lamella of the middle turbinate separates the anterior from the posterior ethmoidal air cells and is an important landmark during FESS.[6] Pneumatization of the basal lamella may be mistaken for an anterior

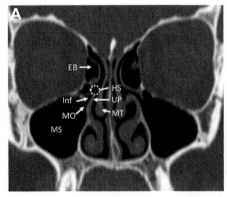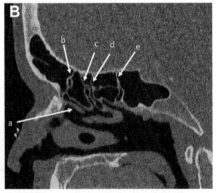

Fig. 1. (*A*) Coronal CT image demonstrating anatomy of the ostiomeatal unit: MS: maxillary sinus, MO: maxillary ostium, Inf: infundibulum, EB, ethmoid bulla; HS, hiatus semilunaris; MT, middle turbinate; UP, uncinate process. (*B*) Sagittal CT image showing the lamellae of the nasal cavity. From anterior to posterior, they include the uncinate process (a), anterior margin of the ethmoid bulla (b), basal lamella (c), lamella of the superior turbinate (d), and the anterior wall of the sphenoid sinus (e).

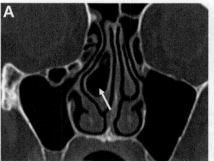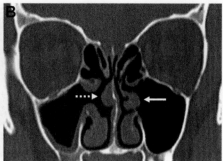

Fig. 2. (*A*) Coronal CT image demonstrating pneumatization of the right middle turbinate consistent with a concha bullosa (*arrow*). (*B*) Coronal CT image demonstrates paradoxical rotation of the left middle turbinate (*solid arrow*). There are postoperative changes from FESS, and there has been medialization of the right middle turbinate (*dotted arrow*).

ethmoidal air cell at the time of surgery.[4] Hypertrophy of the nasal turbinates can also lead to obstruction of nasal passages. During normal physiologic nasal cycling, the mucosa lining the turbinates on one side engorges with blood to become reversibly larger than the contralateral side. The nasal cycle is the periodic alternating pattern of unilateral congestion and decongestion of the erectile tissue within the turbinates and should not be mistaken for pathologic condition.

The lamellae course from the nasal cavity through the ethmoid air cells and attach to the anterior skull base. They are critical surgical landmarks and provide organizational structure for the sinonasal cavity. The lamellae are best understood and visualized in the coronal and parasagittal planes. From anterior to posterior, they include the uncinate process, anterior margin of the ethmoid bulla, basal lamella, lamella of the superior turbinate, occasionally the lamella of the supreme turbinate, and the anterior wall of the sphenoid sinus (see **Fig. 1**).[4]

Understanding the anatomic variants of the anterior skull base is essential to decreasing the risk of surgical complications. The anterior skull base is composed of the fovea ethmoidalis and cribriform plate. The cribriform plate is made up of the medial and lateral lamellae. The medial lamellae forms the floor of the olfactory fossa. The lateral lamella is vertically oriented, forms the lateral wall of the olfactory fossa, and is contiguous with the fovea ethmoidalis superolaterally and medial lamella inferomedially. The olfactory recess is the superomedial portion of the nasal cavity, which abuts the cribriform plate and is medial to the skull base insertion of the middle turbinate. In 1962, Keros[7] classified differences in the heights of the olfactory fossae (**Table 1**) (**Fig. 3**). The height of the olfactory fossa is determined by the length of the lateral lamella. The

lateral lamella is at risk of injury during FESS, which can result in a cerebrospinal fluid (CSF) leak or an encephalocele (**Fig. 4**).[4,8] Risk of injury is greatest with Keros type 3 because of the increased length of the thinness of the bone. There can be asymmetry in the depths of the bilateral olfactory fossae, with the risk of injury being higher on the lower side.[1]

Determining skull base height and evaluating for osseous dehiscence of the cribriform plate preoperatively will decrease the risk of injury. Cribriform plate defects can occur following surgery, traumatic insult, or can be congenital (see **Fig. 4**).[9] Multiple classification systems have been developed to assess the ethmoid skull base height.[10–12] A low-lying anterior skull base can mimic a posterior ethmoid air cell during surgery, resulting in unintended penetration.[11] The methodology proposed by Rudmick and Smith[11] is depicted in **Fig. 5**. The height of the ethmoid skull base is determined on a coronal CT image at the level of the anterior ethmoidal artery. A line is drawn through the midorbital plane and used as the inferior extent of the measurement. The height of the ethmoid skull base is measured from the midorbital plane to the midportion of the fovea ethmoidalis. Their study found that the average height was 8.5 mm, and 70% of patients were greater than

Table 1 Keros classification	
Keros Classification of the Olfactory Fossa	
Type	**Length of Lateral Lamella (mm)**
Type 1	1–3
Type 2	4–7
Type 3	>7

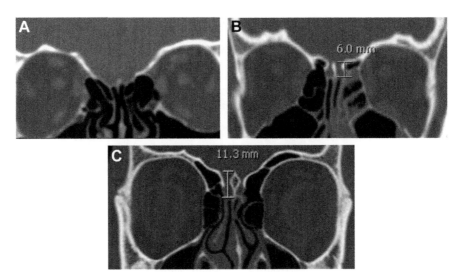

Fig. 3. Coronal CT images in 3 different patients demonstrating the different anatomic variations for the depth of the olfactory fossa. The depth of the olfactory fossa is determined by the height of the lateral lamella, which can be classified using the Keros classification. Type 1 configuration is when the olfactory fossa is shallow and is less than 4 mm deep (as seen in A). Type 2 configuration is when the olfactory fossa is between 4 and 7 mm deep (as seen in B). Type 3 configuration is when the olfactory fossa is greater than 7 mm deep (as seen in C).

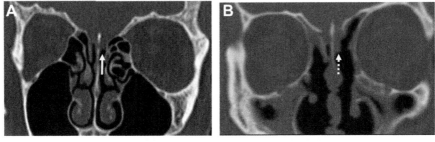

Fig. 4. Coronal CT image (A) demonstrating dehiscence of the cribriform plate with possible associated encephalocele (arrow). Coronal CT image (B) in a different patient status post FESS showing a defect of the cribriform plate. This patient had a confirmed CSF leak and encephalocele (dashed arrow).

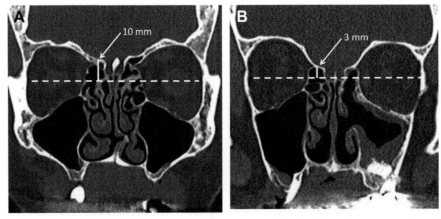

Fig. 5. To assess the ethmoid skull base height, a coronal image at the level of the anterior ethmoidal artery is obtained (A). A line is drawn through the midorbital plane (dashed line). The height is then measured from the midorbital plane to the midportion of the fovea ethmoidalis (solid line). The patient in A has a safe ethmoid skull base height (greater than 7 mm). Coronal CT image (B) in a different patient shows a low-lying ethmoid skull base height.

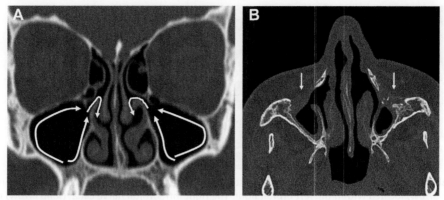

Fig. 6. (*A*) Coronal CT image demonstrating the mucociliary drainage pattern of the maxillary sinus. The cilia of the maxillary sinuses sweep mucous and debris toward the maxillary ostium. The mucous then travels through the maxillary infundibulum, into the region of the hiatus semilunaris, and then into the middle meatus. (*B*) Axial CT image demonstrating osseous defects of the anterior walls of the maxillary sinuses bilaterally (*arrows*) secondary to prior Caldwell-Luc procedure.

7 mm, which is considered safe for surgery. A moderate height of 4 to 7 mm was seen in 25% of patients and is moderately safe. A low height of less than 4 mm was seen in 5% of patients and poses the highest risk for complication.[11]

MAXILLARY SINUS AND OSTIOMEATAL UNIT

The maxillary sinus has several recesses, the most prominent being the alveolar recess, which points inferiorly, and the zygomatic recess, which points laterally.[13] Mucosal thickening or small cysts are common in the alveolar recess and often incidental. The maxillary alveolar ridge forms the floor of the maxillary sinus. The sinuses' natural mucous drainage pattern is the basis for FESS. The anterior group of paranasal sinuses, which include the maxillary sinuses, anterior ethmoid air cells, and frontal sinus, drain toward the OMU. The cilia within the maxillary sinus propel mucous and debris along the sinus walls toward the maxillary ostium, even though it is at the highest point of the medial maxillary wall (**Fig. 6**). Before the development of FESS, the Caldwell-Luc procedure was performed to create a window along the anterior maxillary sinus wall assuming that gravity would assist in mucosal drainage (see **Fig. 6**). However, the mucociliary apparatus drains upwards toward the maxillary ostium and bypasses the surgically created fenestrations.[13] The goal of modern FESS is to reestablish normal ventilation and drainage, remove foci of disease, and preserve the mucosa and mucociliary clearance.[14]

Maxillary sinus variants may affect the sinus drainage pattern or result in increased surgical risk. Some variants include hypoplasia, internal septations, or accessory ostia.[15] Variations in

the orientation and attachment of the uncinate process can be a factor in narrowing the OMU.[3]

Haller cells, or infraorbital ethmoid air cells, are located inferomedial to the orbit and lateral to the infundibulum. If large or inflamed, they may narrow or obstruct the maxillary ostium and ethmoidal infundibulum (**Fig. 7**). Haller cells can also restrict surgical access to the maxillary sinus or the anterior ethmoidal cells.[15]

The infraorbital nerve runs in the infraorbital canal, a bony canal located along the maxillary sinus roof. An anatomic variant is when the nerve protrudes into the sinus or the bony canal is dehiscent. Failure to recognize this variant may lead to injury of the infraorbital nerve (**Fig. 8**).

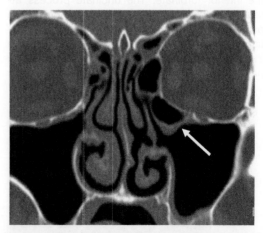

Fig. 7. Coronal CT images showing an air cell located along the inferior surface of the orbital floor consistent with a Haler cell (*arrow*).

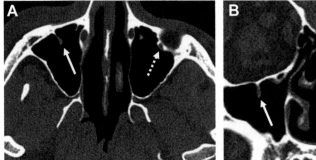
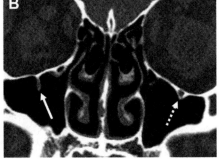

Fig. 8. Axial CT (*A*) and coronal CT (*B*) images demonstrate a normal course of the infraorbital nerve canal on the left (*dotted arrow*) located within the left orbital floor. The right infraorbital nerve canal (*solid arrow*) protrudes into the right maxillary sinus and is at increased risk of injury during surgery.

ANTERIOR ETHMOID AIR CELLS

The anterior ethmoid air cells are located anterior to the basal lamella and drain through the OMU. The ethmoid bulla is the largest and least varying cell of the anterior ethmoid air cells and, if hyperpneumatized, can displace the uncinate process medially.[3] The lamina papyracea forms the lateral walls of the ethmoid air cells. Integrity and position of the lamina papyracea are important during FESS to avoid orbital penetration and orbital injuries such as orbital hematoma, extraocular muscle injury, injury to the optic nerve, and blindness.[16] Dehiscence of the lamina papyracea may be congenital, posttraumatic, or postoperative (**Fig. 9**).[17]

A study by Herzallah and colleagues[18] describes a grading system that can be used to grade the position of the lamina papyracea. The plane of the planned middle meatal antrostomy is identified on the coronal CT by drawing a vertical line at the location of the lateral attachment of the inferior turbinate. The uncinate process attaches at this point. The location of the lamina papyracea is then graded with respect to this vertical plane. Type I lamina papyracea lies within 2 mm on either side of this plane. Type II lamina papyracea lies medial to this vertical plane by

more than 2 mm, and type III lamina papyracea lies lateral by more than 2 mm (**Fig. 10**). Increased risk of injury to the lamina papyracea was described in types II and III.

The anterior ethmoidal artery is a branch of the ophthalmic artery. It traverses from the orbit to the anterior cranial fossa by passing along the roof of the anterior ethmoid air cells.[19] It can be located on coronal CT by identifying the anterior ethmoid notch along the medial orbital wall.[20] When the anterior ethmoidal artery travels within the bone of the ethmoid roof, it is more protected during surgery. When the anterior ethmoidal artery traverses freely through the ethmoid air cells suspended on a "mesentery," it is at higher risk of injury during FESS (**Fig. 11**).[19,20] If the artery is transected, it can retract into the orbit leading to an intraorbital hematoma.[16,20]

FRONTAL SINUS AND FRONTAL RECESS

The frontal sinuses drain to the OMU through the frontal sinus outflow tract comprises the frontal ostium and the frontal recess. The frontal recess is an inverted funnel, with the frontal ostium representing the tip of the funnel and the frontal recess flaring out inferiorly.[21] The frontonasal process of the maxilla, also known as the frontal beak, can

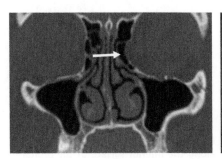
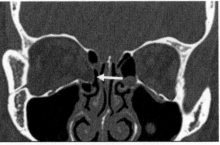

Fig. 9. Coronal CT images in 2 different patients demonstrating dehiscence of the lamina papyracea (*arrows*).

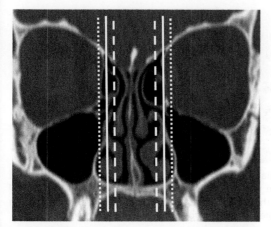

Fig. 10. Utilizing the coronal CT, one can grade the position of the lamina papyracea before surgery. An imaginary vertical axis can be drawn at the level of the insertion of the inferior turbinate to the lateral nasal wall (*solid arrow*). Imaginary lines can be drawn 2 mm medial (*large dashed line*) and 2 mm lateral (*small dashed line*). Type I positioning is within 2 mm on either side of the vertical axis. Type II positioning is medial to the vertical axis by greater than 2 mm. Type III positioning is lateral to the vertical axis by greater than 2 mm.

be visualized on sagittal CT images and demarcates the level of the frontal ostium (**Fig. 12**). The frontal recess anatomy is highly variable and may be pneumatized by various anterior ethmoid cells. Preoperative recognition of anatomic variants is vital if a frontal sinusotomy is planned.

The agger nasi cell is the anterior-most ethmoid air cell located anterior to the frontal recess and along the posterior margin of the frontal beak. The incidence of agger nasi cells has been reported in 78% to 98.5% of patients.[22] There are varying degrees of pneumatization of the agger nasi cell, and if it is hyperpneumatized can narrow

the frontal recess (**Fig. 13**). In addition to the agger nasi cell, the frontal recess may be pneumatized by several other types of frontal recess cells. Multiple classification systems have been developed to describe these additional frontal recess cells, the 2 most common being the Kuhn classification[23] and the International Frontal Sinus Anatomy Classification (IFAC).[24] The frontal recess cells can be categorized into anterior, posterior, and medial groups. Studies have shown a significantly higher interrater reliability utilizing IFAC compared with the Kuhn classification.[25–27] Therefore, for the purposes of this article, the IFAC will be presented. **Table 2** summarizes IFAC and the Kuhn classification. According to IFAC, the anterior-based cells are composed of the agger nasi cell, supra agger cells, and supra agger frontal cells. Supra agger cells are anterolateral ethmoid cells that are located above the agger nasi cell but inferior to the frontal ostium (**Fig. 14**). Supra agger frontal cells are anterolateral ethmoid cells that are above the agger nasi cell and pneumatize into the frontal sinus (see **Fig. 14**).

The posterior group of frontal recess cells is located along the posterior wall of the frontal recess and bordered posteriorly and/or superiorly by the anterior skull base. They are composed of the supraorbital ethmoid cells, supra bulla cells, and supra bulla frontal cells.[21] These cells can also narrow the frontal recess. The supraorbital ethmoid cell extends superiorly and laterally over the orbit from the frontal recess (**Fig. 15**). Supra bulla frontal cells lie above the ethmoid bulla, form the posterior boundary of the frontal recess, and extend superiorly into the posterior aspect of the frontal sinus (**Fig. 16**). Supra bulla cells are similar to supra bulla frontal cells, except they are located entirely below the level of the frontal ostium (see **Fig. 16**). During FESS, supra bulla cells and supra bulla frontal cells can be mistaken as

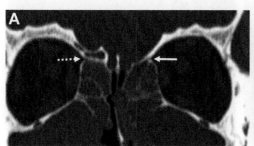
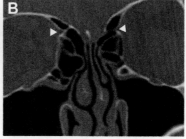

Fig. 11. Coronal CT (*A*) shows the course of the anterior ethmoidal artery passing through the anterior ethmoidal canal, which is normally positioned directly inferior to the fovea ethmoidalis (*arrow*). However, an anatomic variation is when there is pneumatization between the skull base and anterior ethmoidal canal. This is referred to as the artery being on a "mesentery" (*dashed arrow*). Coronal CT (*B*) demonstrating the anterior ethmoidal arteries on a mesentery bilaterally (*arrow heads*).

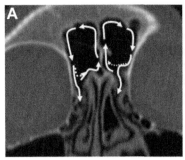
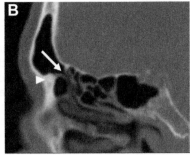
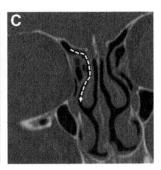

Fig. 12. Coronal CT image (*A*) demonstrating the mucociliary drainage pattern of the frontal sinus. The cilia of the frontal sinuses sweep mucous and debris toward the frontal ostium (*solid arrow*) as seen on the sagittal CT (*B*). The level of the frontal ostium is demarcated by the frontal beak (*arrow head* in *B*). The mucous then travels through the frontal recess and then into the middle meatus as shown by the dashed line in (*C*).

the skull base resulting in incomplete resection and failure to relieve obstruction of the frontal recess.[21] The medial group is composed of a frontal septal cell. The frontal septal cell is an aerated cell attached to or located within the interfrontal sinus septum and is an additional variant air cell that can narrow the frontal ostium (**Fig. 17**).

POSTERIOR ETHMOID AIR CELLS, SPHENOID SINUS, AND SPHENOETHMOIDAL RECESS

The sphenoethmoidal recess is the drainage pathway for the posterior ethmoid air cells and sphenoid sinuses located posterior to the basal lamella. An important anatomic variant of the posterior ethmoid air cells is the sphenoethmoidal air cell (Onodi cell). Sphenoethmoidal air cells occur when an ethmoid air cell extends posteriorly and superiorly over the sphenoid sinus. Sphenoethmoidal air cells are best visualized on coronal

reformatted images where a horizontal septation is seen between the sphenoethmoidal air cell superiorly and the sphenoid sinus inferiorly (**Fig. 18**). It is important to recognize this variant to avoid intracranial penetration and injury to the optic nerve, which is in close approximation and may traverse through this cell.

Sphenoid sinus pneumatization is best categorized utilizing the sagittal plane as conchal, presellar, or sellar.[20] The conchal variant is an underpneumatized sphenoid sinus with a bony margin between the sphenoid sinus and the sella. The presellar variant is when pneumatization of the sphenoid sinus extends to the anterior margin of the sella. The sellar variant is when pneumatization extends inferior and posterior to the sella extending to the clivus. Identification of the intersphenoid sinus septum attachment is important because resection of its attachment to the thin bony covering of the internal carotid artery may result in carotid injury.

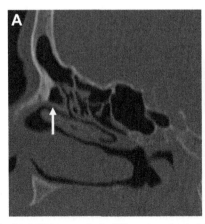
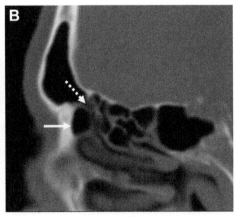

Fig. 13. Sagittal CT images in 2 different patients (*A* and *B*) showing an air cell located anterior to the frontal recess consistent with the agger nasi cell (*solid white arrows*). The agger nasi cell in (*B*) is prominent and results in narrowing of the frontal recess (*dashed arrow*).

Table 2
Frontal sinus anatomy

Cell Type	IFAC	Kuhn	Definition
Anterior	Agger nasi cell	Agger nasi cell	The agger nasi cell is the anterior most ethmoid air cell and is located anterior to the frontal recess and along the posterior margin of the frontal beak
	Supra agger cell	Type 1 frontal cell Type 2 frontal cell	Anterolateral ethmoid cells that are located above the agger nasi cell but inferior to the frontal ostium (Kuhn differentiation: Type 1 is a single cell above the agger nasi. Type 2 is 2 or more cells above the agger nasi.)
	Supra agger frontal cell	Type 3 frontal cell Type 4 frontal cell	Anterolateral ethmoid cells that are above the agger nasi cell and pneumatize into the frontal sinus (Kuhn differentiation: Type 4 is an air cell, which is isolated within the frontal sinus along the anterior wall.)
Posterior	Supraorbital ethmoid cell	Supraorbital ethmoid cell	Extend superiorly and laterally over the orbit from the frontal recess
	Supra bulla cell	Suprabullar cell	Air cells that lie above the ethmoid bulla, form the posterior boundary of the frontal recess, and do not enter the frontal sinus
	Supra bulla frontal cell	Frontobullar cell	Air cells that lie above the ethmoid bulla, form the posterior boundary of the frontal recess, and extend superiorly into the posterior aspect of the frontal sinus
Medial	Frontal septal cell	Interfrontal sinus septal cell	Medially based air cell, which is attached to or is located in the interfrontal sinus septum

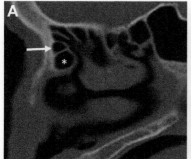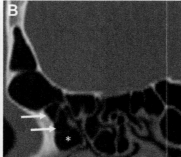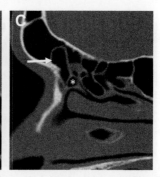

Fig. 14. Sagittal CT image (*A*) demonstrates a single air cell (*arrow*) above the agger nasi cell (*asterisk*) and below the frontal sinus ostium consistent with a supra agger cell. Sagittal CT image (*B*) demonstrates 2 adjacent supra agger cells above the agger nasi cell (*asterisk*) and below the frontal ostium. Sagittal CT image (*C*) demonstrates a single air cell (*arrow*) sitting above the agger nasi cell (*asterisk*) and pneumatizing into the frontal sinus consistent with a supra agger frontal cell.

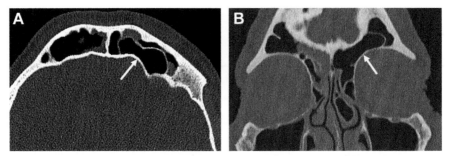

Fig. 15. Axial (*A*) and coronal (*B*) CT images demonstrate an anterior ethmoid air cell that extends superiorly and laterally over the orbit from the frontal recess consistent with a supraorbital ethmoid cell (*arrow*).

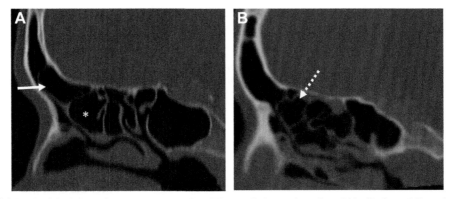

Fig. 16. (*A*) Sagittal CT image demonstrates an air cell located above the ethmoid bulla (*asterisk*) and extending into the frontal sinus consistent with a supra bulla frontal cell (*arrow*). This forms the posterior boundary of the frontal recess and frontal sinus. (*B*) In contrast, sagittal CT image demonstrates a supra bulla cell (*dashed arrow*), which is similar except it lies entirely below the level of the frontal sinus ostium.

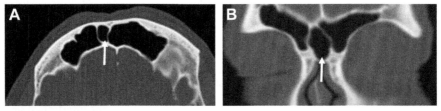

Fig. 17. Axial (*A*) and coronal (*B*) CT images demonstrate pneumatization of the frontal sinus septum consistent with a frontal septal cell (*arrow*).

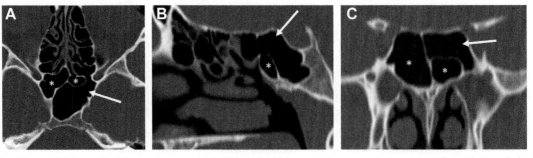

Fig. 18. Axial (*A*), sagittal (*B*), and coronal (*C*) CT images demonstrating a posterior most ethmoid air cell that extends posteriorly to lie superolateral to the sphenoid sinus consistent with a sphenoethmoidal air cell, also known as an Onodi cell (*arrows*). These images show the relationship with the sphenoid sinuses (*asterisks*).

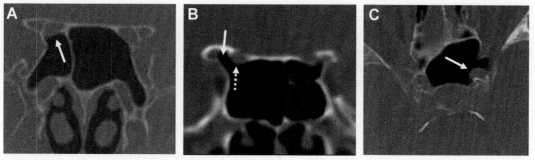

Fig. 19. (*A*) Coronal CT image demonstrates osseous dehiscence of the optic nerve canal (*arrow*), which increases the risk of injury during surgery. (*B*) Coronal CT image demonstrates pneumatization of the anterior clinoid process (*arrow*). This can potentially place the optic nerve at risk as the optic canal can project into the sinus lumen. In this patient, the optic canal is also dehiscent (*dashed arrow*). (*C*) Axial CT image demonstrates osseous dehiscence of the bony covering of the internal carotid artery (*arrow*).

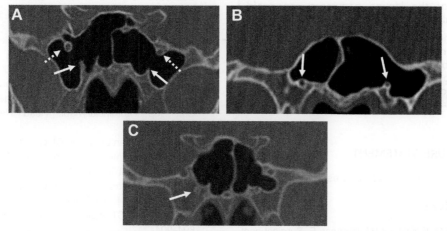

Fig. 20. Coronal CT images in 3 different patients demonstrating the different anatomic variations for the course of the vidian canal (*arrows*). Type 1 configuration is when the vidian canal is completely within the sphenoid sinus (*solid arrows* as seen in *A*). Of note, also in A the foramen rotundum is seen traversing through the sphenoid sinuses connected by thin bony stalks (*dotted arrows*). Type 2 configuration is when the vidian canal is on the floor of the sphenoid sinus or partially protruding into the sphenoid sinus (as seen in *B*). Type 3 configuration is when the vidian canal is completely embedded in the sphenoid bone (as seen in *C*).

Identification of the optic nerves and internal carotid arteries is essential to assess for dehiscence of the bony covering with respect to the sphenoid sinus and to avoid potential injury at the time of surgery (**Fig. 19**). Pneumatization of the anterior clinoid process can lead to the optic canal passing through the superolateral aspect of the sphenoid sinus with associated bony dehiscence (see **Fig. 19**).

Smaller neurovascular canals traverse along the sphenoid sinus walls should also be evaluated, including the vidian canal and the foramen rotundum. Hyperpneumatization of the sphenoid sinuses can result in osseous dehiscence of these canals or can cause the structures to be exposed traversing through the sphenoid sinus (**Fig. 20**). A study by Lee and colleagues[28]

categorizes the configuration of the vidian canal into 3 types (see **Fig. 20**). Type 1 configuration is when the vidian canal is completely within the sphenoid sinus. Type 2 configuration is when the vidian canal is on the floor of the sphenoid sinus or partially protruding into the sphenoid sinus. Type 3 configuration is when the vidian canal is completely embedded in the sphenoid bone.

SUMMARY

Knowledge of sinonasal normal anatomy is essential to understand and effectively treat the gamut of inflammatory and neoplastic pathology, which involves the nasal cavity and paranasal sinuses. There is much variability among individuals in normal sinus anatomy, and these normal variants can have significant ramifications in the cause of disease and treatment outcomes. A thorough understanding of these variants and their potential clinical sequelae is necessary to provide optimal outcomes and avoid complications.

CLINICS CARE POINTS

- The surgeon must understand anatomic variants of the skull base to avoid complications such as CSF leak and encephalocele.
- Knowledge of the course of the anterior ethmoidal artery and the integrity and position of the lamina papyracea can avoid orbital complications.
- The normal sinus drainage pathways and anatomic variants that affect those pathways must be understood to effectively treat pathologic condition obstructing normal sinonasal drainage.

DISCLOSURE STATEMENT

The authors have no disclosures.

REFERENCES

1. Ogle EO, Weinstock RJ, Fiedman E. Surgical anatomy of the nasal cavity and paranasal sinuses. Oral Maxillofacial Surg Clin N Am 2012;24:155–66.
2. Capello Z.J., Minutello K. and Dublin A.B., Anatomy, head and neck, nose paranasal sinuses, 2022, StatPearls, Orlando, FL.
3. Papadopoulou AM, Chrysikos D, Samolis A, et al. Anatomical variations of the nasal cavities and paranasal sinuses: a systematic review. Cureus 2021; 13(1):e12727.
4. Vaid S, Vaid N. Normal anatomy and anatomic variants of the paranasal sinuses on computed tomography. Neuroimaging Clin N Am 2015;25(4):527–48.
5. Azila A, Irfan M, Rohaizan Y, et al. The prevalence of anatomical variations in osteomeatal unit in patients with chronic rhinosinusitis. Med J Malaysia 2011; 66(3):191–4.
6. Eördögh M, Baksa G, Grimm A, et al. Three-dimensional structure of the basal lamella of the middle turbinate. Sci Rep 2021;11(1):17960.
7. Keros P. On the practical value of differences in the level of the lamina cribrosa of the ethmoid. Z Laryngol Rhinol Otol 1962;41:809–13.
8. Kainz J, Stammberger H. Das Dach des vorderen Siebbeines: Ein Locus minoris resistentiae an der Schädelbasis [The roof of the anterior ethmoid: a locus minoris resistentiae in the skull base]. Laryngol Rhinol Otol 1988;67(4):142–9.
9. Tolley NS, Lloyd GA, Williams HO. Radiological study of primary spontaneous CSF rhinorrhoea. J Laryngol Otol 1991;105(4):274–7.
10. Meyers RM, Valvassori G. Interpretation of anatomic variations of computed tomography scans of the sinuses: a surgeon's perspective. Laryngoscope 1998;108(3):422–5.
11. Rudmik L, Smith TL. Evaluation of the ethmoid skull-base height prior to endoscopic sinus surgery: a preoperative computed tomography evaluation technique. Int Forum Allergy Rhinol 2012;2(2): 151–4.
12. Ramakrishnan VR, Suh JD, Kennedy DW. Ethmoid skull-base height: a clinically relevant method of evaluation. Int Forum Allergy Rhinol 2011;1(5): 396–400.
13. Whyte A, Boeddinghaus R. The maxillary sinus: physiology, development and imaging anatomy. Dentomaxillofac Radiol 2019;48(8):20190205.
14. Weber RK, Hosemann W. Comprehensive review on endonasal endoscopic sinus surgery. GMS Curr Top Otorhinolaryngol, Head Neck Surg 2015;14:Doc08.
15. Sarna A, Hayman LA, Laine FJ, et al. Coronal imaging of the osteomeatal unit: anatomy of 24 variants. J Comput Assist Tomogr 2002;26(1):153–7.
16. Bhatti MT, Schmalfuss IM, Mancuso AA. Orbital complications of functional endoscopic sinus surgery: MR and CT findings. Clin Radiol 2005;60(8): 894–904.
17. Moulin G, Dessi P, Chagnaud C, et al. Dehiscence of the lamina papyracea of the ethmoid bone: CT findings. AJNR Am J Neuroradiol 1994;15(1): 151–3.
18. Herzallah IR, Marglani OA, Shaikh AM. Variations of lamina papyracea position from the endoscopic view: a retrospective computed tomography analysis. Int Forum Allergy Rhinol 2015;5(3): 263–70.
19. Simmen D, Raghavan U, Briner HR, et al. The surgeon's view of the anterior ethmoid artery. Clin Otolaryngol 2006;31(3):187–91.
20. O'Brien WT Sr, Hamelin S, Weitzel EK. The preoperative sinus CT: avoiding a "CLOSE" call with surgical complications. Radiology 2016;281(1):10–21.
21. Huang BY, Lloyd KM, DelGaudio JM, et al. Failed endoscopic sinus surgery: spectrum of CT findings in the frontal recess. Radiographics 2009;29(1): 177–95.
22. DelGaudio JM, Hudgins PA, Venkatraman G, et al. Multiplanar computed tomographic analysis of frontal recess cells: effect on frontal isthmus size and frontal sinusitis. Arch Otolaryngol Head Neck Surg 2005;131(3):230–5.

23. Bent JP, Cuilty-Siller C, Kuhn FA. The frontal cell as a cause of frontal sinus obstruction. Am J Rhinol 1994; 8(4):185–91.

24. Wormald PJ, Hoseman W, Callejas C, et al. The international frontal sinus anatomy classification (IFAC) and classification of the extent of endoscopic frontal sinus surgery (EFSS). Int Forum Allergy Rhinol 2016;6(7): 677–96.

25. Choby G, Thamboo A, Won TB, et al. Computed tomography analysis of frontal cell prevalence according to the International Frontal Sinus Anatomy Classification. Int Forum Allergy Rhinol 2018;8(7):825–30.

26. Langille M, Walters E, Dziegielewski PT, et al. Frontal sinus cells: identification, prevalence, and association with frontal sinus mucosal thickening. Am J Rhinol Allergy 2012;26(3):e107–10.

27. Villarreal R, Wrobel BB, Macias-Valle LF, et al. International assessment of inter- and intrarater reliability of the International Frontal Sinus Anatomy Classification system. Int Forum Allergy Rhinol 2019;9(1): 39–45.

28. Lee JC, Kao CH, Hsu CH, et al. Endoscopic transsphenoidal vidian neurectomy. Eur Arch Oto-Rhino-Laryngol 2011;268(6):851–6.

Infectious and Inflammatory Sinonasal Diseases

Marcus J. Lacey, MD, Margaret N. Chapman, MD*

KEYWORDS

- Acute rhinosinusitis • Chronic rhinosinusitis • Sinonasal inflammatory disease • Fungal sinusitis
- Sinonasal manifestations of systemic disease

KEY POINTS

- Rhinosinusitis is a commonly encountered condition. Although often treated clinically, a thorough understanding of the role of diagnostic imaging is crucial to diagnosing alternative causes and complications. CT and MRI are often complementary in the evaluation of sinonasal infectious and inflammatory processes.
- Rhinosinusitis exists on a spectrum ranging from acute to chronic defined by symptoms, disease duration, and sometimes radiologic findings. Treatment implications, complications, and prognosis will vary along this spectrum.
- Fungal rhinosinusitis is classified into invasive and noninvasive subtypes affecting different patient populations. The acute invasive subtype has high morbidity and is suspected in the setting of rapidly progressive symptoms and certain complications such as vascular and cranial nerve compromise.
- Various inflammatory conditions can manifest as rhinosinusitis both clinically and radiographically and should be considered as differential diagnoses in the appropriate clinical context.

INTRODUCTION

Rhinosinusitis affects approximately 12% of adults in the United States per year.[1] As one of the most common conditions encountered by clinicians, a large proportion of ambulatory office and emergency room visits and a similarly large proportion of adult antibiotic prescriptions are attributed to sinonasal disease each year.[2] Perhaps more important than the direct health care costs of diagnosing and treating sinusitis is the significant impact on quality of life experienced by those affected, which can contribute to the indirect costs of the disease from lost productivity and days away from work.[2,3]

Sinusitis is defined as a *symptomatic* inflammatory process of the paranasal sinuses. As inflammation of the sinuses is generally accompanied by inflammation of the nasal mucosa, the term rhinosinusitis is preferred.[2] Rhinosinusitis can be classified by the duration of symptoms and further subclassified by the cause of disease and responsible pathogen. The diagnosis and treatment of uncomplicated sinusitis—where inflammation is confined to the sinonasal spaces—does not usually require imaging and can be made by (duration of) symptoms and physical examination findings.[2,4]

Imaging can assist clinicians in surgical planning, reaching a correct diagnosis when an alternative process is suspected, and evaluating for rare but serious complications. In addition to neoplastic processes that may affect the sinonasal region, some systemic and inflammatory processes have a predilection for the nasal cavity and paranasal sinuses. Although these cases can present with nonspecific symptoms mimicking rhinosinusitis, they will occasionally have more onerous signs leading the clinician to pursue imaging to confirm their suspicion of an alternate cause.[5,6]

M.J. Lacey and M.N. Chapman: No relevant financial disclosures.
Department of Radiology, Virginia Mason Medical Center, 1100 Ninth Avenue, C5-XR, Seattle, WA 98101, USA
* Corresponding author.
E-mail address: margaret.n.chapman@gmail.com

Oral Maxillofacial Surg Clin N Am 35 (2023) 359–376
https://doi.org/10.1016/j.coms.2023.02.005

Abbreviations	
CT	Computed tomography
MR	Magnetic Resonance
MRI	Magnetic resonance imaging
OMC	Ostiomeatal complex
OMU	Ostiomeatal unit
CSF	Cerebral spinal fluid
DWI	diffusion weighted imaging
FLAIR	Fluid attenuation inversion recovery
IgG4-RD	IgG4 related disease
GPA	Granulomatosis with polyangiitis
ANCA	Antineutrophil cytoplasmic antibodies
CST	cavernous sinus thrombosis

This article discusses the role of diagnostic radiology, the imaging features, and differential diagnoses of infectious and inflammatory sinonasal diseases. Neoplastic processes are covered in another article in this issue.

ROLE OF IMAGING

Imaging evaluation of patients presenting with uncomplicated rhinosinusitis may not be indicated if clinical diagnostic criteria are met.[4] Acute uncomplicated rhinosinusitis is medically managed with antibiotic therapy.[7] The clinical scenario in combination with imaging recommendation guidelines can be used to direct the appropriate imaging modality (or modalities) on a patient-specific basis when sinonasal symptoms are present and an alternative diagnosis or complications of sinonasal inflammatory disease are suspected.

Computed tomography (CT) is the modality of choice in the evaluation of inflammatory disease given its wide availability and ability to provide high spatial resolution for evaluating the fine osseous and anatomic detail of the paranasal sinuses. CT images are usually acquired with thin-slice technique in the axial plane with coronal and sagittal reformations provided for interpretation. Images are reviewed in both osseous and soft tissue algorithms. Iodinated contrast is generally not necessary unless there is concern for a complicated extrasinus process. High-resolution CT is also the modality of choice in preoperative planning for endoscopic sinus surgeries.[8]

MRI offers improved soft tissue contrast resolution and affords accurate delineation of suspected extrasinus soft tissue and intracranial complications and allows for sensitive characterization of soft tissue masses. MRI is infrequently used in the diagnosis of rhinosinusitis unless complications are suspected. The field of view for standard multiplanar multisequence MRI technique of the paranasal sinuses should include the orbits, skull base, and adjacent intracranial structures. Multiplanar fat-suppressed T1-weighted images acquired after the administration of intravenous gadolinium are used to evaluate the extent of an extrasinus process and enhancement patterns of soft tissue masses. High-resolution MRI also allows for detailed evaluation of small anatomic structures such as the skull base foramina, cranial nerves, and vessels.[8]

MRI and CT imaging are often complementary in the complete characterization of sinonasal processes, in particular when atypical or complicated processes are suspected. With the increasing availability of cross-sectional imaging modalities providing superior anatomic detail of the paranasal sinuses and sinonasal pathologies, radiography has become relatively obsolete with its lower sensitivity and specificity in detection of disease.[9]

RELEVANT ANATOMY

A detailed review of paranasal sinus anatomy and physiology is outside of the scope of this article, and the reader is directed to Richard D. Beegle and colleagues' article, "Normal and Variant Sinonasal Anatomy," in this issue. However, a discussion of paranasal sinus disease would not be complete without a brief review of mucociliary clearance physiology and sinus drainage pathways.

The sinonasal cavity is lined by ciliated pseudostratified columnar epithelium with mucinous and serous glands that aid in directing secretions through the drainage pathways.[8] Mucociliary clearance is an important defense mechanism against inhaled pathogens. The cilia act in a concerted fashion to direct secretions through the sinus ostium (sometimes in an antidependent manner), to the nasal cavity, where they then travel to the nasopharynx and are eventually swallowed.[10]

The frontal recess is an anatomically variable portion of the frontal sinus outflow tract that drains the frontal sinuses (**Fig 1**A). Depending on the

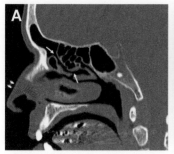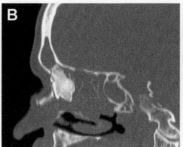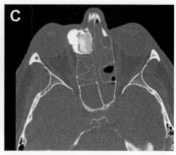

Fig. 1. Frontal recess. Sagittal CT of the paranasal sinuses in osseous algorithm (*A*) shows the frontal recess (*yellow arrows*). The agger nasi is anterior to the frontal recess and the ethmoid air cells are located posteriorly. Sagittal (*B*) and axial (*C*) CT images demonstrate an osteoma centered in the right frontal recess resulting in obstruction and complete opacification of the right frontal, ethmoid, and sphenoid sinuses.

attachment point of the uncinate process to either the anterior skull base medial to the frontal recess or to the lamina papyracea and agger nasi cell, the frontal recess may drain into either the ethmoid infundibulum or the middle meatus, respectively.[8,11-14] Rhinosinusitis may occur when the frontal recess is obstructed (**Fig. 1**B, C).

The ostiomeatal complex (OMC) or ostiomeatal unit (OMU) is the common drainage pathway of the frontal and maxillary sinuses and the anterior ethmoid air cells.[8] The maxillary infundibulum, hiatus semilunaris, middle meatus, and frontal recess comprise the OMC (**Fig. 2**A). Anatomic variants may result in narrowing of the OMC with the potential to contribute to obstruction.[14,15] Pneumatization of the middle turbinate (concha bullosa) or a paradoxic curvature of the middle turbinate may distort the uncinate process and narrow the infundibulum[8,16] (**Fig. 2**B). Other variants such as infraorbital or uncinate air cells, prominent ethmoid bulla, and nasal septal deviation may also alter the OMC.[14,15] An OMC pattern of obstruction will be seen on imaging as opacification of the anterior ethmoid air cells and frontal and maxillary sinuses (**Fig. 2**C and D).

The basal lamella, the coronal attachment the middle turbinate, separates the anterior and the posterior ethmoid air cells.[10,14] The anterior ethmoid air cells drain through the OMC and the middle meatus. The posterior ethmoid air cells drain via the superior or supreme meati, and with the sphenoid sinus, into the sphenoethmoidal recesses to the nasal cavity.[8,14]

Rhinosinusitis arises when there is retention of mucous secretions due to apposition of mucous membranes and resultant unproductive mucociliary clearance with obstruction of outflow.[10] This condition can lead to superimposed bacterial infection due to an increase in oxygen tension in the local environment.[9] The frontal recess, the infundibulum, the middle meatus, and the sphenoethmoidal recess are anatomic "tight spots" where obstruction may occur.[11] A list of common pathogens responsible for rhinosinusitis can be found in **Table 1**.[17-19]

The nasal cycle refers to physiologic congestion and subsequent decongestion of unilateral nasal mucosa occurring in a reciprocal pattern where congestion of one side is accompanied by decongestion on the other.[20] On imaging, mucosal

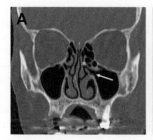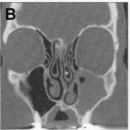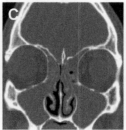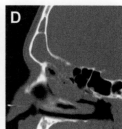

Fig. 2. OMC. The OMC is the common drainage pathway of the frontal and maxillary sinuses and the anterior ethmoid air cells. Coronal CT image of the paranasal sinuses (*A*) shows a patent maxillary infundibulum (*yellow arrow*) and hiatus semilunaris (below the *asterisk*). These two structures, together with the middle meatus and frontal recess, comprise the OMC. (*B*) An opacified OMC and left maxillary sinus. A concha bullosa (*asterisk*) may distort the uncinate process and result in narrowing of the infundibulum. Coronal (*C*) and sagittal (*D*) images of another patient show an ostiomeatal unit pattern of obstruction with opacification of the frontal sinuses, anterior ethmoid air cells, and maxillary sinuses.

Table 1
Common pathogens in rhinosinusitis

Viral	Acute Bacteria	Chronic Bacteria	Allergic Fungal	Invasive Fungal	Chronic Invasive Fungal

• Rhinovirus
• Parainfluenza
	• S. Pneumonia
	• Haemophilus influenzae
	• Moraxella catarrhalis
	• Gram-negative (nosocomial)
	• Pseudomonas
	• Anaerobes (dental infection)
		• Staphylococcus
		• Anaerobes
		  ○ Peptostreptococcus
		  ○ Fusobacterium
		  ○ Prevotella
			• Aspergillus
			  ○ Alternaria
			  ○ Bipolaris
			  ○ Curvularia
				• Mucormycosis
				• Rhizopus
					• Aspergillus
					• Mucorales
					• Candida
					• Pseudallescheria boydii
					• Sporothrix schenckii

thickening of approximately 2 to 3 mm is seen in the nasal cavity and anterior ethmoid air cells with accompanying hyperemia and swelling of the ipsilateral turbinates.[8,20,21] It is important to recognize this process and its imaging features as a normal physiologic phenomenon that should not be confused with a pathologic source of nasal obstruction.[21]

As CT is often obtained for surgical planning, the radiologist should be familiar with (and report) anatomic variations that may have implications for surgical misadventure. Variants that affect critical structures that place the patient at risk for cerebrospinal fluid leaks or for major arterial, orbital, optic nerve, or nasolacrimal duct injuries must be described.[7,16]

INFECTIOUS AND INFLAMMATORY PROCESSES
Rhinosinusitis

Rhinosinusitis is considered acute if characteristic symptoms are present for less than 4 weeks in duration and chronic if symptoms are present for greater than 12 weeks. Subacute sinusitis occurs in the time frame between 4 and 12 weeks.[2] Bacterial, viral, and fungal pathogens may be responsible culprits and can also serve as further classification criteria (see **Fig. 17**, **Table 1**). Uncomplicated rhinosinusitis refers to inflammation confined to the paranasal sinuses without extension into adjacent structures such as the intracranial vault, orbits, or adjacent soft tissues.[2,8]

Acute Rhinosinusitis

Imaging is generally not necessary in patients who meet the clinical criteria for acute rhinosinusitis unless an alternative diagnosis or intracranial, orbital, or other extrasinus soft tissue complications of sinusitis are suspected. Acute rhinosinusitis is diagnosed clinically in patients who present with cardinal symptoms of the disease; patients with acute rhinosinusitis may experience up to 4 weeks of purulent nasal drainage in combination with nasal obstruction and/or facial pain, pressure, or fullness. A distinction between bacterial and viral causes may be made based on clinical improvement (presumed viral origin) or failure to improve (presumed bacterial origin) within a 10-day period. This distinction helps to guide appropriate use of antibiotic therapy.[2,22]

CT findings of acute rhinosinusitis are relatively nonspecific and include mucosal thickening, air fluid levels, and bubbly or aerated opacification (**Fig. 3**). The imaging findings should be taken in the context of clinical symptoms to arrive at the correct diagnosis. An odontogenic source of sinusitis occurs in approximately 20% of cases and can be suspected radiographically in the presence of adjacent dental caries, periapical lucency, and/or focal osseous dehiscence between the affected tooth and sinus[8,23] (**Fig. 4**).

Chronic Rhinosinusitis

Chronic rhinosinusitis is a commonly diagnosed otolaryngologic disease occurring after 12 weeks duration of sinonasal symptoms and usually resulting from repeated episodes of acute or subacute sinusitis.[9] A Task Force on Rhinosinusitis published a consensus report in 1997 to standardize clinical diagnostic criteria of this process requiring either 2 major or 1 major and 2 minor criteria for diagnosis. Major criteria include facial pain, congestion, obstruction, nasal discharge, purulence, and olfactory disturbances. Minor criteria include headache, fever, fatigue, cough, ear pain, halitosis, and dental pain.[8]

CT is the most used imaging modality for the diagnosis of chronic rhinosinusitis, although as in the case of its acute counterpart, imaging features are not specific for the disease and must be interpreted in the appropriate clinical context.[8] For example, mucosal thickening has been shown to be present in greater than 90% of patients with a viral upper respiratory illness.[11]

Repeated episodes of inflammation may result in mucosal hypertrophy and retention cysts in the affected sinus with these findings often visualized on CT (**Fig. 5**). Mucosal thickening of up to 3 mm may be seen in normal individuals.[24,25] Sinonasal polyps and bony changes including hyperostosis and sclerosis of the sinus walls can also be seen and may be used to confirm a chronic process because these signs generally are not present in the true acute setting.[8,9] Hyperdense sinus opacification may represent inspissated mucus or proteinaceous debris, calcification, or an atypical fungal process. Calcifications related to chronic rhinosinusitis generally show a peripheral pattern, whereas calcifications located centrally suggest fungal disease.[8]

On MRI, paranasal sinus mucosal thickening and opacification usually demonstrate T1-hypointense and T2-hyperintense signal due to its dominant water content, although the signal characteristics are variable in chronic obstruction and depend on proteinaceous content. One potential MRI pitfall is a completely opacified sinus appearing as a signal void in the setting of high protein content and viscosity, mimicking a normally aerated sinus on MRI.[9] Although MRI is not typically used to evaluate uncomplicated sinonasal disease, imaging findings of rhinosinusitis

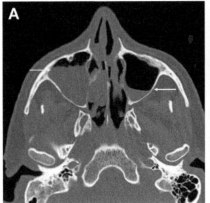
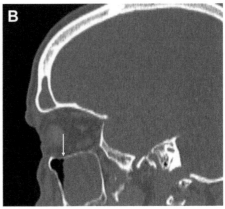

Fig. 3. Acute rhinosinusitis. Axial (*A*) and coronal (*B*) CT images of the paranasal sinuses demonstrate imaging features of acute rhinosinusitis. Air fluid levels are seen in the bilateral maxillary sinuses, more pronounced on the left (*arrows* in *A* and *B*). There is also "bubbly" opacification in the anterior aspect of the right maxillary sinus.

are often seen on MRI performed for other purposes.

A combination of features of acute and chronic rhinosinusitis can be seen on imaging and may raise the suspicion of acute on chronic rhinosinusitis in patients with the appropriate clinical scenario of acute symptoms in a background of known chronic sinonasal disease (see **Fig. 5**).

Retention Cysts and Polyps

Retention cysts are commonly encountered lesions in the setting of chronic sinus disease. Both mucous or serous retention cysts can occur either from obstruction of the seromucinous glands or submucosal accumulation of serous fluid respectively.[9] These cysts cannot be differentiated from each other or from polyps on imaging.[24] These cysts are most often seen in the maxillary sinuses and on CT as circumscribed hypodense lesions with rounded or domed morphology (**Fig. 6**). On MRI, they are T1 hypointense and T2 hyperintense.[9,24]

Sinonasal polyps are also a commonly encountered finding in patients with chronic sinonasal disease and represent the most common sinonasal mass lesion.[8] These polyps result from chronic mucosal inflammation and infection resulting in hypertrophic mucosal protrusions with submucosal accumulation of fluid. Expansion of the nasal cavity and sinuses from polypoid soft tissue may also be seen (**Fig. 7**). CT may demonstrate hyperdense central material with peripheral hypodensity in the affected sinus. The density on CT and intensity on

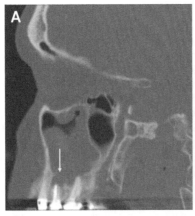
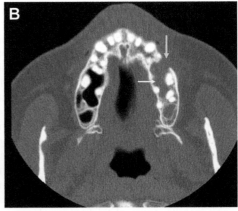

Fig. 4. Odontogenic rhinosinusitis. Sagittal CT image of the paranasal sinuses (*A*) demonstrates near-complete opacification of the left maxillary sinus. There are no air fluid levels present. An axial CT image through the floor of the maxillary sinuses shows periapical lucencies about the roots of the left first and second maxillary molars (*yellow arrows* in *A* and *B*). A focal dehiscence of the buccal surface of the maxilla is also present (*blue arrow* in *B*), also related to apical periodontal disease.

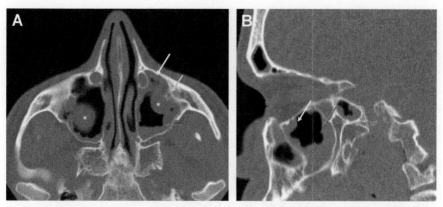

Fig. 5. Acute on chronic rhinosinusitis. Axial (*A*) and sagittal (*B*) CT images through the maxillary sinuses demonstrate retention cysts (*asterisks* in *A*), mucosal thickening (*yellow arrows* in *A* and *B*), and peripheral calcification (*blue arrow* in *A*), all features of chronic rhinosinusitis. An air fluid level is present in the left maxillary sinus (*pink arrows* in *A* and *B*) indicative of an acute on chronic rhinosinusitis in the appropriate clinical context.

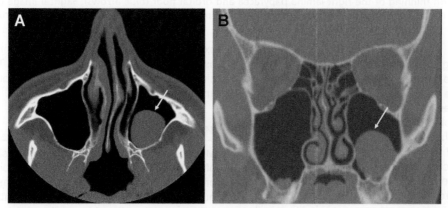

Fig. 6. Retention cyst. Axial (*A*) and coronal (*B*) CT images through the sinuses reveal a circumscribed dome-shaped lesion in the left maxillary sinus (*yellow arrows* in *A* and *B*) compatible with a retention cyst; these are commonly encountered lesions seen with chronic sinus disease and most often in the maxillary sinuses.

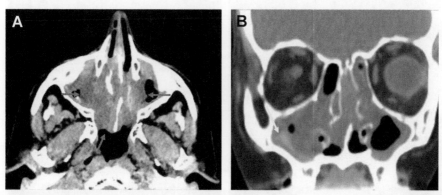

Fig. 7. Sinonasal polyposis. Axial (*A*) and coronal (*B*) CT images through the nasal cavity and maxillary sinuses demonstrate polypoid soft tissue expanding the nasal cavity and involving the maxillary sinuses (*pink arrows* in *A*), left more so than right. There is some hyperdense attenuation present in the right maxillary sinus (*yellow arrow* in *B*) with variable density depending on the proteinaceous content.

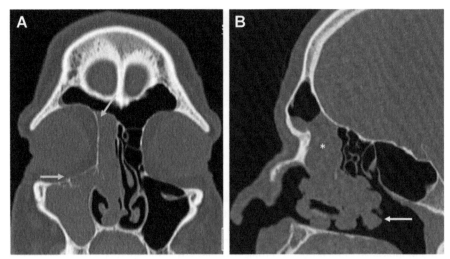

Fig. 8. Sinonasal polyposis. Coronal (*A*) CT image through the paranasal sinuses in a different patient with sino-nasal polyposis reveals complete opacification of the right OMC and maxillary sinus. There are associated osseous changes with thinning of the right lamina papyracea and orbital floor (*blue arrows*). Sagittal image (*B*) shows expansion of the frontal recess (*asterisk*) and the polypoid morphology in the nasal cavity (*yellow arrow*).

T1- and T2-weighted MRI may be variable depending on the proteinaceous content. Expansion of the nasal cavity and sinuses from polypoid soft tissue as well as osseous remodeling and/or erosion can be seen (**Fig. 8**). Polyps may be indistinguishable from retention cysts and mucoceles on unenhanced imaging, although contrast-enhanced images will show enhancement of polyps in contradistinction to absent enhancement of the latter 2 lesions.[8,9]

An antrochoanal polyp is a solitary polypoid lesion that arises most commonly in the maxillary sinus (with less common involvement of the sphenoid and ethmoid sinuses). Soft tissue opacification extends to the maxillary antrum with extension through and expansion of the maxillary ostium to involve the nasal cavity (**Fig. 9**). The opacification may extend into to the posterior choana and involve the nasopharynx[8,9] (**Fig. 10**).

Mucoceles

Mucoceles are the most common expansile lesion of the paranasal sinuses resulting from obstruction of the sinus ostia.[8] In order of decreasing frequency these most often affect the frontal sinus, followed by the ethmoid, maxillary, and sphenoid sinuses. As these lesions are expansile, symptoms are generally related to mass effect with orbital symptoms most common.

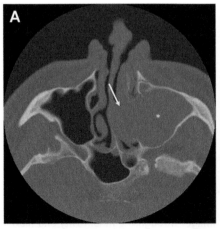
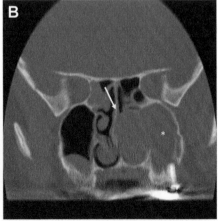

Fig. 9. Antrochoanal polyp. Axial (*A*) and coronal (*B*) CT images through the maxillary sinuses demonstrate complete opacification of the left maxillary sinus (*asterisk* in *A* and *B*). There is extension through and expansion of the maxillary ostium with soft tissue involving the left nasal cavity (*yellow arrows* in *A* and *B*).

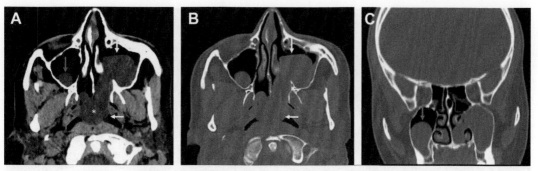

Fig. 10. Antrochoanal polyp. Axial CT images in soft tissue (*A*) and osseous (*B*) algorithms demonstrate a lobulated hypodense soft tissue mass lesion (*yellow arrows* in *A* and *B*) arising from the left maxillary sinus and extending through the posterior nasal cavity into the nasopharynx (*asterisk* in *A*). Note the retention cyst in the right maxillary sinus on the coronal CT image (*pink arrow* in *C*), partially visualized on the axial image (*pink arrow*, *A*). Polyps are sometimes difficult to distinguish from retention cysts on unenhanced imaging, although contrast-enhanced images will reveal enhancement of the former and not the latter.

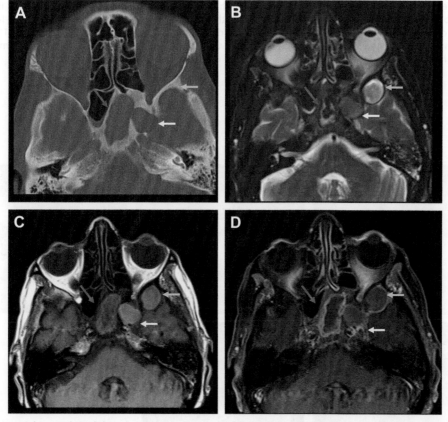

Fig. 11. Mucocele. Axial CT (*A*) and corresponding axial fat-suppressed T2-weighted images through the sphenoid sinuses and middle cranial fossa demonstrate a completely opacified left sphenoid sinus (*pink arrows* in *A* and *B*). There is hyperostosis of the sinus walls compatible with a chronic process, best seen on CT. A focal area of osseous dehiscence is seen along the lateral wall of the left sphenoid sinus (*yellow arrow* in *A*). There is scalloping of the left greater sphenoid wing of the middle cranial fossa (*blue arrow* in *A*). On corresponding axial magnetic resonance images including precontrast T1-weighted image (*C*) and postcontrast fat-suppressed T1-weighted image (*D*) there is nonenhancing intrinsic T1-hyperintense material in the lateral sphenoid sinus (*yellow arrows* in *B*, *C*, and *D*) and adjacent to the sphenoid wing and left temporal pole (*blue arrows* in *B*, *C* and *D*, compatible with a mucocele. Note the signal in the medial left sphenoid sinus (*pink arrows*), with an area of "signal void" on magnetic resonance images in a completely opacified sinus seen on CT.

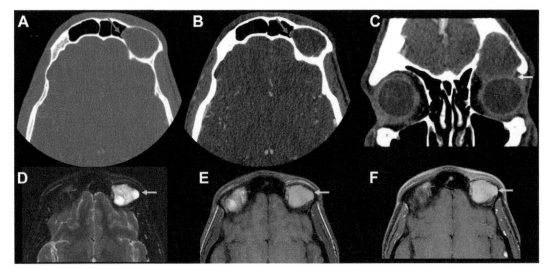

Fig. 12. Cholesterol granuloma. Axial contrast-enhanced CT images (*A* and *B*) demonstrate complete opacification of the left frontal sinus with a low-density nonenhancing expansile mass (*pink arrows*). There is erosion of the floor of the left frontal sinus with extension into the left superior orbit and mass effect on the left globe seen on a coronal CT image (*yellow arrow, C*). Corresponding axial T2 fat-suppressed (*D*), precontrast T1 (*E*), and postcontrast fat-suppressed T1-weighted images (*F*) show a T1- and T2-hyperintense nonenhancing mass (*blue arrows*), similar in appearance to a mucocele. Pathology revealed a cholesterol granuloma.

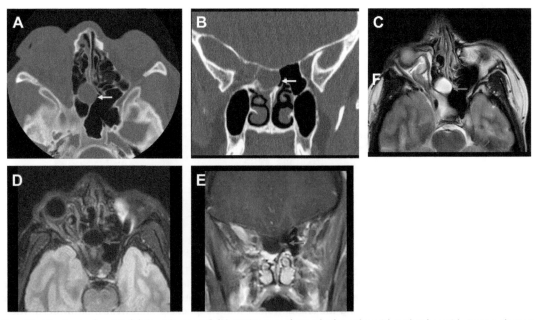

Fig. 13. Meningocele. Axial (*A*) and coronal (*B*) CT images through the ethmoid and sphenoid sinuses demonstrate a circumscribed expansile mass in a right posterior ethmoid air cell (*yellow arrows*). The lesion is hyperintense on axial T2-weighted image (*pink arrow, C*). Complete suppression of signal on an axial fluid-attenuated inversion recovery image (*D*) is compatible with cerebrospinal fluid. No brain tissue or enhancement was seen on a coronal postcontrast fat-suppressed T1-weighted image (*pink arrow, E*). Findings are compatible with a meningocele—a skull base defect was seen on another image from the CT (not shown).

On CT, mucoceles will appear as an expansile nonenhancing low-attenuation mass with adjacent osseous thinning and/or erosion, but no destructive-appearing osseous changes. There may be remodeling of the inner wall of the sinus with new reactive outer wall formation (**Fig. 11**A). MRI will similarly show an expansile mass, although the signal intensity is rather variable depending on the hydration status, proteinaceous content, and viscosity of the mucocele. Although these lesions can demonstrate variable T1 and T2 signal intensities, they are most commonly T1 and T2 hyperintense or T1 and T2 hypointense (**Fig. 11**B–D). Contrast-enhanced images will reveal thin peripheral enhancement distinguishing mucoceles from neoplastic process that may demonstrate solid enhancement[8,9,26] (see **Fig. 11**D). Cholesterol granuloma is a differential consideration, although they rarely occur in the paranasal sinuses[27] (**Fig. 12**). Cephaloceles are also an important diagnosis to consider and exclude so as not to perform an unwarranted biopsy (**Fig. 13**).

Complications

Complicated rhinosinusitis occurs when an infectious sinonasal process extends from the sinuses into the adjacent extrasinus soft tissues or structures. The ethmoid sinuses are the most frequent source of infection because the thin lamina papyracea is all that separates the ethmoid air cells from the orbit and intraorbital structures. Infection may extend through this thin osseous barrier or through the valveless anterior or posterior ethmoidal veins. Extrasinus infection arising from the sphenoid, frontal, and maxillary sinuses is less common but also occurs.[8]

Orbital complications that may be encountered from a sinus origin include preseptal or postseptal cellulitis, subperiosteal and orbital abscesses, and/or superior ophthalmic vein thrombosis. CT and MRI may show subtle fat stranding or enhancement in the orbits, as well as rim-enhancing collections in the setting of abscesses. Diffusion restriction on diffusion-weighted imaging may be seen on MRI when an abscess is present.[8,9,24]

Intracranial complications of sinus disease include meningitis, epidural or subdural abscesses/empyemas, cerebritis, or cerebral abscesses. The frontal sinus is the most common source of intracranial infections via bone defects or emissary veins (**Fig. 14**). MRI is preferred to CT for evaluation of orbital and intracranial complications owing to its superior ability to reveal (1) leptomeningeal or pachymeningeal enhancement and abnormal extra-axial fluid-attenuated inversion recovery signal with meningitis; (2) rim-enhancing parenchymal, epidural, or subdural collections with restricted diffusion with abscesses; and (3) parenchymal rim-enhancing collections with restricted diffusion with cerebral abscesses.[8] Cavernous sinus thrombosis is seen as areas of nonenhancement in the cavernous sinus on

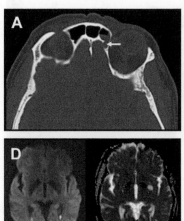
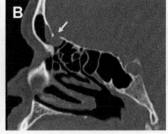
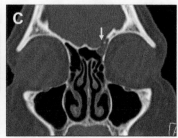

Fig. 14. Meningitis and ventriculitis. Axial (*A*), sagittal (*B*), and coronal (*C*) CT images through the frontal sinuses in a patient with meningitis show a focal defect in the posterior wall of the left frontal sinus (*yellow arrows*) leading to the anterior cranial fossa. An air-fluid level is seen on the axial CT image. Diffusion-weighted imaging (DWI) with a corresponding apparent diffusion coefficient map (*D*) shows restricted diffusion in the posterior horns of the lateral ventricles, compatible with pyogenic ventriculitis (*pink arrows*). A few additional areas of restricted diffusion were seen over the convexities in leptomeningeal distribution (not shown). The frontal sinus defect was considered the source of the infection and was surgically repaired.

contrast-enhanced CT and MRI, most often in the context of sphenoid sinus disease (**Fig. 15**).

Osteomyelitis can occur in the bones adjacent to the paranasal sinuses. Imaging findings include osseous erosion, sclerosis, and periosteal bone formation on CT, as well as marrow edema and enhancement of the involved bones and adjacent soft tissues on MRI. Pott puffy tumor refers to the unique scenario of outer table osteomyelitis with an associated subgaleal abscess and edema in the context of frontal sinusitis[8] (**Fig. 16**).

Neurosurgical consultation is warranted when life-threatening intracranial complications are encountered.

Silent Sinus Syndrome

Silent sinus syndrome refers to asymptomatic unilateral atelectasis of a maxillary sinus that occurs in the setting of chronic obstruction of the maxillary ostium. Enophthalmos and hypoglobus with facial asymmetry may be visible on physical examination. Imaging will show a completely opacified and asymmetrically small maxillary sinus with hyperostosis of the sinus walls.[8,28–30]

Fungal Rhinosinusitis

Fungal sinusitis is categorized into noninvasive and invasive forms (**Fig. 17**). Allergic fungal rhinosinusitis and mycetomas (fungus balls) comprise the noninvasive category of fungal sinonasal disease. These processes generally occur in immunocompetent individuals. Invasive fungal rhinosinusitis demonstrates involvement of the mucosa, submucosa, and bone on histologic analysis and can be further categorized into acute, chronic, and granulomatous types with the acute and chronic invasive types affecting immunocompromised hosts. The granulomatous form affects immunocompetent individuals in North Africa, the Middle East, and Southeast Asia.[8,9]

Allergic fungal rhinosinusitis
Allergic fungal rhinosinusitis affects immunocompetent children and young adults with a history of

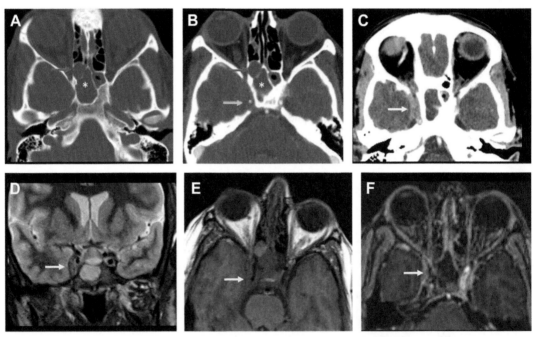

Fig. 15. CST. Axial CT images in bone (*A*) and soft tissue (*B*) algorithms through the ethmoid and sphenoid sinuses and the cavernous sinuses performed as a CT angiogram in a patient with a prolonged severe headache demonstrates complete opacification of the right posterior ethmoid and sphenoid sinuses (*asterisks*). There is a focal dehiscence of the lateral wall of the sinus at the level of the right orbital apex (*pink arrows*). Narrowing of the right cavernous internal carotid artery is seen (*blue arrow, B*). There is also relative nonopacification of the right cavernous sinus when compared with the left in arterial phase (*blue arrow, B*), and on delayed venous phase (*yellow arrow, C*). A subsequent MRI shows expansion with lateral bulging of the cavernous sinus on a coronal T2 fat-suppressed image (*yellow arrow, D*). An axial T1-weighted image (*E*) demonstrates infiltrative T1-isointense soft issue tissue in the right cavernous sinus (*yellow arrow*). There are regions of nonenhancement present on an axial postcontrast 3D T1-weighted image (*yellow arrow, F*) confirming CST. CST, cavernous sinus thrombosis.

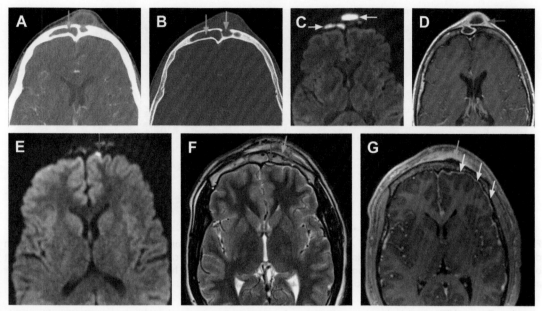

Fig. 16. Pott puffy tumor. Axial CT images (*A* and *B*) demonstrate complete opacification of the frontal sinuses (*green arrows*) with a bony defect in the calvarium (*blue arrow*). There is pus within the frontal sinus and soft tissue collection seen as restricted diffusion on DWI (*yellow arrows* in *C*) with extension of abscess in the adjacent frontal extracranial soft tissues (*red arrow* in *D*) through the bony defect. In another patient with Pott puffy tumor (*E* and *F*) intracranial complications are seen with small epidural abscess on axial DWI (*E*) and T2-weighted images (*F*) (*red arrows*). A small subperiosteal abscess is seen on the axial T2-weighted images (*F*) and a postcontrast 3D T1-weighted image (*G*) (*blue arrows*). Adjacent pachymeningeal enhancement (*yellow arrows*) is also seen (*G*). (Case courtesy of Emilio Supsupin, M.D.)

atopy, recurrent sinusitis, and polyposis. *Aspergillus* is the most common responsible pathogen. CT demonstrates hyperdense sinus opacification and a peripheral hypodense rim within the affected sinuses. The sinuses may be expanded with associated osseous remodeling and regions of erosion, thinning, or dehiscence of sinus walls. Central calcifications may be present (**Fig. 18**). MRI reveals T2-hypointense signal corresponding to hyperdense areas seen on CT. T1-weighted images

demonstrate isointense or slightly hypointense signal. T1-hyperintense signal is rare.

Mycetoma (fungus balls) typically involves a single sinus in an immunocompetent individual. The maxillary sinus is most often involved. Patients are usually asymptomatic, although facial pressure may be experienced. On CT, a well-defined hyperdense mass with calcifications is seen often superimposed on a background of chronic sinus disease. Mycetoma demonstrates hypointense

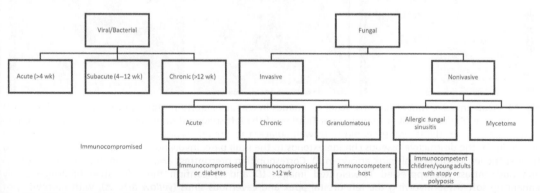

Fig. 17. Categorization of sinus disease.

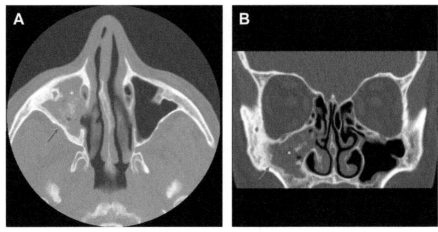

Fig. 18. Chronic fungal rhinosinusitis. Axial (*A*) and coronal (*B*) images from a low-dose unenhanced CT scan demonstrate near-complete opacification of the right maxillary sinus. Calcifications are seen in the central aspect of the sinus cavity (*yellow asterisk*), suggesting a fungal rhinosinusitis. The hyperostosis of the sinus walls (*pink arrows*) is most compatible with a chronic process.

signal on T1- and T2-weighted images with "signal void" appearing like a normal unaffected sinus.

Acute invasive fungal rhinosinusitis

Acute invasive rhinosinusitis is a rapidly progressive, highly morbid, and often fatal infection that affects immunocompromised hosts or patients with poorly controlled diabetes mellitus. Early recognition is crucial to guide appropriate management. The nasal cavity and middle turbinate are usually the first sites of infection.[8,31–33] Mucormycosis and *Rhizopus* are responsible pathogens.[3,31] The fungal organisms

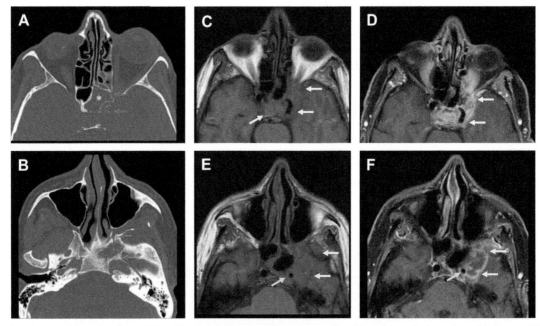

Fig. 19. Acute invasive fungal sinusitis. Axial CT images in osseous algorithm through the sphenoid sinuses (*A*) and skull base (*B*) demonstrate complete opacification of the left sphenoid sinus (*asterisk* in *A*). There is permeative destruction of the lateral sphenoid sinus wall adjacent to the left orbital apex and cavernous sinus (*pink arrows* in *A*). The destructive osseous change extends to the skull base, involving the vidian canal and extending to near the left carotid canal (*pink arrows* in *B*). Corresponding precontrast axial T1-weighted images (*C* and *E*) and postcontrast fat-suppressed T1-weighted images (*D* and *F*) confirm the infiltrative heterogeneously enhancing soft tissue involving the left orbital apex and cavernous sinus (*yellow arrows*), with narrowing of the left internal carotid artery flow void (*blue arrows*) in this patient with acute invasive fungal sinusitis.

rapidly propagate and result in ischemic necrosis of the mucosa with rapid progression and extension into the adjacent structures including the facial soft tissues, orbits, skull base, cavernous sinus, and intracranial vault. Extension can be direct or via perivascular channels or hematogenous spread.[31,32]

Stranding or soft tissue density in the premaxillary or retroantral fat may be the only subtle imaging findings on CT during the early phase of acute invasive fungal rhinosinusitis.[31,32,34] Nonspecific mucosal thickening or abnormal soft tissue density in the sinus or nasal cavity with subtle osseous erosion can also be seen on CT early in the disease course. The mucosal thickening may demonstrate T2 hypointensity on MRI. An aggressive enhancing mass outside of the confines of the sinus with osseous erosion is seen in the fulminant form. Cranial nerve and vasculature involvement can occur with enhancement extending through skull base foramina and along cranial nerves.[31,32] Vascular invasion may result in vessel occlusion and resultant ischemia and infarction[8,9,31,35] (**Fig. 19**).

Chronic invasive fungal rhinosinusitis

The chronic invasive form of fungal rhinosinusitis is a slowly progressive process affecting immunocompromised individuals with symptoms present for greater than 12 weeks. The symptoms may be similar to those of chronic rhinosinusitis, but atypical features, such as focal neurologic deficits, visual symptoms, and extrasinus soft tissue swelling, may be encountered.[8,9,31] Common pathogens include *Aspergillus*, *Mucorales*, *Pseudomonas*, *Altemarias*, and *Candida* species.[36] The ethmoid and sphenoid sinuses are most often involved. CT may reveal a hyperdense intrasinus soft tissue mass with adjacent osseous erosions. As with the other fungal processes, a T2-hypointense and T1-hypointense intrasinus mass is demonstrated on MRI. Local invasion with minimal surrounding inflammation may also be present.[8,31,34]

Systemic Inflammatory Processes

Several systemic inflammatory processes may result in clinical symptoms and imaging features of rhinosinusitis.

Sarcoidosis

Sinonasal sarcoidosis affects up to 5% of patients with sarcoidosis; it may be an isolated finding or may present as part of the systemic process.[37] Patients may experience nasal stuffiness or crusting, rhinorrhea, anosmia, epistaxis,

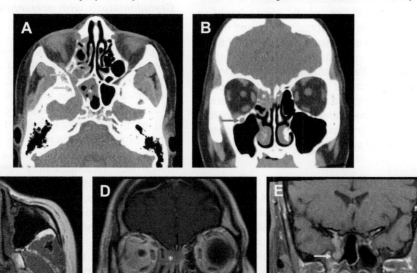

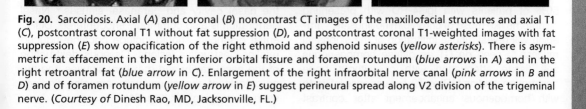

Fig. 20. Sarcoidosis. Axial (*A*) and coronal (*B*) noncontrast CT images of the maxillofacial structures and axial T1 (*C*), postcontrast coronal T1 without fat suppression (*D*), and postcontrast coronal T1-weighted images with fat suppression (*E*) show opacification of the right ethmoid and sphenoid sinuses (*yellow asterisks*). There is asymmetric fat effacement in the right inferior orbital fissure and foramen rotundum (*blue arrows* in *A*) and in the right retroantral fat (*blue arrow* in *C*). Enlargement of the right infraorbital nerve canal (*pink arrows* in *B* and *D*) and of foramen rotundum (*yellow arrow* in *E*) suggest perineural spread along V2 division of the trigeminal nerve. (*Courtesy of* Dinesh Rao, MD, Jacksonville, FL.)

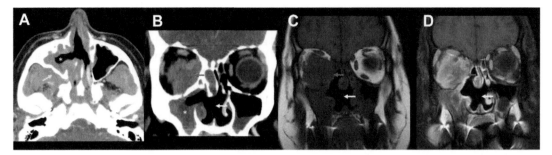

Fig. 21. GPA. An axial CT image through the maxillary sinuses (*A*) in a patient with granulomatosis with poly-angiitis demonstrates thickened soft tissue in the right maxillary sinus (*yellow asterisk*). Note the effacement of the right retroantral fat (*blue arrow*). A coronal CT image (*B*) shows extension of the infiltrative soft tissue into the right orbit with displacement and mass effect on the right medial and inferior rectus muscles and encasement of the right optic nerve (*pink arrow*). There is asymmetric right proptosis. Coronal precontrast (*C*) and postcontrast fat-suppressed (*D*) T1-weighted images show T1-isointense enhancing soft tissue corre-sponding to the CT findings (*pink arrows* in *C* and *D*). Note the nasal septal perforation (*yellow arrows* in *B–D*).

or facial pain. On direct inspection, purplish mu-cosa with granulations and/or mucosal hypertro-phy, nasal polyps, septal perforation, or a saddle nose deformity may be seen. Imaging may reveal nodular lesions of the nasal septum and inferior turbinates, mucosal thickening, and partial or complete opacification of the paranasal sinuses with possible adjacent osseous sclerosis. Careful evaluation of skull base foramina including along the infraorbital, vidian, and maxil-lary nerve for perineural spread is required if there is cranial nerve or other atypical symptoms (**Fig. 20**). Differential considerations include infec-tious causes such as aspergillosis, actinomy-cosis, or tuberculosis or other systemic processes such as granulomatosis with polyan-giitis. Neoplastic process should also be consid-ered if perineural spread is present.[37–39]

IgG4-related disease

Head and neck manifestations of IgG4-related dis-ease (RD) are common, with the salivary glands and orbits the most often affected sites.[40] Sino-nasal involvement is common and usually not pre-sent in isolation. Two patterns of involvement have been described in the literature—mucosal infiltra-tion and an invasive mass. Symptoms are nonspe-cific and include nasal obstruction, epistaxis, and facial pain.[41]

The mucosal infiltration pattern is seen in 30% to 50% of patients with IgG4-RD with presenting symptoms like those of chronic rhinosinusitis.[41] Im-aging will reveal diffuse infiltration of the sinonasal mucosa,[41] seen on CT as diffuse homogeneous soft tissue attenuation with or without bone destruction, and on MRI as T2-hypointense infiltrate with homogenous enhancement after contrast

administration.[40] IgG4-RD may also appear as a locally invasive and destructive sinonasal mass that can mimic malignancy.[41–43] Differential consid-erations include fungal rhinosinusitis, granulomato-sis with polyangiitis, lymphoma, and in the case of an invasive mass, squamous cell carcinoma.[40,41]

Granulomatosis with polyangiitis and other vasculitides

Several systemic vasculitides produce clinical manifestations in the sinonasal regions. Granulo-matosis with polyangiitis (GPA) and eosinophilic granulomatosis with polyangiitis affect small and medium-sized arteries and comprise the majority of vasculitic sinonasal disease cases (up to 90% and up to 69%, respectively). Like many of the other processes described in this review, the symptoms are nonspecific and include epistaxis, rhinorrhea, nasorespiratory insufficiency, and hyposmia or anosmia. Nasal septal perforation, ul-cerations, scabs, or polyps are demonstrated on direct inspection. Histopathology may reveal the characteristic antineutrophil cytoplasmic anti-bodies with cytoplasmic antineutrophil cytoplas-minc antibodies (c-ANCA) indicative of GPA and peripheral antineutrophil cytoplasmic antibodies (p-ANCA) indicative of eosinophilic granulomato-sis with polyangiitis, although these may not be positive until late in the disease.[6,44] Imaging will demonstrate nonspecific mucosal thickening in the nasal cavity and paranasal sinuses.[5] Nasal perforation is also commonly encountered. Differ-ential diagnosis should include cocaine-induced midline destructive lesions. Osseous destruction of the nasal cavity and maxillary sinuses and hy-perostosis of the sinus walls are also findings seen on imaging[45,46] (**Fig. 21**).

SUMMARY

Imaging of sinonasal infectious and inflammatory diseases is generally reserved for clinical scenarios in which acute complications or diagnoses other than uncomplicated rhinosinusitis are suspected. CT is the modality of choice in the evaluation of sinonasal inflammatory disease due to its high spatial resolution and fine osseous detail of anatomic structures. MRI provides improved soft tissue resolution in the characterization of soft tissue masses and in the evaluation of intracranial complications. As symptoms and imaging features of various infectious, inflammatory, and systemic sinonasal processes may be nonspecific, imaging is used in combination with the clinical context and laboratory and histopathologic analysis to arrive at the correct diagnoses.

CLINICS CARE POINTS

- Rhinosinusitis is a clinical diagnosis. Imaging is usually reserved for surgical planning or in cases in which complications or alternative diagnoses are suspected.

- The imaging features of rhinosinusitis are nonspecific and must be used in combination with the clinical context, including the duration of symptoms, to arrive at the correct diagnosis.

- Recognition of subtle early signs of acute invasive fungal sinusitis is critical to guide early management because progression is rapid and mortality is high.

- Some systemic inflammatory and vasculitic processes have a predilection for the sinonasal region and may present with symptoms similar to rhinosinusitis. Imaging can be used with laboratory and/or histopathologic analysis to arrive at the correct diagnosis.

REFERENCES

1. Villarroel MA, Blackwell DL, Jen A. Tables of Summary Health Statistics for U.S. Adults: 2018 National Health Interview Survey. National Center for Health Statistics. 2019. 2018. Available at: http://www.cdc.gov/nchs/nhis/SHS/tables.htm.

2. Rosenfeld RM, Piccirillo JF, Chandrasekhar SS, et al. Clinical practice guideline (update): Adult sinusitis. Otolaryngol Head Neck Surg 2015;152:S1–39. https://doi.org/10.1177/0194599815572097.

3. Momeni AK, Roberts CC, Chew FS. Imaging of chronic and exotic sinonasal disease: Review. Am J Roentgenol 2007;189(6 SUPPL). https://doi.org/10.2214/AJR.07.7031.

4. Mari Hagiwara M, Bruno Policeni MM, Amy F, et al. ACR Appropriateness Criteria® Sinonasal Disease. Available at: https://acsearch.acr.org/docs/69502/Narrative/. Accessed January 23, 2023.

5. Armengot M, Gárcia-Lliberós A, Gómez MJ, et al. Sinonasal Involvement in Systemic Vasculitides and Cocaine-Induced Midline Destructive Lesions: Diagnostic Controversies. Allergy & Rhinology 2013;4(2). https://doi.org/10.2500/ar.2013.4.0051. ar.2013.4.0051.

6. Fuchs HA, Tanner Sb. Granulomatous disorders of the nose and paranasal sinuses. Curr Opin Otolaryngol Head Neck Surg 2009;17:23–7.

7. O'Brien WT, Hamelin S, Weitzel EK. The preoperative sinus CT: Avoiding a "cLOSE" call with surgical complications. Radiology 2016;281(1):10–21. https://doi.org/10.1148/radiol.2016152230.

8. Mossa-Basha M, Blitz AM. Imaging of the Paranasal Sinuses. Semin Roentgenol 2013;48(1):14–34. https://doi.org/10.1053/j.ro.2012.09.006.

9. Rao VM, El-Noueam KI. Sinonasal Imaging. Radiol Clin 1998;36(5):921–39.

10. Whyte A, Boeddinghaus R. The maxillary sinus: Physiology, development and imaging anatomy. Dentomaxillofacial Radiol 2019;48(8). https://doi.org/10.1259/dmfr.20190205.

11. Huang BY, Lloyd KM, DelGaudio JM, et al. Failed endoscopic sinus surgery: Spectrum of CT findings in the frontal recess. Radiographics 2009;29(1):177–95. https://doi.org/10.1148/rg.291085118.

12. Daniels DL, Mafee MF, Smith MM, et al. The frontal sinus drainage pathway and related structures. AJNR Am J Neuroradiol 2003;24:1618–27.

13. Kantarci M, Karasen RM, Alper F, et al. Remarkable anatomic variations in paranasal sinus region and their clinical importance. Eur J Radiol 2004;50:296–302.

14. Beale TJ, Madani G, Morley SJ. Imaging of the paranasal sinuses and nasal cavity: normal anatomy and clinically relevant anatomical variants. Semin Ultrasound CT MR 2009;30(1):2–16. https://doi.org/10.1053/j.sult.2008.10.011.

15. Shpilberg KA, Daniel SC, Doshi AH, et al. CT of anatomic variants of the paranasal sinuses and nasal cavity: Poor correlation with radiologically significant rhinosinusitis but importance in surgical planning. Am J Roentgenol 2015;204(6):1255–60. https://doi.org/10.2214/AJR.14.13762.

16. Beale TJ, Madani G, Morley SJ. Imaging of the paranasal sinuses and nasal cavity: Normal anatomy and clinically relevant anatomical variants. Semin Ultrasound CT MR 2009;30:2–16.

17. Aring AM, Chan MM. Current Concepts in Adult Acute Rhinosinusitis. Am Fam Physician 2016;94(2):97–105.

18. Scheid DC, Hamm RM. Acute bacterial rhinosinusitis in adults: part I. Evaluation. Am Fam Physician 2004; 70(9):1685–92.

19. Eloy JA, Govindaraj S. Microbiology and Immunology of Rhinosinusitis. In: Rhinosinusitis. New York: Springer; 2008. p. 1–12. https://doi.org/10.1007/978-0-387-73062-2_2.

20. Pendolino AL, Lund VJ, Nardello E, et al. The nasal cycle: a comprehensive review. Rhinol Online 2018; 1(1):67–76. https://doi.org/10.4193/rhinol/18.021.

21. Zinreich SJ, Kennedy DW, Kumar AJ, et al. MR imaging of normal nasal cycle: comparison with sinus pathology. J Comput Assist Tomogr 1988;12(6):1014–9. https://doi.org/10.1097/00004728-198811000-00019.

22. Peters AT, Spector S, Hsu J, et al. Diagnosis and management of rhinosinusitis: A practice parameter update. Ann Allergy Asthma Immunol 2014;113(4): 347–85. https://doi.org/10.1016/j.anai.2014.07.025.

23. Chapman MN, Nadgir RN, Akman AS, et al. Periapical lucency around the tooth: Radiologic evaluation and differential diagnosis. Radiographics 2013; 33(1). https://doi.org/10.1148/rg.331125172.

24. Joshi VM, Sansi R. Imaging in Sinonasal Inflammatory Disease. Neuroimaging Clin 2015;25(4): 549–68. https://doi.org/10.1016/j.nic.2015.07.003.

25. Thayil N, Chapman MN, Saito N, et al. Magnetic Resonance Imaging of Acute Head and Neck Infections. Magn Reson Imag Clin N Am 2016;24(2): 345–67. https://doi.org/10.1016/j.mric.2015.11.003.

26. van Tassel P, Lee YY, Jing BS, et al. Mucoceles of the paranasal sinuses: MR imaging with CT correlation. AJR Am J Roentgenol 1989;153(2):407–12. https://doi.org/10.2214/ajr.153.2.407.

27. Kim TH, Lim EJ, Kim S, et al. Cholesterol Granuloma of the Maxillary Sinus Misdiagnosed as Nasal Polyp or Mucocele: Four Cases. J Craniofac Surg 2021;32(6):e600–2. https://doi.org/10.1097/SCS.0000000000007899.

28. Hourany R, Aygun N, della Santina CC, et al. Silent sinus syndrome: An acquired condition. AJNR Am J Neuroradiol 2005;26:2390–2.

29. Brandt MG, Wright ED. The silent sinus syndrome is a form of chronic maxillary atelectasis: A systematic review of all reported cases. Am J Rhinol 2008;22: 68–73.

30. Illner A, Davidson HC, Harnsberger HR, et al. The silent sinus syndrome: clinical and radiographic findings. AJR Am J Roentgenol 2002;178(2):503–6. https://doi.org/10.2214/ajr.178.2.1780503.

31. Aribandi M, McCoy VA, Bazan C. Imaging Features of Invasive and Noninvasive Fungal Sinusitis: A Review. Radiographics 2007;27(5):1283–96. https://doi.org/10.1148/rg.275065189.

32. Kamalian S, Avery L, Lev MH, et al. Nontraumatic Head and Neck Emergencies. Radiographics 2019;39(6):1808–23. https://doi.org/10.1148/rg.2019190159.

33. Gillespie MB, O'Malley Bert W, Francis HW. An Approach to Fulminant Invasive Fungal Rhinosinusitis in the Immunocompromised Host. Arch Otolaryngol Head Neck Surg 1998;124(5):520. https://doi.org/10.1001/archotol.124.5.520.

34. Fatterpekar G, Mukherji S, Arbealez A, et al. Fungal diseases of the paranasal sinuses. Semin Ultrasound CT MR 1999;20:391–401.

35. deShazo RD, Chapin K, Swain RE. Fungal sinusitis. N Engl J Med 1997;337:254–9.

36. Wang T, Zhang L, Hu C, et al. Clinical Features of Chronic Invasive Fungal Rhinosinusitis in 16 Cases. Ear Nose Throat J 2020;99(3):167–72. https://doi.org/10.1177/0145561318823391.

37. Chapman MN, Fujita A, Sung EK, et al. Sarcoidosis in the head and neck: An Illustrative review of clinical presentations and imaging findings. Am J Roentgenol 2017;208(1):66–75. https://doi.org/10.2214/AJR.16.16058.

38. Aubart FC, Ouayoun M, Brauner M, et al. Sinonasal involvement in sarcoidosis: a case-control study of 20 patients. Medicine 2006;85(6):365–71. https://doi.org/10.1097/01.md.0000236955.79966.07.

39. Kirsten AM, Watz H, Kirsten D. Sarcoidosis with involvement of the paranasal sinuses - a retrospective analysis of 12 biopsy-proven cases. BMC Pulm Med 2013;13(1):59.

40. Fujita A, Sakai O, Chapman MN, et al. IgG4-related disease of the head and neck: CT and MR imaging manifestations. Radiographics 2012;32(7):1945–58. https://doi.org/10.1148/rg.327125032.

41. Thompson A, White A. Imaging of IgG4-related disease of the head and neck. Clin Radiol 2018;73: 106–20.

42. Song BH, Baiyee D, Liang J. A Rare and Emerging Entity: Sinonasal IgG4–related Sclerosing Disease. Allergy Rhinol 2015;6(3). https://doi.org/10.2500/ar.2015.6.0136. ar.2015.6.0136.

43. Inoue A, Wada K, Matsuura K, et al. IgG4-related disease in the sinonasal cavity accompanied by intranasal structure loss. Auris Nasus Larynx 2016; 43(1):100–4. https://doi.org/10.1016/j.anl.2015.05.005.

44. Kohanski MA, Reh DD. Chapter 11: Granulomatous diseases and chronic sinusitis. Am J Rhinol Allergy 2013;27(Suppl 1):S39–41. https://doi.org/10.2500/ajra.2013.27.3895.

45. Lohrmann C, Uhl M, Warnatz K, et al. Sinonasal computed tomography in patients with Wegener's granulomatosis. J Comput Assist Tomogr 2006;30(1):122–5. https://doi.org/10.1097/01.rct.0000191134.67674.c6.

46. Benoudiba F, Marsot-Dupuch K, Rabia MH, et al. Sinonasal Wegener's granulomatosis: CT characteristics. Neuroradiology 2003;45(2):95–9. https://doi.org/10.1007/s00234-002-0885-9.

Malignant and Nonmalignant Sinonasal Tumors

Natalya Nagornaya, MD*, Gaurav Saigal, MD, Rita Bhatia, MD

KEYWORDS

- CT • MRI • Sinonasal • Tumors • Classification • Staging

KEY POINTS

- It is vital for surgeons and radiologists to be familiar with imaging findings that raise suspicion of a sinonasal tumor given the nonspecific clinical presentation that mimics inflammatory rhinosinusitis.
- Although there is considerable overlap in the imaging findings of sinonasal tumors, certain diagnostic features on computed tomography (CT) and MRI can help narrow the differential and assist in preoperative diagnosis.
- CT is better in the assessment of the osseous matrix and cortical bone involvement of the skull base.
- MRI is superior for evaluation of the tissue components of the tumor, bone marrow involvement, and extension along skull base foramen and intracranial extension.

INTRODUCTION

The sinonasal tract can be involved by a variety of neoplasms. The authors have adopted a simplified classification of sinonasal neoplasms that divides sinonasal tumors based on benignity versus malignancy and tissue of origin in accordance with the World Health Organization classification scheme (**Table 1**).

CLINICAL PRESENTATION

The diagnosis of sinonasal tumors is often delayed because of nonspecific and subtle symptoms that can be similar to rhinosinusitis, such as purulent nasal discharge, epistaxis, nasal obstruction, headache, and facial pain.[1] Clinical suspicion is the most important factor in the accurate diagnosis of sinonasal malignancy.[1]

The relative age of the patient (>50 years) and the insidious onset of unilateral symptoms or recurrent epistaxis should alert the possibility of neoplasm as a cause of the patient's symptoms. Approximately 40% are discovered at a locally advanced stage with presenting symptoms that include anosmia, epiphora, facial pain and swelling, visual disturbances, exophthalmos, diplopia, trismus, loose teeth, and cranial neuropathy. Shooting neuropathic pain along the distribution of the trigeminal nerve is typical of perineural spread. Orbital involvement at presentation is typically associated with worse prognosis.[1,2]

IMAGING

Computed tomography (CT) and magnetic resonance imaging (MRI) are complementary in the assessment of tumor size, morphology, invasion, and disease extent. CT is superior for evaluation of anatomic details, presence and type of calcifications and matrix of the tumor, and pattern of bone invasion, provides a bony map for surgery, and may help define the origin of the tumor.[3]

MRI provides better contrast resolution and characterization of the soft tissue components of sinonasal tumors, evaluation of multicompartmental extension, detection of bone marrow infiltration, perineural spread, and intracranial extension. CT

Department of Radiology, University of Miami Miller School of Medicine, Jackson Memorial Hospital, 1611 NW12th Avenue, WW- 279, Miami, FL 33136, USA
* Corresponding author.
E-mail address: nnagornaya@med.miami.edu

Oral Maxillofacial Surg Clin N Am 35 (2023) 377–398
https://doi.org/10.1016/j.coms.2023.03.002
1042-3699/23/© 2023 Elsevier Inc. All rights reserved.

Table 1
Simplified classification of sinonasal neoplasms

Benign Tumors	Malignant Tumors

1. Sinonasal papillomas
  a. Inverted type
  b. Oncocytic type
  c. Exophytic type
	1. Epithelial tumors
	  a. Keratinizing and nonkeratinizing SCC
	  b. NUT carcinoma
	  c. SWI/SNF deficient sinonasal carcinoma
	  d. Sinonasal lymphoepithelial carcinoma
	  e. SNUC
	  f. HPV-related multi-phenotypic sinonasal carcinoma

2. Respiratory epithelial lesions
  a. Respiratory epithelial adenomatoid hamartoma
  b. Seromucinous hamartoma
	2. Adenocarcinoma
	  a. Intestinal type
	  b. Nonintestinal sinonasal adenocarcinoma/renal cell carcinoma

3. Salivary gland tumors
  a. Pleomorphic adenoma
	3. Salivary gland neoplasm
	  a. Adenoid cystic carcinoma

4. Benign soft tissue tumors
  a. Leiomyoma
  b. Schwannoma
  c. Neurofibroma
  d. Hemangioma
  e. Angiofibroma (JNA)
	4. Hematolymphoid neoplasms/lymphoproliferative
	  a. Sinonasal lymphoma
	  b. Plasmacytoma

5. Fibro-osseous lesions
  a. Ossifying Fibroma
  b. Osteoma
  c. Fibrous dysplasia
	5. Vascular tumors with low malignant potential
	  a. Hemangiopericytoma

6. Other tumors
  a. Meningioma
  b. Sinonasal ameloblastoma
	6. Mesenchymal tumors/sarcomas
	  a. Rhabdomyosarcoma
	  b. Biphenotypic sinonasal sarcoma
	  c. Chondrosarcoma
	  d. Osteosarcoma

	7. Neuroectodermal malignancies
	  a. Olfactory neuroblastoma/ Esthesioneuroblastoma
	  b. Mucosal melanoma

Abbreviation: SWI/SNF, switch/sucrose nonfermenting.

angiography or magnetic resonance angiography can be used to determine the relationship of the tumor to the intracranial course of the internal carotid artery and its branches and feeding vessels for hypervascular tumor.[2]

PET/CT is a useful tool in the detection of nodal disease and distant metastatic spread in the setting of aggressive malignancies, evaluation of response to therapy, and detection of residual or recurrent tumor. More recently, 68-Ga DOTATATE PET/CT plays an important role in the evaluation and management of the rare somatostatin receptor expression sinonasal neuroendocrine tumors.[4]

BENIGN NEOPLASMS
Sinonasal Papilloma

Sinonasal papillomas are benign sinonasal tumors also known as Schneiderian papillomas, as they arise from the Schneiderian epithelium of the nasal cavity and the paranasal sinuses.[5,6] These account for approximately 2.5% of all sinonasal tumors and are histologically subdivided into 3 subtypes: inverted, oncocytic, and exophytic types.[7] Of these, inverted papilloma (IP) is the most frequent type, seen 2.5 to 3 times more frequently in men compared with women and commonly occurring in the fifth and sixth decades of life.[7] The inverted and oncocytic types usually arise from the lateral wall of the nasal cavity, whereas the exophytic type arises from the lower anterior nasal septum. The inverted and oncocytic types have a high incidence of recurrence with up to a 15% risk of malignant transformation to squamous cell carcinoma (SCC).[8,9]

It is difficult to differentiate the 3 subtypes from each other on imaging; however, IP, the most common type, has a characteristic imaging appearance, which suggests the histologic subtype. On CT, IP is seen as a lobulated soft tissue mass centered along the lateral nasal wall and middle meatus. A cone-shaped focus of hyperostosis is often seen and points to the origin of the lesion (**Fig. 1**A).[10] Identification of this hyperostotic stalk is helpful in localizing and determining the extent of tumor during surgery, complete resection of which is necessary to prevent local recurrences. Intralesional calcifications are frequently seen. On MRI, a "convoluted cerebriform pattern" (CCP), seen as alternating lines of high and low signal intensity on T2 and postcontrast T1-weighted images, resembling cerebral gyri has been described (**Fig. 1**B, C).[11] A focal loss of this CCP, necrosis within the mass, bone destruction, or

extrasinonasal extension, is suggestive of malignant transformation to SCC (**Fig. 1**D–F).[10,12]

Respiratory Epithelial Adenomatoid Hamartoma

Respiratory epithelial adenomatoid hamartoma (REAH) is a benign, polypoidal mass of submucosal glandular proliferation, most commonly found in the anterior half of the olfactory cleft or the posterior nasal septum/posterior nasal cavity.[13] The median age of presentation is the sixth decade, and the tumor is 7 times more commonly seen in men compared with women.[14] It is usually seen as an isolated lesion; however, concomitant association with sinonasal polyposis has also been reported.[7]

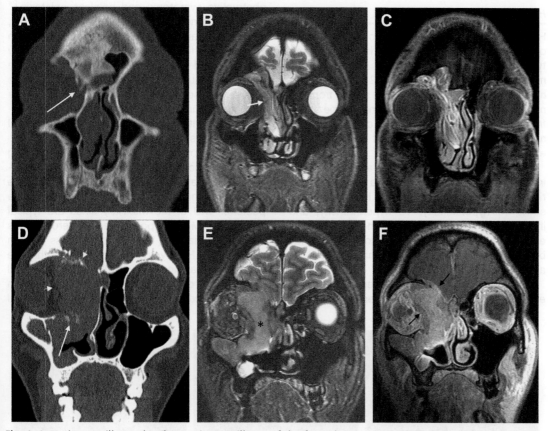

Fig. 1. Inverting papilloma. (*A–C*) Inverting papilloma of the frontal sinus. Coronal CT shows soft tissue density lesion in the right frontal sinus and nasal cavity with localized hyperostosis of the medial wall of the right frontal sinus (*arrow*), which is the origin of the IP (*A*). Classic convoluted "cerebriform pattern" is seen in the mass involving the frontal and ethmoid sinus and nasal cavity in both the T2-weighted imaging (*B*) (*arrow*) and the postgadolinium T1-weighted imaging (*C*). (*D–F*) Inverting papilloma, dedifferentiation into SCC. Expansile lesion with bony destruction on the CT (*D*) (*arrowheads*) and extrasinus tumor extension intracranially and into the orbit (*E, F*) (*arrows*) together with the loss of the normal CCP on the T2-weighted image (*E*) (*asterisk*) and heterogenous enhancement on the T1-weighted image (*F*) indicates malignant transformation. Inspissated postobstructive changes in the remainder of the maxillary sinus. Note cone-shaped hyperostosis of the superior wall of the maxillary sinus (*D*) (*arrow*) indicating the origin of the preexisting inverting papilloma.

Very often incidentally found, the lesion is seen as a homogeneously enhancing, well-defined soft tissue mass centered in the olfactory cleft on CT or MRI.[15] REAH is frequently bilateral (40%) and causes widening of the clefts (**Fig. 2**). Involvement of the anterior half of the olfactory cleft with significant widening is useful in differentiating this lesion from sinonasal polyposis. Absence of bone destruction helps differentiate this lesion from olfactory neuroblastoma, which occurs in a similar location.

BENING SOFT TISSUE TUMORS

Benign soft tissue tumors of the sinonasal cavities are rare and include nerve-sheath tumors, hemangioma, angiofibroma, myxoma, leiomyoma, and meningioma.

Hemangioma

Hemangioma is a benign vascular neoplasm occurring in the nasal cavity and is divided into 2 types, capillary and cavernous, based on the microscopic vessel size.[16] Of the 2 types, capillary hemangiomas are more common, arising from the nasal septum, whereas the cavernous type arises from the lateral wall of the nasal cavity.[17] Almost all intraosseous hemangiomas of the facial skeleton are of the cavernous type.

On CT, capillary hemangiomas are well-defined intensely enhancing masses with a hypodense peripheral rim (**Fig. 3**A).[18] On MRI, lesions demonstrate T1 hypointensity, T2 hyperintensity, and intense enhancement with a peripheral rim of nonenhancement (**Fig. 3**B, C). A washout pattern may be seen on dynamic contrast-enhanced study in approximately 75% of cases.[19]

Because of their large size, cavernous intraosseous hemangiomas produce benign-appearing expansion and thinning of adjacent bone structures.[20] CT is the most useful imaging technique for diagnosing an intraosseous cavernous hemangioma, showing a honeycomb appearance (**Fig. 3**D). Cavernous hemangiomas are predominantly hyperintense on T2-weighted images and heterogenous on all other sequences (**Fig. 3**E, F). Unlike capillary hemangiomas, cavernous hemangiomas demonstrate heterogenous enhancement on CT and MRI owing to bleeding and necrosis.[21]

Nasopharyngeal Angiofibroma

Also known as juvenile nasopharyngeal angiofibroma (JNA), nasopharyngeal angiofibroma masses are almost exclusively found in adolescent and young men (mean age, 9–15 years) accounting for approximately 0.5% of head and neck tumors.[22,23] Clinical presentation is with obstructive symptoms and painless epistaxis.[24] They are nonencapsulated, well-circumscribed, highly vascular polypoidal masses made of both vascular and fibrous stromal tissue.[24] When they are large and extensive, symptoms may include proptosis, visual disturbances, and cranial nerve palsies. These tumors usually arise within the sphenopalatine foramen, close to the pterygopalatine fossa with extension into the posterior nasal cavity and nasopharynx.[25]

On CT, a homogeneously and avidly enhancing well-defined soft tissue mass is seen in the posterolateral nasal cavity.[26] Extension and widening of the pterygopalatine fossa with anterior bowing of the posterior wall of the maxillary sinus are typical (**Fig. 4**A). On MRI, a hypointense T1/heterogeneous T2 avidly enhancing hypervascular mass is seen (**Fig. 4**B, C). Flow voids may be seen within the mass secondary to hypervascularity. MRI is useful in delineation of the tumor extent, especially when large and extending into the orbit, paranasal

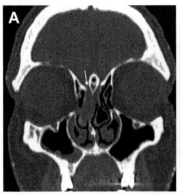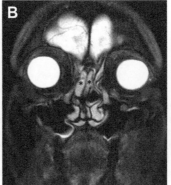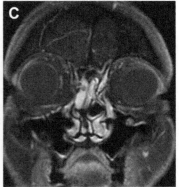

Fig. 2. Sinonasal REAH. Coronal CT shows mass lesions in the olfactory clefts with widening of both olfactory clefts (A) (arrow) and well-delineated hyperintense mass lesions on the coronal T2-weighted image (B) (asterisks) with enhancement on the coronal T1-weighted images with contrast (C).

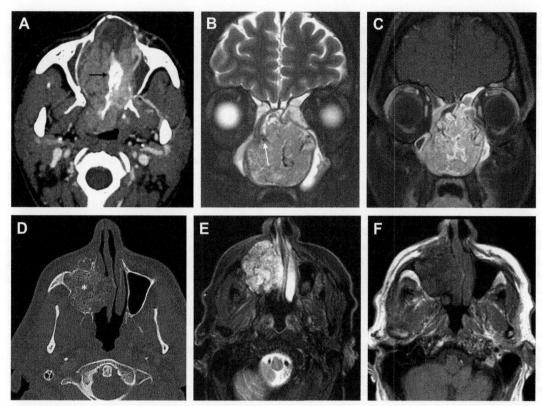

Fig. 3. Hemangioma. (*A–C*) Lobular capillary hemangioma of the nasal cavity. Axial and coronal CT with contrast demonstrates an expansile, lobular heterogeneously enhancing mass lesion with dense central calcifications (*black arrow*) of the nasal cavity (*A*). Prominent flow voids are noted in the lesion on the coronal T2 (*B*) (*white arrow*) and heterogenous enhancement of the lesion postcontrast T1-weighted images with postobstructive changes in the sinuses (*C*). (*D–F*) Intraosseous hemangioma of the maxilla. Axial CT (*D*) demonstrates expansile thinning of the bone with "honeycomb" appearance of the mass in the maxilla (*asterisk*). High T2 signal intensity of the lesion on the axial T2-weighted image (*E*) and heterogenous signal intensity on the T1-weighted image (*F*).

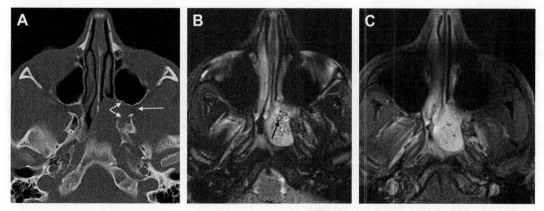

Fig. 4. Juvenile angiofibroma. Axial CT (*A*) demonstrates a polyploid nasal cavity mass, centered within the left sphenopalatine foramen, causing pressure erosion of the pterygoid plates and anterior bowing of the posterior wall of the maxillary sinus (*double arrows*) and widening the pterygopalatine fossa (*A*) (*arrow*). Hyperintense signal intensity of the mass on axial T2-weighted image (*B*) with flow voids (*arrow*) and avid enhancement on postcontrast axial T1-weighted images (*C*) is seen.

sinuses, infratemporal fossa, nasopharynx and intracranially.[25] Angiography is usually performed before surgery for identification and embolization of feeding arterial vasculature to reduce intraoperative blood loss. Arterial supply is most commonly from the internal maxillary and ascending pharyngeal branches of the external carotid artery.[24,27]

FIBRO-OSSEOUS LESIONS

The term "fibro-osseus" refers to a category of benign neoplasms or tumorlike lesions, with ossifying fibroma (OF), osteoma, and fibrous dysplasia being the most common.[28] Osteomas are most common in the frontoethmoid region and appear as well-defined sclerotic lesions (compact bone) with possible trabeculae (cancellous bone) and lucent areas on CT (**Fig. 5**A) and signal void on MR (**Fig. 5**B). Classic fibrous dysplasia typically has an expansile, ground glass appearance on CT with intact cortical bone (**Fig. 5**C), and the pagetoid and cystic variants may demonstrate mixed lucent and sclerotic areas. On MRI, lesions with a high fibrous content show a low to intermediate T1 signal intensity and T2 low signal in mineralized areas and high signal in cystic lesions (**Fig. 5**D). Active lesions markedly enhance.

Ossifying Fibroma

Ossifying fibroma is a rare, expansile benign tumor that arises predominantly from the maxilla or the mandible and is much more common in women aged 20 to 40 years.[29] In rare instances, it may arise in the nasal cavity and paranasal sinuses.[28,30]

On CT, in the early stages, OFs demonstrate a soft tissue density fibrous center surrounded by a thick bony cortex. In later stages, there is progressive filling of the center with mature bone (**Fig. 5**E).[31,32] On MRI, OF is low to intermediate signal on T1-weighted images, hypointense on T2-weighted imaging with the fibrous component demonstrating enhancement (**Fig. 5**F–H).[28] OF has been reported to be associated with aneurysmal bone cysts, in which case, fluid-fluid levels can be seen (see **Fig. 5**F).[33]

OTHER TUMORS
Sinonasal Meningioma

Extracranial meningiomas represent approximately 1% to 2% of all meningiomas.[34] These are seen more commonly as an extension from an intracranial site. Rarely, these can be seen as a primary tumor within the nasal cavity, paranasal sinuses, or the nasopharynx.[35,36] Tumor origin from arachnoid cells present in the nerve or vessel sheath at the exit foramina, or an origin from undifferentiated or multipotent mesenchymal cells have been proposed as possible mechanisms of development of tumor.[35] Histologically, the tumors demonstrate features similar to intracranial meningiomas.[35] Most are grade 1 tumors; however, a few grade 2 and 3 meningiomas have been reported.[37,38] These extracranial tumors are mostly seen in adults around the fifth decade of life, with a few cases described in children.[35,39,40]

CT demonstrates an isodense or hyperdense homogenously and intensely enhancing mass. Underlying calcification may be seen.[41] Adjacent bone erosion or hyperostosis can be seen similar to intracranial meningiomas.[7] MRI features are isointense to hypointense T1 signal, mixed predominantly isointense to hypointense T2 signal, restricted diffusion, and intense homogenous enhancement (**Fig. 6**A–C). Although most of the extracranial meningiomas have similar imaging characteristics as the intracranial type, caution needs to be exerted when interpreting extracranial meningiomas based on signal characteristics on MRI, because different signal intensities between the intracranial and extracranial components can sometimes be present.[42]

Diagnosis is usually straightforward in cases of direct sinonasal extension of intracranial meningioma. In cases of primary sinonasal lesions, typical imaging features of meningioma are helpful in making a diagnosis (**Fig. 6**D–F). However, given the rarity of these lesions, histopathology is often needed for diagnosis.

Sinonasal Ameloblastoma

Ameloblastomas are benign odontogenic tumors with aggressive features, which most commonly arise from the posterior mandible and less frequently (15%) from the maxilla.[43] Rarely, the sinonasal cavity can be a primary site for these tumors.[44] Primary sinonasal ameloblastomas are more frequent in men and present around the sixth decade, occurring later as compared with those in the jaw.[44,45]

On CT, they appear as a solid soft tissue mass occupying the nasal cavity or the paranasal sinuses with bone remodeling or occasionally erosion (**Fig. 7**A). This imaging appearance is different from their counterpart in the jaw where they have a multicystic or "bubble-like" appearance.[46] MRI findings are not pathognomonic, and lesions are usually isointense to muscle and enhance intensely (**Fig. 7**B, C). Primary sinonasal ameloblastoma requires a biopsy for confirmation.[47]

MALIGNANT NEOPLASMS

Sinonasal malignancies are rare, accounting for 3% of head and neck malignancies and 3.6% of

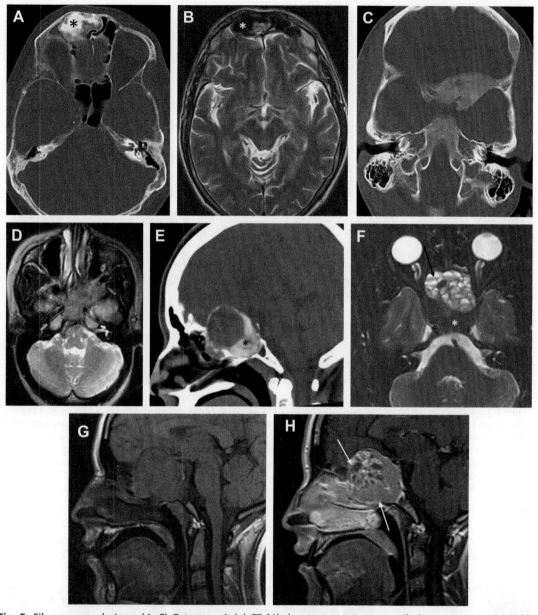

Fig. 5. Fibro-osseous lesions. (*A, B*) Osteoma. Axial CT (*A*) demonstrates an expansile heterogeneous ivory-like lesion with density similar to cortical bone involving the right frontal sinus (*black asterisk*). Axial T2-weighted image (*B*) demonstrates associated low T2 signal intensity that corresponds to the dense sclerotic component of the lesion (*white asterisk*). (*C, D*) Fibrous dysplasia. Axial CT (*C*) on a different patient demonstrates an expansile bony lesion with a ground glass matrix involving the sphenoid bone and the clivus, a typical imaging characteristic of fibrous dysplasia with narrowing of the left optic canal. Axial T2-weighted image (*D*) demonstrates isointense signal intensity of the lesion. (*E–H*) OF and secondary aneurysmal bone cyst (ABC). Noncontrast sagittal CT (*E*) demonstrates a well-circumscribed, expansile cystic lesion remodeling and occupying the sphenoid bone with cortical thinning anteriorly and hyperdensity along the posterior aspect (*black asterisk*). Well-circumscribed lesion with hypointense signal intensity on axial T2-weighted image (*F*) (*white asterisk*) of the posterior fibrous compo-nent and high T2 signal intensity and multiple fluid-fluid levels in the anterior aspect suggestive of ABC (*arrow*). Lesion demonstrates isointensity to low signal intensity on the sagittal T1-weighted image (*G*) and heterogenous enhancement of the cystic component and homogenous enhancement of the fibrous component (*H*) (*arrows*).

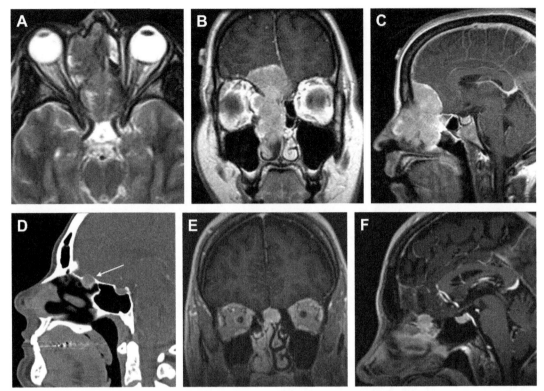

Fig. 6. Sinonasal meningioma. (A–C) Anterior cranial fossa meningioma extending to the sinonasal cavity. Expansile low signal intensity lesion in the right sinonasal cavity on axial T2-weighted image (A). Coronal and sagittal postcontrast T1-weighted images demonstrate homogenous enhancement of the dural-based lesion extending to the nasal cavity and the anterior cranial fossa (B, C). (D–F) Sinonasal meningioma. Sagittal CT with contrast demonstrates a well-circumscribed mildly enhancing lesion in the superior nasal cavity elevating the planum sphenoidale (arrow) (D). Postcontrast coronal (E) and sagittal (F) T1-weighted images show a homogenously enhancing lesion with similar imaging characteristics as intracranial meningioma.

upper aerodigestive tract malignancies.[48] Malignant tumors carry a poor prognosis, despite advances in surgical techniques, radiotherapy, and systemic therapy. Maxillary sinus tumors comprise 20% to 30% of sinonasal malignancies; 20% to 30% arise from the nasal cavity; 10% to 15% from the ethmoid sinuses; and 1% arise from the frontal and sphenoid sinuses.[2] Malignancies of

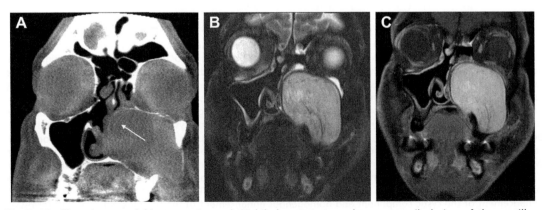

Fig. 7. Maxillary sinus ameloblastoma. Coronal CT (A) demonstrates a large expansile lesion of the maxillary antrum with bony remodeling and medial displacement of the nasal wall (A) (arrow). Well-circumscribed lobulated mass with slightly higher signal intensity to muscle on coronal T2-weighted image (B) and homogenous and intense enhancement on postcontrast coronal T1-weighted image (C) is noted.

the sinonasal cavity represent a heterogeneous group of aggressive tumors with highly variable histology, which include epithelial malignancies, salivary gland tumors, lymphoproliferative neoplasms, neuroectodermal malignancies, and various types of sarcomas.

The majority of malignant neoplasms share nonspecific CT and MRI characteristics and cannot be differentiated based on imaging alone. CT typically demonstrates a heterogeneously enhancing mass with irregular margins, areas of necrosis, and osseous destruction.[49] On MRI, lesions demonstrate variable enhancement with heterogeneous hypointense to mildly hyperintense T2 signal. T1 signal is typically isointense but may demonstrate increased signal owing to the presence of hemorrhage.[49–51] On DWI, most malignant tumors demonstrate significantly lower mean apparent diffusion coefficient (ADC) values compared with benign tumors and inflammatory lesions. ADC values of SCC and undifferentiated carcinomas have been reported to be the lowest among the epithelial sinonasal malignancies but higher than in sarcomas, neuroendocrine cancers, and lymphomas.[52,53] Skull base, intracranial, and orbital extension is common.[50,54] Neurotropic cancers, such as adenoid cystic carcinoma (ACC), SCC, sinonasal undifferentiated carcinomas (SNUC), and lymphoma, have a propensity to perineural spread. On fluorodeoxyglucose (FDG)-PET, lesions are typically FDG-avid, which helps in the accurate staging and evaluation of distant metastatic disease. However, the utility of FDG-PET in differentiation between different types of malignant sinonasal tumors remains low.[49,55]

Despite the significant overlap in imaging features, the diagnosis can be suggested in some cases based on the location (**Table 2**) and specific imaging characteristics of the lesion. In addition to suggesting a specific histologic diagnosis, imaging plays an important role in the mapping of tumor extent, which has important implications in staging and treatment planning and prediction of clinical outcome. Key anatomic sites to evaluate include the cribriform plate, clivus, pterygopalatine fossa, retroantral fat, orbital fissures, palate, nasopharynx, cranial nerves, dura, brain parenchyma, cavernous sinus, and the internal carotid artery.[3] Overall, dural and intracranial extension and orbital apex invasion are the most adverse prognostic factors in malignant sinonasal malignant tumors.[56]

EPITHELIAL MALIGNANCIES

SCC is the most common epithelial malignancy of the nasal cavity and paranasal sinuses and represents approximately 50% to 60% of all sinonasal tumors. SCC is histologically subdivided into keratinizing and nonkeratinizing types.[57] Of these, the nonkeratinizing type is more frequently associated with the human papillomavirus (HPV).[58] The causative role and prognostic significance of this association are not clear but may imply a better prognosis.[57,59] In approximately 15% of the cases, SCC is associated with or arises from a preexisting Schneiderian papilloma.[57,60,61] Sinonasal SCC is more frequently seen in male patients, 55 years or older, and is observed at a slightly younger age in patients with HPV-associated sinonasal SCC (50 years and older).[57] This is in contrast to HPV-associated oropharyngeal SCC, with an average age of presentation of 59 years.[61] The maxillary sinus is the most commonly affected site (**Fig. 8**).[57] Regional metastatic disease can be seen in 15% of patients at the presentation; distant metastases are uncommon.[57,62]

Adenocarcinoma is the second most common primary sinonasal neoplasm, accounting for 10% to 20% of cases.[50,63] These tumors can be further classified as intestinal and nonintestinal types, with various histologic grades.[58] Among these, survival rates appear to correlate with the grade of differentiation, but not the histologic subtypes.[63] Intestinal-type adenocarcinomas have a strong association with occupational dust exposure and more commonly occur in male patients during the sixth decade.[50,63,64] Approximately

Table 2
Sinonasal tumors classified based on location

Maxillary Sinus	Ethmoid Sinus	Nasal Cavity
Squamous cell carcinoma	Adenocarcinoma	Esthesioneuroblastoma
Adenoid cystic carcinoma	SNUC	Melanoma
DLBC lymphoma	NUT	NK-T cell lymphoma
Rhabdomyosarcoma		SNUC
Chondrosarcoma		NUT
Osteosarcoma		

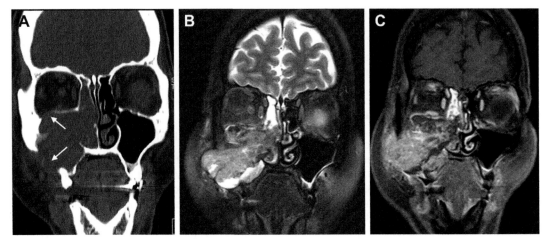

Fig. 8. SCC of the maxillary sinus. Coronal CT without contrast demonstrates an expansile, destructive lesion with erosion of the lateral wall of the maxillary sinus and orbital floor (*A*) (*arrows*). Heterogenous predominantly low T2 signal intensity mass lesion with extension to the nasal cavity, along the orbital floor and infraorbital foramen on coronal T2-weighted image (*B*) and heterogenous enhancement on postcontrast T1-weighted image (*C*) is noted. Postobstructive changes in the right maxillary and ethmoid sinuses are seen.

20% of intestinal-type adenocarcinomas are sporadic and more commonly are seen in women.[58]

Sinonasal adenocarcinomas show a strong predilection to the ethmoid sinus, with less frequent involvement of the nasal cavity and maxillary sinus.[50,63] Skull base invasion is common, more frequently occurring at the level of the cribriform plate (**Fig. 9**).[50,63] These tumors are locally aggressive, typically present at advanced stages, and show a high local recurrence rate, but rarely metastasize.[50,63,64]

ACC is the most common minor salivary gland carcinoma involving the sinonasal cavity. Clinical course is characterized by indolent growth with frequent local recurrences and distant metastases, which can occur many years after the initial presentation.[65–67] It often presents in advanced stages and is known for its high propensity for perineural spread.[66–68] The tumor most commonly arises in the maxillary sinuses.[68] Imaging appearance depends on the histologic grade, with low-grade tumors typically demonstrating homogenous enhancement, high T2 signal intensity, and bone remodeling (**Fig. 10**A–C), whereas high-grade tumors are indistinguishable from other aggressive sinonasal malignancies, showing heterogeneous enhancement with tumor necrosis, low T2 signal intensity, and bone destruction (**Fig. 10**D–F).[69,70]

NUT carcinoma is defined by the mutation of the NUTM1 gene and is considered to be the most undifferentiated type of sinonasal SCC, with a dismal prognosis.[57,58,71,72] The neoplasm occurs in a younger age group with diagnosis between 16 and 30 years and a median survival time of less than 10 months.[71–73] On imaging, tumors are characterized by rapid growth, orbital, and intracranial invasion, with half of the cases demonstrating regional or distant metastases at presentation.[71] On CT, hyperostosis and tumor mineralization have been described (**Fig. 11**A).[71] MRI appearance is nonspecific, similar to other high-grade malignancies (**Fig. 11**B, C).[71,73] Given the high incidence of metastatic disease, PET/CT plays an important role in staging.[71,72]

SNUC is an aggressive carcinoma characterized by a lack of squamous, glandular, or neuroendocrine features.[58] Tumors are typically large and locally destructive, with a predilection for the nasoethmoidal region and a high propensity for skull base, intracranial, and orbital involvement (**Fig. 12**A, B).[74,75] CT demonstrates erosive or expansile bone changes (**Fig. 12**C), with calcifications in up to half of the cases, and may show an aggressive "hair-on-end" type of periosteal reaction (**Fig. 12**D).[75] Among other sinonasal malignancies, SNUC has been reported to demonstrate the highest standardized uptake value (SUV) uptake on FDG-PET (**Fig. 12**E).[55]

HEMATOLYMPHOID/LYMPHOPROLIFERATIVE NEOPLASMS
Sinonasal Lymphoma

Lymphomas are the most common nonepithelial malignancies arising in the sinonasal tract, representing approximately 6% to 13% of all extranodal head and neck lymphomas and 12% to 17% of all sinonasal cancers.[49,76] The most common types of sinonasal lymphomas are natural killer (NK) T-cell lymphoma and diffuse large B-cell (DLBC) lymphoma. Among these, DLBC lymphomas are

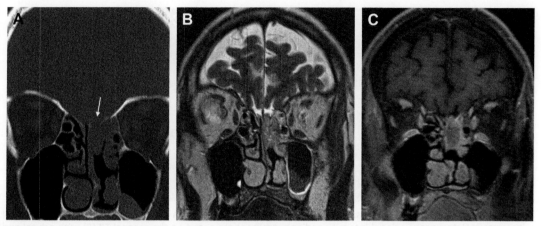

Fig. 9. Sinonasal nonintestinal type adenocarcinoma. Coronal CT (*A*) demonstrates soft tissue mass in the left nasal cavity and ethmoid sinus with erosion of the cribriform plate and fovea ethmoidalis (*arrow*). Heterogenous signal intensity and enhancement are noted on the coronal T2 (*B*) and T1 postcontrast (*C*) images. Postobstructive changes of the ethmoid sinus.

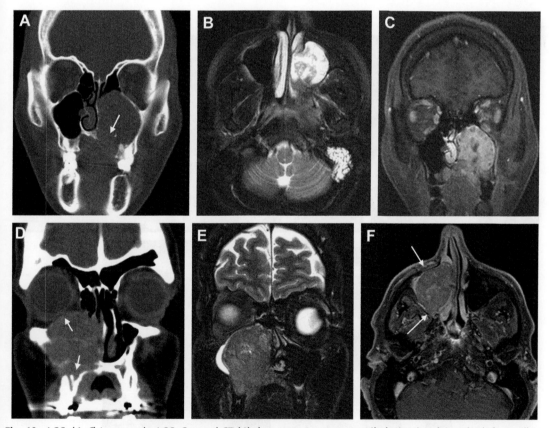

Fig. 10. ACC. (*A–C*) Low-grade ACC. Coronal CT (*A*) demonstrates an expansile lesion involving the left maxillary sinus, nasal cavity, hard and soft palate with bony erosion (*arrow*). High T2 signal intensity of the lesion on the axial T2-weighted image (*B*) and heterogenous enhancement on postcontrast coronal T1-weighted image (*C*). (*D–F*) High-grade ACC. Coronal CT without contrast (*D*) demonstrates an expansile destructive lesion involving the right maxillary sinus and nasal cavity with erosion of the hard palate and orbital floor (*arrows*). Predominantly hypointense T2 signal intensity on the coronal T2-weighted image (*E*) suggests a high-grade tumor. Heterogenous enhancement on the postcontrast T1-weighted image (*F*) and perineural extension to the pterygopalatine fossa and right infraorbital foramen (*arrows*).

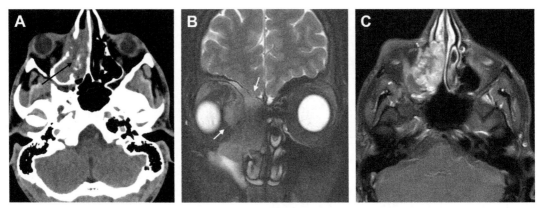

Fig. 11. NUT carcinoma. Noncontrast axial CT (*A*) demonstrates a mass lesion with calcification in the right nasal cavity (*arrow*). Heterogenous signal intensity and enhancement are noted on the coronal T2 (*B*) with orbital and intracranial extension (*arrows*). Postcontrast axial T1-weighted images (*C*) with postobstructive changes in the right maxillary sinus are noted posterior and lateral to the enhancing mass.

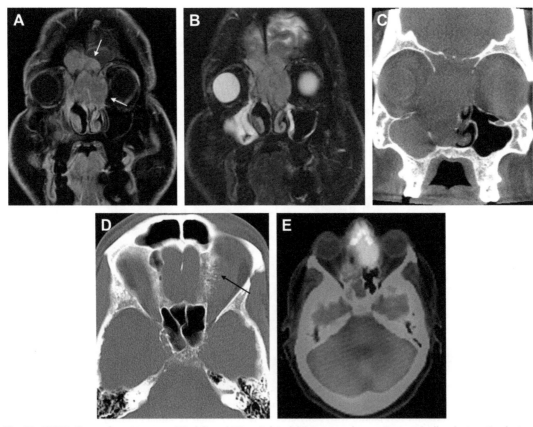

Fig. 12. SNUC. Coronal postcontrast T1- (*A*) and T2-weighted (*B*) images demonstrate a bulky destructive heterogeneously enhancing intermediate T2 signal intensity mass invading the lamina papyracea and cribriform plate with intraorbital and intracranial extension along the anterior cranial fossa (*arrows*). Coronal noncontrast CT (*C*) demonstrates erosive expansile bone changes. Axial noncontrast CT (*D*) in another patient with SNUC demonstrates aggressive "hair-on-end" type of periosteal reaction (*arrow*). FDG-PET demonstrates very high SUV in the lesion (*E*).

the predominant type in the Western hemisphere, typically affecting patients during the sixth and seventh decade.[49,76] NK T-cell lymphomas are common in Asia and strongly associated with Epstein-Barr virus.[76,77] NK T-cell lymphomas present at a younger age than DLBC lymphomas and tend to have a worse prognosis.[76,78]

DLBC lymphomas more commonly involve the paranasal sinuses.[76] On imaging, they typically present as large bulky homogenous lesions, slightly hyperdense on CT, with more bone remodeling than bone destruction (**Fig. 13**A).[49,79] On MRI, lesions demonstrate homogenous intermediate T1 and T2 signal intensity, low ADC values correlating to high tumor cellularity, and homogenous enhancement (**Fig. 13**B–E).[52,75,76,79] ADC values of lymphomas were found to be the lowest among other benign and malignant sinonasal lesions, helping to differentiate them from other malignancies.[49,52] Intracranial and orbital extension occurs in up to two-thirds of cases.[76–78] NK T-cell lymphomas typically present as midfacial destructive lesions with a predilection for involvement of the nasal cavity.[76,77] They typically cause destruction of the nasal septum (**Fig. 13**F) and turbinates. Large lesions may demonstrate tumor necrosis with heterogeneous signal and enhancement (**Fig. 13**G–J). Tumor extension into the hard palate, alveolar ridge, nasopharynx, paranasal sinuses, and subcutaneous soft tissue of the face and buccal space can occur.[77,78]

MESENCHYMAL TUMORS: SARCOMAS

Malignant mesenchymal tumors of sinonasal regions include rare soft tissue and bone sarcomas.

Rhabdomyosarcoma

Rhabdomyosarcoma (RMS) is the most common soft tissue sarcoma in the pediatric population, frequently arising in the sinonasal region. Tumors can also be seen in young adults between 20 and 40 years of age and subdivided based on location into orbital, parameningeal, and non-parameningeal subtypes.[80] Parameningeal subtype carries a worse prognosis and includes tumors arising in the sinonasal cavity, nasopharynx, temporal bone, and skull base.[81] They demonstrate widespread regional and distant nodal metastases as well as distant metastatic disease to the lungs and bones.[82] The prognosis is worse in adults compared with children.[82,83]

Sinonasal RMS commonly arises in the paranasal sinuses, with a tendency for local spread throughout the sinonasal cavity, orbital and intracranial extension. On CT, tumors demonstrate an expansile appearance with bone erosions

(**Fig. 14**A) and inhomogeneous enhancement, hypointense T1 signal, and heterogenous hyperintense T2 signal on MRI (**Fig. 14**B, C)[80,82] On DWI, RMS typically demonstrates low ADC signal (**Fig. 14**D, E).[81,84]

Chondrosarcoma

Chondrosarcoma is a malignant mesenchymal tumor of cartilaginous origin that accounts for less than 2% of all head and neck cancers. Most patients present during the third and fourth decades.[85] There are known associations with bone dysplasias and benign skeletal disorders, including Ollier disease, Maffucci syndrome, and Paget disease.[86] Sinonasal chondrosarcomas are locally aggressive tumors with a high recurrence rate that rarely metastasize.

The maxillary sinus is the most commonly affected site.[85] Chondrosarcomas typically show locally aggressive growth patterns with frequent skull base and orbital extension. Tumors are usually well-defined, lobulated masses with bone erosion or destruction, sharp zone of transition, and absent periosteal reaction.[87] CT demonstrates a characteristic chondroid matrix, with areas of speckled, coarse, or curvilinear "arc and ring calcification" (**Fig. 15**A).[85,88] Peripheral eggshell calcifications can be seen.[87] On MRI, lesions show typical hyperintense T2 signal of the chondroid matrix owing to high water content with underlying low signal intensity septations (**Fig. 15**B) and heterogenous enhancement of the fibrovascular core (**Fig. 15**C, D).[86,88]

Osteosarcoma

Osteosarcoma is a primary malignant bone tumor, which rarely affects the sinonasal tract and accounts for less than 10% of all osteosarcomas and less than 1% of all head and neck malignancies.[89,90] The disease usually presents in the third and fourth decades. Sinonasal osteosarcomas can arise de novo or in association with prior craniofacial radiation.[90,91] Radiation-induced osteosarcomas can develop after a latent period following the initial therapeutic radiation ranging between 5 and 24 years. Other known predisposing factors include preceding bone disorders, such as Paget disease. Distant metastatic disease is uncommon compared with osteosarcomas arising outside of the head and neck.[89,92]

Osteosarcomas most commonly involve the maxillary and ethmoid sinuses.[90] Radiation-induced osteosarcomas tend to arise along the margins of the radiation field and may involve multiple bones.[91] Radiologically, most sinonasal osteosarcomas present as aggressive destructive

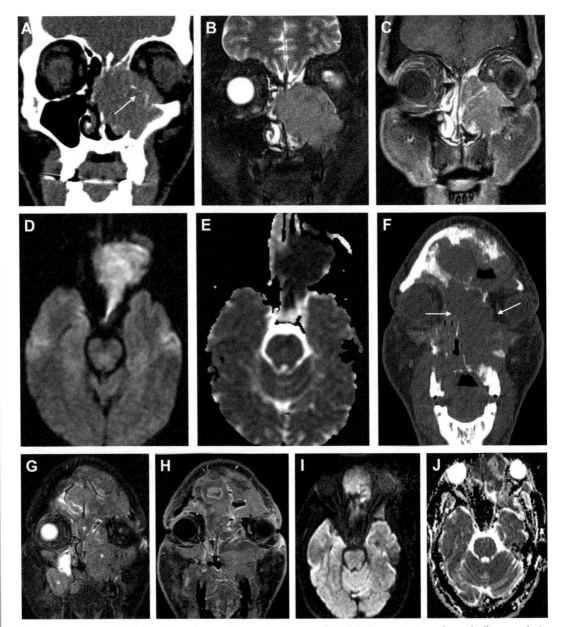

Fig. 13. Lymphoma. (*A–E*) B-cell lymphoma. Noncontrast coronal CT (*A*) demonstrates a large bulky mass lesion within the left maxillary sinus with significant bony destruction with intraorbital extension (*arrow*). Homogenous intermediate signal intensity on coronal T2-weighted image (*B*) and homogenous enhancement on postcontrast coronal T1-weighted image (*C*) is noted. Corresponding diffusion restriction and low ADC are consistent with high tumor cellularity (*D, E*). (*F–J*) T-cell lymphoma. Noncontrast CT (*F*) demonstrates a very large midfacial destructive lesion involving the nasal cavity and paranasal sinuses with extensive bone erosions, soft tissue, and intraorbital extension (*arrows*). Heterogenous signal intensity with enhancement and tumor necrosis on coronal T2 (*G*) (*asterisks*) and postcontrast coronal T1-weighted images (*H*) and corresponding diffusion restriction and low ADC (*I, J*) are seen.

osteolytic lesions, with heterogenous enhancement on MRI, a wide zone of transition, and no periosteal reaction.[91] On CT, tumor matrix is typically with either osteoid or less frequently chondroid-type calcifications (**Fig. 16**). Most cases demonstrate soft tissue extension.

NEUROECTODERMAL MALIGNANCIES

Neuroectodermal tumors of the sinonasal tract include neuroendocrine carcinomas and nonepithelial neuroectodermal neoplasms.[89] They include esthesioneuroblastoma (ENB) and primary mucosal melanoma.

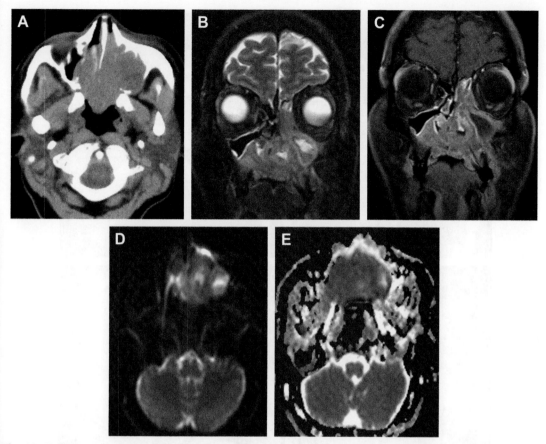

Fig. 14. RMS. Noncontrast axial CT (*A*) demonstrates a large bulky soft tissue mass in the sinonasal cavity with extensive bony erosion and hard palate involvement. Isointensity on the coronal T2-weighted image (*B*) and heterogenous enhancement on the coronal post-contrast T1-weighted image (*C*) are noted. Diffusion images typically demonstrate restricted diffusion with low ADC (*D, E*).

Esthesioneuroblastoma

ENB, also known as olfactory neuroblastoma, is a rare malignant neoplasm of neuroendocrine origin arising from the olfactory neuroepithelium in the olfactory recess of the superior nasal cavity. It accounts for 3% to 6% of all sinonasal malignancies.[58] The disease can be seen at any age, with most patients presenting in the fifth and sixth decades.[93] Patients usually require long-term follow-up owing to the propensity of ENB for delayed locoregional recurrences, including cerebrospinal fluid seeding. Among other sinonasal malignancies, ENBs have a relatively favorable prognosis.[93]

Small tumors typically present as circumscribed intranasal polypoid lesions with an epicenter in a unilateral olfactory recess. They cause asymmetric osseous remodeling and widening of the olfactory recess, with extension to the cribriform plate.[94] Locally advanced tumors can extend throughout the paranasal sinuses and demonstrate skull base, orbital, and brain invasion. On noncontrast CT,

lesions are typically homogeneously isodense to slightly hyperdense, occasionally with tumoral calcifications (**Fig. 17**A).[94–96] CT can help identify remodeling or erosion of the cribriform plate and lamina papyracea. On MRI, most lesions demonstrate intermediate T2 signal and low ADC signal owing to high cellularity, variable enhancement with occasional areas of necrosis and hemorrhage (**Fig. 17**B, C), and, rarely, the presence of flow voids owing to high vascularity.[69,94,96] When intracranial extension is present, characteristic peritumoral cysts can be seen along the intracranial margins of the lesion (**Fig. 17**D).[95] Although uncommon at presentation, cervical nodal metastases and distant metastatic disease can occur (**Fig. 17**E).[97,98]

18-FDG-PET/CT has been routinely used for diagnosis, staging, and evaluation of treatment response and detection of local recurrence.[97,99] Evaluation of local recurrence, however, is often limited by the normal intense 18-FDG uptake of brain tissue. To overcome this, 68Ga-DOTATATE, a somatostatin analogue, is now being more

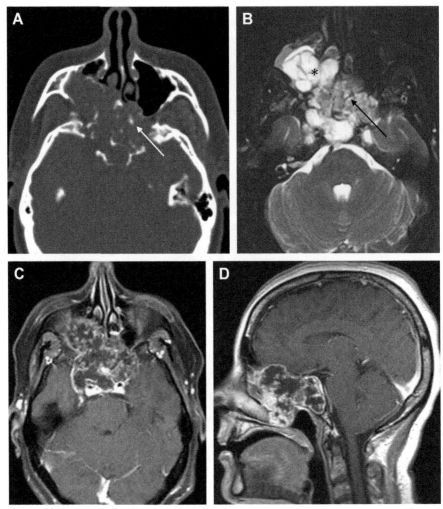

Fig. 15. Chondrosarcoma. Noncontrast axial CT (*A*) shows an expansile, destructive, bulky mass of the sphenoid, right maxillary, and ethmoid sinuses with internal "ringlike" chondroid calcifications (*arrow*). The mass is heterogeneous on T2 with typical areas of high T2 signal corresponding to water content of the chondroid matrix (*asterisk*). Low T2 signal intensity areas are noted on the axial T2-weighted image (*B*) owing to mineralization and septations (*arrow*). Lesion demonstrates heterogeneous curvilinear septal enhancement on the axial and sagittal postcontrast T1-weighted images (*C*, *D*).

increasingly used in the evaluation of local skull base and intracranial recurrences.[100,101]

Sinonasal mucosal melanoma

Primary mucosal melanoma of the sinonasal tract is rare and highly malignant, accounting for 0.6% of all invasive melanomas and 3.5% of all sinonasal malignancies.[102–104] Most patients present in the seventh decade. The melanotic variety is more common.[105] Sinonasal mucosal melanomas tend to be more aggressive than cutaneous and ocular melanomas.[102]

Sinonasal melanoma has a predilection for the nasal cavity, most commonly arising from the nasal septum. Tumors originating in the maxillary and ethmoid sinuses constitute 20% and tend to carry a worse prognosis.[103] CT appearance is typically a soft tissue density lobulated polypoid mass with well-defined margins either remodeling or eroding bone (**Fig. 18**A).[69] On MRI, most tumors enhance and demonstrate heterogeneous hypointense to hyperintense T1 and T2 signal.[105] The presence of melanin is characterized by hyperintense T1 and hypointense T2 signal (**Fig. 18**B, C). Enhancement may be mild and difficult to appreciate owing to intrinsic T1 shortening of the melanin (**Fig. 18**D).[104,106] Rarely, sinonasal melanomas may demonstrate perineural spread, which can occur after a long latent period following the initial diagnosis.[102,107]

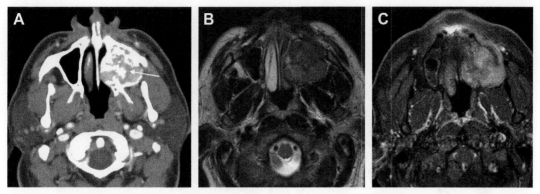

Fig. 16. Osteosarcoma. Axial CT with contrast (*A*) demonstrates an aggressive destructive lesion with heterogenous osteoid matrix within the left maxillary sinus (*arrow*). The mass is predominantly hypointense on the axial T2-weighted image (*B*) with heterogenous enhancement on postcontrast axial T1-weighted image (*C*).

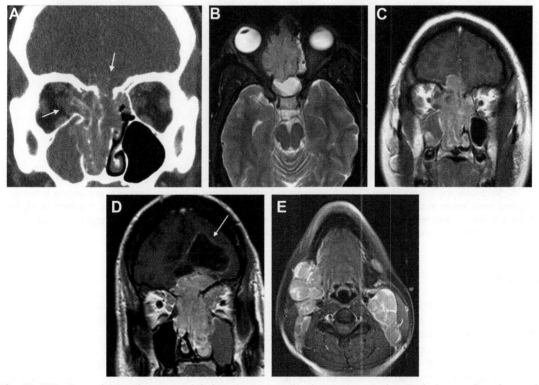

Fig. 17. ENB. Coronal CT with contrast (*A*) shows an expansile, destructive nasal cavity lesion eroding the nasal septum, cribriform plate, and lamina papyracea (*arrows*). The mass involves both nasal cavities and right orbit and demonstrates intermediate signal intensity on the axial T2-weighted image (*B*) and heterogenous enhancement on coronal postcontrast T1-weighted image with characteristic "waist "at the level of the cribriform plate (*C*). In another case, coronal T1-weighted postcontrast image (*D*) demonstrates a heterogeneously enhancing lesion in both nasal cavities with orbital and parenchymal invasion along the anterior cranial fossa and the pathognomonic "peritumoral cysts" along the intracranial margins of the lesion (*arrow*). Extensive and bulky lymphadenopathy is noted in the neck (*E*).

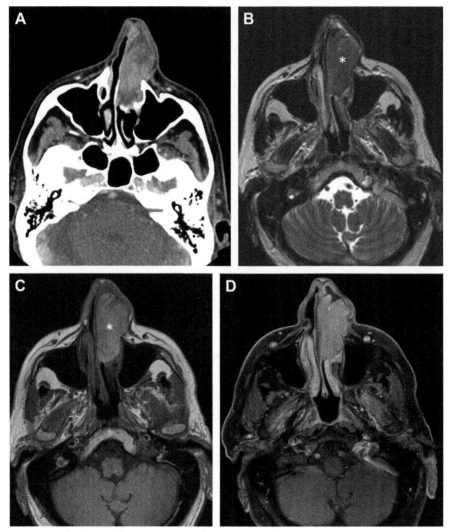

Fig. 18. Sinonasal melanoma. Axial CT with contrast (*A*) demonstrates a heterogeneously enhancing lobulated polyploid mass lesion in the left anterior nasal cavity with bony remodeling. Heterogenous, predominantly iso-intensity to low T2 and high T1 signal intensity owing to melanin on the axial T2- and T1-weighted images (*B, C*) (*asterisks*) with homogenous enhancement on postcontrast axial T1-weighted image (*D*).

SUMMARY

In this article, the authors provide an overview of the imaging features of benign and malignant sinonasal tumors. Although there is a significant imaging overlap among the different pathologic conditions, familiarity with the CT and MRI features can enable the radiologist to provide a realistic differential, identify disease extension, and guide therapeutic strategies for the best outcome.

DISCLOSURES

The authors have nothing to disclose.

REFERENCES

1. Famuyide A, Juliano A, Moonis G. MRI of sinonasal malignancies. Top Magn Reson Imaging 2021; 30(3):139–49.
2. Som PM, brandwein-gensler MS, kassel EE, et al. Tumors and tumor-like conditions of the sinonasal cavities. In: Som PM, Curtin HD, editors. Head and neck imaging. 5th edition. St louis: Elsevier; 2011. p. 253–410.
3. Connor SEJ. The skull base in the evaluation of sinonasal disease: Role of computed tomography and MR imaging. Neuroimaging Clin N Am 2015; 25(4):619–51.
4. Zlochower AB, Steinklein JM. Doing great with DO-TATATE: update on GA-68 DOTATATE positron

emission tomography/computed tomography and magnetic resonance imaging for evaluation of sinonasal tumors. Top Magn Reson Imaging 2021;30(3): 151–8.

5. Batsakis JG, suarez P. Schneiderian papillomas and carcinomas: A review. Adv Anat Pathol 2001; 8(2):53–64.

6. Cheng T-Y, ueng S-H, chen Y-L, et al. Oncocytic Schneiderian papilloma found in a recurrent chronic paranasal sinusitis. Chang gung Med J 2006;29(3):336–41.

7. Tatekawa H, Shimono T, Ohsawa M, et al. Imaging features of benign mass lesions in the nasal cavity and paranasal sinuses according to the 2017 WHO classification. Jpn J Radiol 2018;36(6): 361–81.

8. Nudell J, Chiosea S, Thompson LDR. Carcinoma ex-Schneiderian papilloma (malignant transformation): A clinicopathologic and immunophenotypic study of 20 cases combined with a comprehensive review of the literature. Head Neck Pathol 2014; 8(3):269–86.

9. Eggesbo HB. Imaging of sinonasal tumours. Cancer Imag 2012;12:136–52.

10. Lee DK, Chung SK, Dhong H, et al. Focal hyperostosis on CT of sinonasal inverted papilloma as a predictor of tumor origin. AJNR Am J Neuroradiol 2007;28(4):618–21.

11. Ojiri H, Ujita M, Tada S, et al. Potentially distinctive features of sinonasal inverted papilloma on MR imaging. AJR Am J Roentgenol 2000;175(2):465–8.

12. Jeon TY, Kim H, Chung S, et al. Sinonasal inverted papilloma: Value of convoluted cerebriform pattern on MR imaging. AJNR Am J Neuroradiol 2008; 29(8):1556–60.

13. Wenig BM, Heffner DK. Respiratory epithelial adenomatoid hamartomas of the sinonasal tract and nasopharynx: a clinicopathologic study of 31 cases. Ann Otol Rhinol Laryngol 1995;104(8): 639–45.

14. Lee JT, Garg R, Brunworth J, et al. Sinonasal respiratory epithelial adenomatoid hamartomas: Series of 51 cases and literature review. Am J Rhinol Allergy 2013;27(4):322–8.

15. Hawley KA, Ahmed M, Sindwani R. CT findings of sinonasal respiratory epithelial adenomatoid hamartoma: A closer look at the olfactory clefts. AJNR Am J Neuroradiol 2013;34(5):1086–90.

16. Thompson LDR, bullerdiek J, flucke U, et al. Benign soft tissue tumour. In: El-naggar AK, chan JKC, grandis JR, et al, editors. WHO classification of head and neck tumours. 4th edition. lyon: IARC press; 2017. p. 47–50.

17. Thompson LDR, Fanburg-Smith JC. Update on select benign mesenchymal and meningothelial sinonasal tract lesions. Head Neck Pathol 2016; 10(1):95–108.

18. Lee DG, Lee SK, Chang HW, et al. CT features of lobular capillary hemangioma of the nasal cavity. AJNR Am J Neuroradiol 2010;31(4):749–54.

19. Yang BT, Li SP, Wang YZ, et al. Routine and dynamic MR imaging study of lobular capillary hemangioma of the nasal cavity with comparison to inverting papilloma. AJNR Am J Neuroradiol 2013;34(11):2202–7.

20. Dillon WP, Som PM, Rosenau W. Hemangioma of the nasal vault: MR and CT features. Radiology 1991;180(3):761–5.

21. Kim HJ, Kim JH, Kim JH, et al. Bone erosion caused by sinonasal cavernous hemangioma: CT findings in two patients. AJNR Am J Neuroradiol 1995;16(5):1176–8.

22. Alshaikh NA, Eleftheriadou A. Juvenile nasopharyngeal angiofibroma staging: An overview. Ear Nose Throat J 2015;94(6):E12–22.

23. Lopez F, Triantafyllou A, Snyderman CH, et al. Nasal juvenile angiofibroma: Current perspectives with emphasis on management. Head Neck 2017; 39(5):1033–45.

24. Prasad ML, franchi A, thompson LDR. Soft tissue tumours. In: El-naggar AK, chan JKC, grandis JR, et al, editors. WHO classification of head and neck tumours. 4th edition. lyon: IARC press; 2017. p. 74–5.

25. Szymanska A, Szymanski M, Czekajska-Chehab E, et al. Invasive growth patterns of juvenile nasopharyngeal angiofibroma: Radiological imaging and clinical implications. Acta Radiol 2014;55(6): 725–31.

26. Mishra S, Praveena NM, Panigrahi RG, et al. Imaging in the diagnosis of juvenile nasopharyngeal angiofibroma. J Clin Imaging Sci 2013;3(Suppl 1): 1–7514, 109469. Print 2013.

27. Chawla A, Shenoy J, Chokkappan K, et al. Imaging features of sinonasal inverted papilloma: A pictorial review. Curr Probl Diagn Radiol 2016;45(5): 347–53.

28. Ciniglio Appiani M, Verillaud B, Bresson D, et al. Ossifying fibromas of the paranasal sinuses: Diagnosis and management. Acta Otorhinolaryngol Ital 2015;35(5):355–61.

29. Alawi F. Benign fibro-osseous diseases of the maxillofacial bones. A review and differential diagnosis. Am J Clin Pathol 2002;118(Suppl):S50–70.

30. Choi YC, Jeon EJ, Park YS. Ossifying fibroma arising in the right ethmoid sinus and nasal cavity. Int J Pediatr Otorhinolaryngol 2000;54(2–3): 159–62.

31. Eller R, Sillers M. Common fibro-osseous lesions of the paranasal sinuses. Otolaryngol Clin North Am 2006;39(3):585–600, x.

32. Engelbrecht V, Preis S, Hassler W, et al. CT and MRI of congenital sinonasal ossifying fibroma. Neuroradiology 1999;41(7):526–9.

33. Kendi ATK, Kara S, Altinok D, et al. Sinonasal ossifying fibroma with fluid-fluid levels on MR images. AJNR Am J Neuroradiol 2003;24(8):1639–41.

34. Farr HW, Gray GFJ, Vrana M, et al. Extracranial meningioma. J Surg Oncol 1973;5(5):411–20.

35. Thompson LD, Gyure KA. Extracranial sinonasal tract meningiomas: A clinicopathologic study of 30 cases with a review of the literature. Am J Surg Pathol 2000;24(5):640–50.

36. Ro JY, bel LD, nicolai P, et al. Meningioma. In: El-naggar AK, chan JKC, grandis JR, et al, editors. WHO classification of head and neck tumours. 4th edition. lyon: IARC press; 2017. p. 50–1.

37. Perry A. 13 - Meningiomas, In: Perry A, Brat DJ, editors. Practical Surgical Neuropathology: A Diagnostic Approach (Second Edition), Elsevier, 2018, 259-298.

38. Rushing EJ, Bouffard J, McCall S, et al. Primary extracranial meningiomas: An analysis of 146 cases. Head Neck Pathol 2009;3(2):116–30.

39. Mnejja M, Hammami B, Bougacha L, et al. Primary sinonasal meningioma. Eur Ann Otorhinolaryngol Head Neck Dis 2012;129(1):47–50.

40. Petrulionis M, Valeviciene N, Paulauskiene I, et al. Primary extracranial meningioma of the sinonasal tract. Acta Radiol 2005;46(4):415–8.

41. Taori K, Kundaragi NG, Disawal A, et al. Imaging features of extra cranial parapharyngeal space meningioma: Case report. Iran J Radiol 2011;8(3): 176–81.

42. Shimono T, Akai F, Yamamoto A, et al. Different signal intensities between intra- and extracranial components in jugular foramen meningioma: An enigma. AJNR Am J Neuroradiol 2005;26(5): 1122–7.

43. Giraddi GB, Arora K, Saifi AM. Ameloblastoma: A retrospective analysis of 31 cases. Journal of Oral Biology and Craniofacial Research 2017;7(3): 206–11. https://doi.org/10.1016/j.jobcr.2017.08. 007. Available at: https://www.sciencedirect.com/ science/article/pii/S2212426817301069.

44. Schafer DR, Thompson LD, Smith BC, et al. Primary ameloblastoma of the sinonasal tract: A clinicopathologic study of 24 cases. Cancer 1998; 82(4):667–74.

45. El-Naggar AK, Chan JKC, Takata T, et al. The fourth edition of the head and neck World Health Organization blue book: Editors' perspectives. Hum Pathol 2017;66:10–2.

46. WeissmJ L, Snyderman CH, Yousem SA, et al. Ameloblastoma of the maxilla: CT and MR appearance. AJNR Am J Neuroradiol 1993; 14(1):223–6.

47. Tranchina MG, Amico P, Galia A, et al. Ameloblastoma of the sinonasal tract: Report of a case with clinicopathologic considerations. Case Rep Pathol 2012;2012:218156.

48. Surveillance, epidemiology, and end results (SEER) program (www.seer.cancer.gov) SEER*Stat database: Incidence - SEER 9 regs research data, Nov 2017 sub (1973-2015) - linked to county attributes - total U.S., 1969-2016 counties, national cancer institute, DCCPS, surveillance research program, released April 2018, based on the November 2017 submission.

49. Kim S, Mun S, Kim H, et al. Differential diagnosis of sinonasal lymphoma and squamous cell carcinoma on CT, MRI, and PET/CT. Otolaryngol Head Neck Surg 2018;159(3):494–500.

50. Sklar EML, Pizarro JA. Sinonasal intestinal-type adenocarcinoma involvement of the paranasal sinuses. AJNR Am J Neuroradiol 2003;24(6):1152–5.

51. Gomaa MA, Hammad MS, Abdelmoghny A, et al. Magnetic resonance imaging versus computed tomography and different imaging modalities in evaluation of sinonasal neoplasms diagnosed by histopathology. Clin Med Insights Ear, Nose Throat 2013;6:9–15.

52. Sasaki M, Eida S, Sumi M, et al. Apparent diffusion coefficient mapping for sinonasal diseases: Differentiation of benign and malignant lesions. AJNR Am J Neuroradiol 2011;32(6):1100–6.

53. Razek AAKA, Sieza S, Maha B. Assessment of nasal and paranasal sinus masses by diffusion-weighted MR imaging. J Neuroradiol 2009;36(4): 206–11.

54. Raghavan P, Phillips CD. Magnetic resonance imaging of sinonasal malignancies. Top Magn Reson Imaging 2007;18(4):259–67.

55. Felix-Ravelo M, Bey A, Arous F, et al. Relationship between (18)FDG-PET and different types of sinonasal malignancies. Acta Otolaryngol 2017; 137(2):191–5.

56. Lopez F, Shah JP, Beitler JJ, et al. The selective role of open and endoscopic approaches for sinonasal malignant tumours. Adv Ther 2022;39(6):2379–97.

57. Ferrari M, Taboni S, Carobbio ALC, et al. Sinonasal squamous cell carcinoma, a narrative reappraisal of the current evidence. Cancers 2021;13(11):2835.

58. Thompson LDR, Bishop JA. Update from the 5th edition of the World Health Organization classification of head and neck tumors: Nasal cavity, paranasal sinuses and skull base. Head Neck Pathol 2022;16(1):1–18.

59. Cohen E, Coviello C, Menaker S, et al. P16 and human papillomavirus in sinonasal squamous cell carcinoma. Head Neck 2020;42(8):2021–9.

60. Ferrari M, Migliorati S, Tomasoni M, et al. Sinonasal cancer encroaching the orbit: Ablation or preservation? Oral Oncol 2021;114:105185.

61. Lechner M, Liu J, Masterson L, et al. HPV-associated oropharyngeal cancer: Epidemiology, molecular biology and clinical management. Nat Rev Clin Oncol 2022;19(5):306–27.

62. Ozturk K, Gawande R, Gencturk M, et al. Imaging features of sinonasal tumors on positron emission tomography and magnetic resonance imaging including diffusion weighted imaging: A pictorial review. Clin Imaging 2018;51:217–28.

63. Veloso-Teles R, Ribeiro I, Castro-Silva J, et al. Adenocarcinomas of the sinonasal tract: A case series from an oncology centre in northern Portugal. Eur Arch Oto-Rhino-Laryngol 2015;272(8):1913–21.

64. Huber GF, Gengler C, Walter C, et al. Adenocarcinoma of the nasal cavity and paranasal sinuses: Single-institution review of diagnosis, histology, and outcome. J Otolaryngol Head Neck Surg 2011;40(1):34–9.

65. Hopf-Jensen S, Buchalla R, Rubarth O, et al. Unusual spinal metastases from an adenoid cystic carcinoma of the maxillary sinus. J Clin Neurosci 2012;19(5):772–4.

66. Trope M, Triantafillou V, Kohanski MA, et al. Adenoid cystic carcinoma of the sinonasal tract: A review of the national cancer database. Int Forum Allergy Rhinol 2019;9(4):427–34.

67. Lupinetti AD, Roberts DB, Williams MD, et al. Sinonasal adenoid cystic carcinoma: The M. D. Anderson cancer center experience. Cancer 2007; 110(12):2726–31.

68. Michel G, Joubert M, Delemazure AS, et al. Adenoid cystic carcinoma of the paranasal sinuses: Retrospective series and review of the literature. Eur Ann Otorhinolaryngol Head Neck Dis 2013;130(5):257–62.

69. McCollister KB, Hopper BD, Michel MA. Sinonasal neoplasms: Update on classification, imaging features, and management. Appl Radiol 2015;12: 7–15.

70. Kato H, Kanematsu M, Sakurai K, et al. Adenoid cystic carcinoma of the maxillary sinus: CT and MR imaging findings. Jpn J Radiol 2013;31(11):744–9.

71. Dean KE, Shatzkes D, Phillips CD. Imaging review of new and emerging sinonasal tumors and tumor-like entities from the fourth edition of the World Health Organization classification of head and neck tumors. AJNR Am J Neuroradiol 2019;40(4): 584–90.

72. Virarkar M, Saleh M, Ramani NS, et al. Imaging spectrum of NUT carcinomas. Clin Imaging 2020; 67:198–206.

73. Bair RJ, Chick JF, Chauhan NR, et al. Demystifying NUT midline carcinoma: Radiologic and pathologic correlations of an aggressive malignancy. AJR Am J Roentgenol 2014;203(4):W391–9.

74. Vaziri Fard E, Zhang S, Cai Z, et al. Sinonasal undifferentiated carcinoma: Clinicopathological spectrums and diagnosis reappraisal. Hum Pathol 2019;89:62–70.

75. Shatzkes DR, Ginsberg LE, Wong M, et al. Imaging appearance of SMARCB1 (INI1)-deficient sinonasal carcinoma: A newly described sinonasal malignancy. AJNR Am J Neuroradiol 2016;37(10): 1925–9.

76. Chen Y, Wang X, Li L, et al. Differential diagnosis of sinonasal extranodal NK/T cell lymphoma and diffuse large B cell lymphoma on MRI. Neuroradiology 2020;62(9):1149–55.

77. King AD, Lei KI, Ahuja AT, et al. MR imaging of nasal T-cell/natural killer cell lymphoma. AJR Am J Roentgenol 2000;174(1):209–11.

78. Ooi GC, Chim CS, Liang R, et al. Nasal T-cell/natural killer cell lymphoma: CT and MR imaging features of a new clinicopathologic entity. AJR Am J Roentgenol 2000;174(4):1141–5.

79. Maitra M, Singh MK. A comparative study on clinico-radiological differentiation of sino-nasal squamous cell carcinoma (SCC) and sino-nasal non-Hodgkins lymphoma (NHL). Indian J Otolaryngol Head Neck Surg 2022;74(2):142–5.

80. Zeng J, Liu L, Li J, et al. MRI features of different types of sinonasan rhabdomyosarcomas: A series of eleven cases. Dentomaxillofac Radiol 2021; 50(8):20210030.

81. Glosli H, Bisogno G, Kelsey A, et al. Non-parameningeal head and neck rhabdomyosarcoma in children, adolescents, and young adults: Experience of the European paediatric soft tissue sarcoma study group (EpSSG) - RMS2005 study. Eur J Cancer 2021;151:84–93.

82. Saboo SS, Krajewski KM, Zukotynski K, et al. Imaging features of primary and secondary adult rhabdomyosarcoma. AJR Am J Roentgenol 2012; 199(6):W694–703.

83. Thompson CF, Kim BJ, Lai C, et al. Sinonasal rhabdomyosarcoma: Prognostic factors and treatment outcomes. Int Forum Allergy Rhinol 2013;3(8): 678–83.

84. Wang X, Song L, Chong V, et al. Multiparametric MRI findings of sinonasal rhabdomyosarcoma in adults with comparison to carcinoma. J Magn Reson Imaging 2017;45(4):998–1004.

85. Knott PD, Gannon FH, Thompson LDR. Mesenchymal chondrosarcoma of the sinonasal tract: A clinicopathological study of 13 cases with a review of the literature. Laryngoscope 2003;113(5):783–90.

86. Coca-Pelaz A, Rodrigo JP, Triantafyllou A, et al. Chondrosarcomas of the head and neck. Eur Arch Oto-Rhino-Laryngol 2014;271(10):2601–9.

87. Lee YY, Van Tassel P. Craniofacial chondrosarcomas: Imaging findings in 15 untreated cases. AJNR Am J Neuroradiol 1989;10(1):165–70.

88. Chen CC, Hsu L, Hecht JL, et al. Bimaxillary chondrosarcoma: Clinical, radiologic, and histologic correlation. AJNR Am J Neuroradiol 2002;23(4): 667–70.

89. Krishnamurthy A, Palaniappan R. Osteosarcomas of the head and neck region: A case series with a

review of literature. J Maxillofac Oral Surg 2018; 17(1):38–43.

90. Low CM, Gruszczynski NR, Moore EJ, et al. Sinonasal osteosarcoma: Report of 14 new cases and systematic review of the literature. J Neurol Surg B Skull Base 2021;82(Suppl 3):e138–47.

91. Lee YY, Van Tassel P, Nauert C, et al. Craniofacial osteosarcomas: Plain film, CT, and MR findings in 46 cases. AJR Am J Roentgenol 1988;150(6): 1397–402.

92. Smith RB, Apostolakis LW, Karnell LH, et al. National cancer data base report on osteosarcoma of the head and neck. Cancer 2003;98(8):1670–80.

93. Ow TJ, Bell D, Kupferman ME, et al. Esthesioneuroblastoma. *Neurosurg Clin N Am.* 2013;24(1): 51–65.

94. Peckham ME, Wiggins RH3, Orlandi RR, et al. Intranasal esthesioneuroblastoma: CT patterns aid in preventing routine nasal polypectomy. AJNR Am J Neuroradiol 2018;39(2):344–9.

95. Som PM, Lidov M, Brandwein M, et al. Sinonasal esthesioneuroblastoma with intracranial extension: Marginal tumor cysts as a diagnostic MR finding. AJNR Am J Neuroradiol 1994;15(7):1259–62.

96. Dublin AB, Bobinski M. Imaging characteristics of olfactory neuroblastoma (esthesioneuroblastoma). J Neurol Surg B Skull Base 2016;77(1):1–5.

97. Howell MC, BF4 Branstetter, Snyderman CH. Patterns of regional spread for esthesioneuroblastoma. AJNR Am J Neuroradiol 2011;32(5):929–33.

98. Bak M, Wcin RO. Esthesioneuroblastoma: A contemporary review of diagnosis and management. Hematol Oncol Clin North Am 2012;26(6): 1185–207.

99. Broski SM, Hunt CH, Johnson GB, et al. The added value of 18F-FDG PET/CT for evaluation of patients with esthesioneuroblastoma. J Nucl Med 2012; 53(8):1200–6.

100. Dadgar H, Norouzbeigi N, Ahmadzadehfar H, et al. 68Ga-DOTATATE and 18F-FDG PET/CT for the management of esthesioneuroblastoma of the sphenoclival region. Clin Nucl Med 2020;45(8): e363–4.

101. Roytman M, Tassler AB, Kacker A, et al. 68Ga]-DOTATATE PET/CT and PET/MRI in the diagnosis and management of esthesioneuroblastoma: Illustrative cases. J Neurosurg Case Lessons 2021;1(2): CASE2058.

102. Singh SRK, Malapati SJ, Kumar R, et al. NCDB analysis of melanoma 2004-2015: Epidemiology and outcomes by subtype, sociodemographic factors impacting clinical presentation, and real-world survival benefit of immunotherapy approval. Cancers 2021;13(6):1455.

103. Na'ara S, Mukherjee A, Billan S, et al. Contemporary multidisciplinary management of sinonasal mucosal melanoma. OncoTargets Ther 2020;13: 2289–98.

104. Sen S, Chandra A, Mukhopadhyay S, et al. Sinonasal tumors: Computed tomography and MR imaging features. Neuroimaging Clin N Am 2015; 25(4):595–618.

105. Kim Y, Choi JW, Kim H, et al. Melanoma of the sinonasal tract: Value of a septate pattern on precontrast T1-weighted MR imaging. AJNR Am J Neuroradiol 2018;39(4):762–7.

106. Xu Q, Fu L, Wang Z, et al. Characteristic findings of malignant melanoma in the sinonasal cavity on magnetic resonance imaging. Chin Med J (Engl). 2012;125(20):3687–91.

107. Chang PC, Fischbein NJ, McCalmont TH, et al. Perineural spread of malignant melanoma of the head and neck: Clinical and imaging features. AJNR Am J Neuroradiol 2004;25(1):5–11.

Perineural Spread of Tumor in the Skull Base and Head and Neck

Kuang-Chun Jim Hsieh, MD[a,*], Kwasi Addae-Mensah, MD[a],
Yahia Alrohaibani, MD[b], Ashley Goad, PA-C[c], Kim Learned, MD[d]

KEYWORDS

- Perineural tumor spread • Perineural invasion • Trigeminal nerve • Facial nerve
- Head and neck cancer • Skull base imaging

KEY POINTS

- Perineural tumor spread (PNS) is a well-recognized mode of metastasis in head and neck cancers.
- Adenoid cystic carcinoma of the minor or major salivary glands is most likely to develop PNS; however, squamous cell carcinoma represents more cases overall, as it is more common.
- PNS most commonly affects the trigeminal and facial nerves and their connections.
- MRI is the most sensitive modality for detection of PNS.

INTRODUCTION

Perineural tumor spread (PNS) of head and neck cancer was first described in the 1800s.[1,2] However, it was not until 1963 when Ballantyne and colleagues published 80 cases exhibiting this manner of spread that physicians realized that PNS occurred more often than previously thought.[3]

It is important to distinguish between perineural invasion (PNI) and PNS. PNI is a histologic finding, when tumor cells lie within any of the layers of the nerve sheath or when tumor cells surround more than 33% of the circumference of the nerve.[4] However, PNS describes extension of malignancy beyond the confines of the primary tumor via neural conduits and represents gross, radiologically evident large nerve involvement. PNS is a mode of metastasis rather than a histologic feature.[5]

Of the head and neck tumors that spread via the perineural route, ACC of the minor or major salivary glands has the greatest propensity for PNS with a prevalence of up to 56%.[6] However, given that ACC is rare, representing 1% to 3% of head and neck cancers, cutaneous and mucosal squamous cell carcinomas are responsible for the highest number of PNS cases even though they have a relatively lower propensity for neural involvement.[7] Desmoplastic melanoma is also known to have a propensity to invade nerves.[8] Additional tumors that can develop PNS include mucoepidermoid and basal cell carcinomas, sarcomas, lymphoma, and leukemia.[5,7]

The pathogenesis of PNS remains poorly understood.[9] However, it is known that PNS is a dynamic process involving active crosstalk between tumor and nerve cells.[10] Once a tumor cell interacts with a nerve cell, axonal migration may be a key element of PNS. Axonal growth is a complex process that requires neurotrophic growth factors. The best characterized family of neurotrophic factors, or neurotrophins, is that comprising nerve growth and brain-derived neurotrophic factors NT3 and NT4/5.[4]

[a] Department of Radiology, Baylor College of Medicine, One Baylor Plaza – BCM360, Houston, TX 77030, USA;
[b] Batterjee Medical College, Prince Abdulla AlFiasal St Prince Abdullah Al-Faisal Street, North, Jeddah, Saudi Arabia; [c] Texas Children's Hospital, Department of Surgery, 6621 Fannin Street, Houston, TX 77030, USA; [d] Neuroradiology Department, The University of Texas MD Anderson Cancer Center, 1515 Holcombe Boulevard, Unit 1482, Houston, TX 77030, USA
* Corresponding author.
E-mail address: Kuang-chun.Hsieh@bcm.edu

Oral Maxillofacial Surg Clin N Am 35 (2023) 399–412
https://doi.org/10.1016/j.coms.2023.02.004
1042-3699/23/© 2023 Elsevier Inc. All rights reserved.

Clinical symptoms of PNS include pain, paresthesia, dysesthesias, weakness, and paralysis; however, up to 40% of patients with PNS are asymptomatic.[11–13] Patients presenting with multiple cranial neuropathies may suggest more central involvement such as the cavernous sinus, spread from one cranial nerve (CN) to another, or leptomeningeal disease.[14,15]

Diagnosing the presence of PNS is important as it correlates with decreased disease-free survival, increased risk of tumor recurrence, and higher morbidity and mortality.[7] Williams and colleagues proposed a system of classifying PNS based on MRI into 3 zones: zone 1, peripheral; zone 2, central/skull base; and zone 3, cisternal.[16] Surgery combined with radiotherapy portends the best outcome in zone 1 and zone 2, and surgery should be avoided with zone 3 due to a higher likelihood of treatment failure and tumor spread.[17] Bakst and colleagues recommend adjuvant radiation in the following settings:

- Cutaneous SCC of the head and neck with extensive microscopic or involvement of large-caliber nerves
- Aggressive salivary gland cancers such as ACC or salivary duct carcinoma containing microscopic PNI
- Mucosal SCC with extensive microscopic PNI
- Any primary tumor demonstrating clinical or radiographic PNS[18]

PERTINENT ANATOMY

The trigeminal and facial nerves are most likely to be involved with PNS, with the highest prevalence along the maxillary division of CN V.[12,19,20] The trigeminal nerve originates from 4 nuclei located in the lateral pons including 3 sensory nuclei (principal pontine sensory nucleus, the mesencephalic nucleus, and the spinal trigeminal nucleus) and a single motor nucleus.[7] From the lateral pons CN V emerges as separate rootlets and continues as a main trunk on each side within the prepontine cistern to Meckel's cave.[5,7] Meckel's cave, or the trigeminal cavity, is a cerebrospinal fluid–filled dural pouch posterolateral to the cavernous sinus that houses the trigeminal (gasserian) ganglion along the lateral and anterior wall of Meckel's cave. From here, the nerve divides into the ophthalmic (V1), maxillary (V2), and mandibular (V3) divisions (**Fig. 1**).[5]

V1 travels via the lateral cavernous sinus wall and then through the superior orbital fissure to the orbit.[5] V2 travels through the cavernous sinus and exits the skull base through foramen rotundum.[5] The infraorbital nerve travels from the infraorbital cutaneous surface posteriorly in the infraorbital canal in the orbital floor where it connects with the superior alveolar branches and extends through the retro antral fat pad toward the PPF. The greater and lesser palatine nerves integrate into the infraorbital nerve located within the PPF.[7]

V3 exits the skull base through foramen ovale without entering the cavernous sinus into the masticator space. The main trunk divides into a small anterior division (giving off masseteric, deep temporal, lateral pterygoid motor branches, and buccal nerve sensory branch) and large posterior division. The auriculotemporal nerve (sensory to temporal scalp, secretomotor to parotid gland) arises from 2 roots of proximal posterior division. The posterior division then divides into terminal branches: lingual nerve (sensory to tongue) and inferior alveolar nerve (IAN). The IAN traverses the mandibular canal supplying the mandibular teeth and gingiva giving off the mental nerve, which exits via the mental foramen on the lateral aspect of the mandibular body supplying the skin of the chin and lower lip.[5]

The facial nerve or CN VII arises from the posterior pons. Its fibers loop around the ipsilateral abducens nucleus and create the facial colliculus at the anterior wall of the fourth ventricle.[5,7] The nerve then continues through the lateral pons and exits the brainstem at the lateral pontomedullary junction.[7] The cisternal segment then traverses the cerebellopontine angle cistern and enters the internal auditory canal into the temporal bone and advances through the anterior otic capsule as the labyrinthine segment, through the middle ear cavity as the anterior genu and horizontal tympanic segment, posterior genu, and then the descending mastoid segment inside the mastoid section of the temporal bone. The nerve exits the temporal bone via the stylomastoid foramen into the parotid gland, dividing the parotid gland into the deep and superficial lobes. Within the parotid gland, the nerve splits into 5 branches: temporal, zygomatic, buccal, marginal mandibular, and cervical (see **Fig. 1**).[5,7] These branches split up into various branches to innervate the facial muscles to provide motor function and facial expression.[7]

Various interconnections exist between the facial and trigeminal nerves, which enables tumors to travel between them. An important interconnection involves the greater superficial petrosal (GSP) nerve, which provides parasympathetic innervation from fibers that originate from the nervus intermedius, to the lacrimal gland, palate, nasal cavity, and nasopharynx. The GSP nerve then joins with the deep petrosal nerve to form the vidian nerve, also known as the nerve of the pterygoid canal.

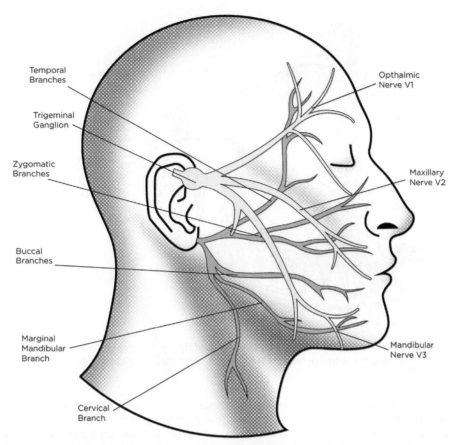

Temporal Branches

Trigeminal Ganglion

Zygomatic Branches

Buccal Branches

Marginal Mandibular Branch

Cervical Branch

Opthalmic Nerve V1

Maxillary Nerve V2

Mandibular Nerve V3

Fig. 1. The trigeminal nerve (*yellow*) divides into the ophthalmic (V1), maxillary (V2), and mandibular (V3) divisions in Meckel cave. Within the parotid gland, the facial nerve (*blue*) splits into 5 branches: temporal, zygomatic, buccal, marginal mandibular, and cervical.

The vidian nerve then travels through the vidian (pterygoid) canal into the pterygopalatine fossa to connect the preganglionic fibers in the pterygopalatine ganglion. Near the PPF assorted postganglionic fibers connect with branches of V2. PNS along the GSP nerve typically occurs after tumor has reached the PPF and can then extend retrograde along the vidian nerve to the GSP nerve (**Fig. 2**). Direct extension of tumor in Meckel cave to the GSP nerve can also occur because of their proximity.[5]

Another important connection between CN V and VII involves the auriculotemporal nerve, which arises as 2 roots from the posterior division of V3 soon after it exits the skull base via foramen ovale. These 2 roots then encircle the middle meningeal artery and merge into a single nerve to pass by the posterior border of the mandibular ramus/condylar head into the parotid gland. Intraparotid secretomotor branches and sensory innervation of the auricle and temporal skin region are provided by this nerve. Within the parotid gland, the auriculotemporal rami crosses with the facial nerve.[5]

PNS has also been described along the sixth CN and greater auricular nerve.[21,22] The greater auricular nerve provides sensory innervation to the skin overlying the parotid gland, mastoid process, and outer ear. It originates from branches of the C2 and C3 spinal nerves (**Figs. 3** and **4**).[5]

IMAGING MODALITIES AND FEATURES

MRI is the most sensitive modality for detecting perineural spread of tumor due to its superior soft tissue contrast resolution. In Nemzek and colleagues, the sensitivity for detecting PNS with 1.5 T MRI was 95%, although sensitivity for identifying the entire extent of involvement was less at 63%.[11] In Hanna and colleagues, the sensitivity and specificity for detecting PNS of ACC at the skull base for MRI were 100% and 85%, respectively, compared with 88% (sensitivity) and 89% (specificity) for computed tomography (CT).[23]

CT is less sensitive than MRI in detecting PNS because it relies on indirect/secondary features such as neural foramen enlargement and erosions

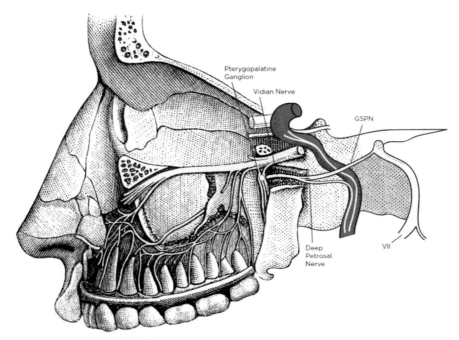

Fig. 2. GSPN anatomy. The GSPN arises from the anterior genu of the facial nerve and travels anteriorly to join the deep petrosal nerve to form the vidian nerve. The vidian nerve connects with V2 branches via the pterygopalatine ganglion in the PPF.

that occur in later disease stages. CT is, however, more sensitive than MRI to detect the neural foramen bony enlargement and erosions.[9] CT is useful to guide biopsy of suspected PNS and helpful as an alternative to MRI if the patient has implants that preclude MRI.[24]

PET/CT can detect PNS; however, it generally has low sensitivity due to lower spatial resolution and partial-volume effects and false-positive results secondary to inflammation and treatment effects.[25] PNS appears as a linear or curvilinear area of F-fluorodeoxyglucose (FDG) uptake along the course of CNs (**Fig. 5**).[26]

There are key features that enable identification of PNS, and they can be separated into 2 major categories: primary or direct findings and secondary or indirect findings. Direct findings describe the features that demonstrate the infiltration of nerve fibers or nerve sheath by tumor such as nerve thickening/enlargement and nerve enhancement. Indirect findings are those that develop after there has been tumor accumulation along a nerve, which then result in neural foramen widening and/or erosion, loss of fat around a nerve, and denervation changes in muscles (**Table 1**).

Nerve Enhancement

Disruption of the blood-nerve barrier by tumor results in increased vascular permeability and

capillary leakage of contrast, resulting in enhancement on imaging.[27] An enhancing nerve can be compared with the contralateral nerve to detect asymmetries, as PNS typically occurs unilaterally. False-positive enhancement can occur for several reasons including asymmetries from patient head positioning and normal enhancement along a nerve due to perineural venous plexus, which may mimic PNS.[13] In these cases, the proximity of a nerve to the primary malignancy should be considered to ascertain if additional features of PNS are present to increase diagnostic confidence. Normal nerve ganglia enhancement such as that of the gasserian (CN V) and geniculate (CN VII) ganglia can be confounded with PNS.[9]

Nerve Thickening/Enlargement and Loss of Fat Around Nerve

The diameter of a nerve enlarges as tumor cells infiltrate and proliferate along the nerve; this enables detection of PNS by comparing the thickness of a nerve versus the contralateral (normal) nerve. Coronal images are particularly helpful for assessing CN V branches. Fat surrounds cranial nerves along much of their extracranial courses and within neural foramina. Increased size of a nerve progressively obliterates the surrounding fat pad, and this serves as another feature of PNS. Both features, nerve enlargement and loss

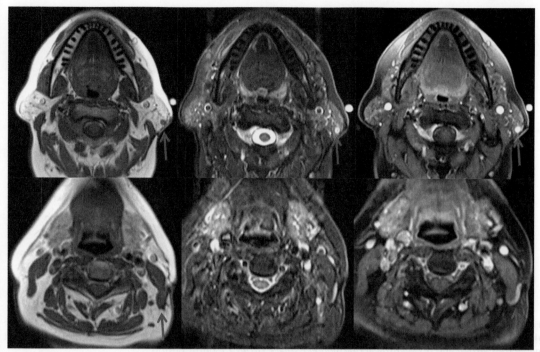

Fig. 3. Skin SCC. Axial T1 and T2 fat-saturated noncontrast and T1 postcontrast fat-saturated images demonstrate thickened, enhancing PNS from superficial parotid along the greater auricular nerve down on surface of sterno-cleidomastoid muscle (SCM) curving along posterior mid-SCM Erb point to cervical plexus (*red arrows*).

of fat around a nerve, can be appreciated well on both CT and MRI (**Figs. 6** and **7**).[9]

Neural Foramen Widening and/or Erosions

Osseous erosions and neural foramen widening are secondary features that result from nerve enlargement from tumor proliferation along a nerve. This finding occurs later in the disease course because its presence requires considerable tumor accumulation and growth. As the tumor accumulates and grows around the nerve, the nerve becomes thickened and the fat planes surrounding the nerve progressively become effaced. Continued tumor growth causes remodeling of surrounding bony foramina, which become eroded and/or widened from the pressure effects. This feature is more easily detected by CT than by

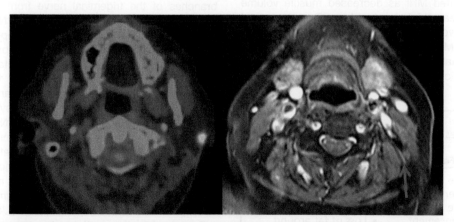

Fig. 4. Skin SCC. Axial T1 postcontrast fat-saturated and PET-CT images demonstrate thickened, enhancing, and FDG-avid PNS from superficial parotid along the greater auricular nerve down on surface of SCM curving along posterior mid-SCM Erb point to cervical plexus (*red arrows*).

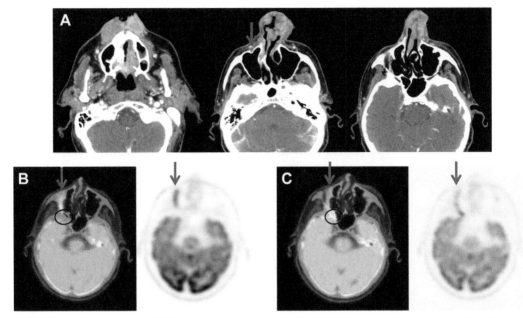

Fig. 5. Axial contrast-enhanced CT images demonstrate (*A*) skin SCC of the upper lip, nose, maxilla with tumor at right infraorbital foramen (*red arrow*). (*B*) PET-CT 3 months postop demonstrating PNS along the infraorbital nerve (*red arrow*) and (*C*) eventually reaching PPF (*black circle*) 7 months postop.

MRI (**Fig. 8**).[13] A principal example of the use of this feature occurs in PNS involving CN VII by evaluating the stylomastoid foramen and mastoid segment of the facial nerve for widening on CT.

Muscle Denervation

Denervation occurs when tumor damages a motor branch of a nerve and results in muscle paresis and eventual atrophy. The signal changes on MRI include hyperintense T2 signal and enhancement in the acute phase (see **Fig. 8**). Features of chronic denervation include atrophy and fatty infiltration of the muscle, which can be identified on T1-weighted MRI as decreased muscle volume and increased fat signal and on CT as decreased muscle volume and fat density throughout the muscle. Muscles that are affected by denervation of the mandibular nerve (V3) include muscles of mastication. There are rare indirect consequences

of PNS related to muscle denervation; for example, V3 denervation of tensor veli palatini can result in ipsilateral middle ear and mastoid effusion due to eustachian tube dysfunction.[24]

Important Checkpoints in Surveying Perineural Tumor Spread Along Cranial Nerves V and VII

The trigeminal and facial nerves are the most commonly involved nerves in PNS. Tumor spread is typically retrograde but anterograde perineural spread can occur.

Tumor typically spreads along the 3 main branches of the trigeminal nerve from sources that are proximal to each respectively. PNS along V1 is typically found in forehead and upper facial cutaneous tumors with spread via the supraorbital and supratrochlear branches of the frontal nerve, the largest branch of V1 (**Figs. 9** and **10**). The orbital roof just above the superior ocular muscle complex should be scrutinized for an asymmetrically thickened and enhancing nerve. PNS along the nasociliary branch of the ophthalmic nerve can also occur (**Fig. 11**).[28] Further retrograde spread via V1 extends through the superior orbital fissure into the intracranial compartment and thus superior orbital fissure should be an important checkpoint for extent of spread (see **Fig. 9**).

Tumor originating in the anterior premaxillary cutaneous surface, sinonasal, and upper pharyngeal mucosal spaces may spread along V2

Table 1 Features of perineural tumor spread	
Direct Features	**Indirect Features**
• Nerve thickening and enlargement • Nerve enhancement	• Neural foramen widening and/or erosions • Loss of fat around nerve • Denervation of muscle

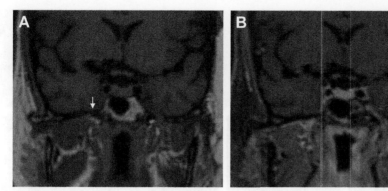

Fig. 6. Left facial basal cell carcinoma status after excision and radiation therapy. (*A*) Coronal T1-weighted and (*B*) coronal T1-weighted fat-saturated images demonstrating normal right foramen ovale (*white arrow*) and contralateral left foramen ovale PNS with nerve thickening and enhancement (*dashed arrows*).

branch such as infraorbital nerve, within the infraorbital canal. Primary oral cavity lesions can spread via V2 branches such as greater and lesser palatine nerves (see **Fig. 5**; **Fig. 12**). A less common route of V2 spread is via the zygomatic nerve, and spread can be noted along the inferior orbital fissure.[29] V2 PNS commonly involves the PPF with subsequent retrograde involvement of foramen rotundum into the cavernous sinus (**Fig. 13**).

Tumor spread along V3 typically occurs in the setting of pharyngeal mucosal, cutaneous, and sinonasal malignancies and can be identified along the IAN and auriculotemporal nerve. The IAN travels through the inferior alveolar canal within the mandible and exits the mandibular bone through the mental foramen. Tumor in the lower face and gingiva frequently involve these branches. The auriculotemporal nerve is an important route of spread for tumors from the side of the head/scalp and parotid gland (see **Fig. 10**; **Fig. 14**). Tumor can spread retrograde along the auriculotemporal and IAN into foramen ovale along the main trunk of V3 (**Fig. 15**). As the 3 trigeminal nerve divisions unite at the gasserian ganglion in Meckel's cave,

it serves as an important checkpoint for assessing intracranial extension of tumor.

The most common causes of PNS along the facial nerve are parotid and cutaneous malignancies arising within the vicinity of main facial nerve trunk and peripheral branches (**Fig. 16**); this can be identified as tumor spread via the main facial nerve segment within the parotid gland, through the stylomastoid foramen, retrograde spread to the geniculate ganglion, and further extension along the facial nerve intracranially. The stylomastoid foramen is an important checkpoint for PNS and should be assessed for abnormal widening on CT or abnormal enhancement within the canal on MRI. Retrograde PNS may reach as far as the GSP nerve.[29]

IMAGING PROTOCOLS AND TECHNIQUES

There are several important considerations when assessing for PNS, and there are techniques that can be used to optimize imaging. The field of view (FOV) should include the entire course of the cranial nerves, from peripheral branches to their respective nuclei, to help identify the full extent of nerve involvement, as this may affect disease prognosis and

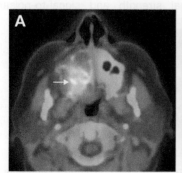
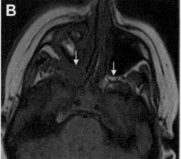
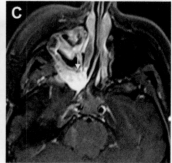

Fig. 7. Right palate ACC. (*A*) Axial FDG-PET demonstrates FDG avid primary tumor. (*B*) Axial unenhanced T1-weighted and (*C*) axial contrast-enhanced T1-weighted fat-saturated images demonstrate normal left PPF (*white arrow*) and PNS in the right PPF with loss of T1 bright fat, expansion, and enhancement (*yellow arrows*).

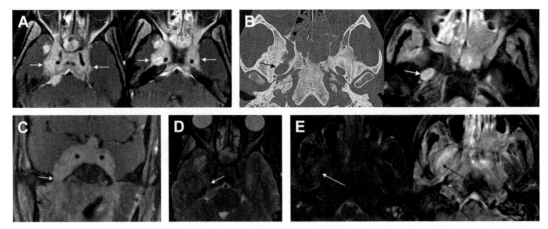

Fig. 8. Nasopharyngeal carcinoma. (*A*) Axial T1 postcontrast image demonstrates bilateral cavernous sinus PNS (*arrows*). (*B*) Axial CT bone kernel and axial T1 postcontrast fat-saturated images demonstrating asymmetric enlargement of right foramen ovale (*arrows*). (*C*) Coronal T1 fat-saturated postcontrast image with right foramen ovale PNS (*arrow*). (*D*) Axial T2 fat-saturated image with right trigeminal nerve PNS (*arrow*). (*E*) Axial T2 and T1 postcontrast fat-saturated images demonstrate T2 hyperintensity and enhancement of right pterygoid muscle denervation (*arrows*).

treatment planning. Another important reason to image the full course of a nerve is because skip lesions can occur in SCC and basal cell carcinoma.[30] As nuclei for CN I and II are in the supratentorium and nuclei for CN III to XII are in the brainstem, imaging must be optimized for each nerve.

Optimizing Techniques for Perineural Tumor Spread Imaging

The anatomy of the skull base foramina is complex with numerous confounding factors when trying to diagnose pathology. A small FOV should be used to increase sensitivity for detection of PNS by increasing spatial and contrast resolution and minimizing scanning of irrelevant anatomy. The largest FOV should be 18 cm,[29] and this should be done for both CT and MRI.

Slice thickness—image slice thickness of 3 mm or less is recommended to enable careful assessment along the course of an affected nerve.[7] Three-dimensional (3D) imaging is another technique in

MRI that enables thin-slice thickness as well as data that can be reformatted into axial, sagittal, and coronal planes to help improve diagnostic confidence.

High-resolution matrix for MRI—another important technique to optimize MRI images is to use high-resolution matrix (320 x 192) to enhance spatial resolution when assessing for PNS.[31]

High-resolution bone algorithm for CT—this technique produces thin-section images with high-spatial-frequency bone reconstruction, superior to the standard algorithm, and produces images with superior spatial resolution and bone detail, which is important to help detect subtle findings such as osseous erosions and remodeling.

MRI

1.5 T versus 3T—1.5 T MRI is usually sufficient to image PNS involving large nerve branches. 3T MRI provides better spatial resolution due to increased signal strength and signal-to-noise

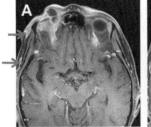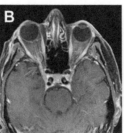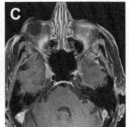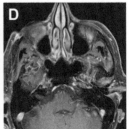

Fig. 9. Supraorbital skin SCC. Axial T1 fat-saturated post-contrast images demonstrate (*A*) PNS along V1 and temporal branch (*blue arrows*) extending retrograde along (*B*) supraorbital fissure (*blue arrow*) and (*C*) and inferior orbital fissure to foramen rotundum and cavernous sinus (*blue arrows*). (*D*) PNS in inferior orbital fissure (*blue arrow*) and GSPN to geniculate ganglion of CN VII (*red arrow*).

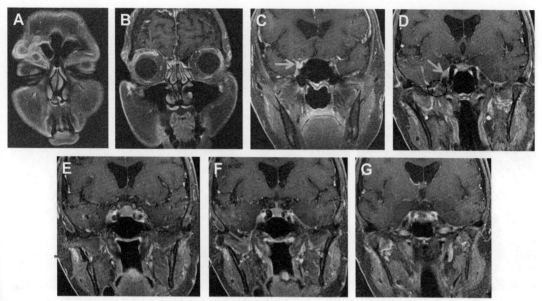

Fig. 10. Supraorbital SCC. Coronal T1 fat-saturated postcontrast images demonstrate (*A*) primary SCC (*blue arrow*) with (*B*) retrograde PNS along V1 (*blue arrow*) (*C*) continuing to orbital apex and superior and inferior orbital fissures (*yellow arrow*) and foramen rotundum (*purple arrow*) to (*D*) cavernous sinus (*green arrow*) and V3 mandibular nerve (*blue arrow*) underneath foramen ovale (*circle*). (*E*) Enhancing tumor is seen at right mandibular foramen (*blue arrow*) and parotid facial nerve (*red arrow*). (*F*) Contrast enhancing PNS right V3 mandibular nerve underneath foramen ovale (*blue arrow*) and facial nerve in parotid (*red arrow*). (*G*) PNS auriculotemporal nerve (*red arrow*), a connection between CN V and VII.

ratio[32] and provides better assessment of PNS of smaller nerve branches.[7] Another benefit of 3T is shorter scan times and thus fewer artifacts from motion. A disadvantage of 3T MRI is that it produces more susceptibility artifacts at air-tissue interfaces, which can make skull base imaging of patients with extensive pneumatization a challenge, and in such cases 1.5 T is recommended.[33]

MRI SEQUENCES
T1 Sequences

- Noncontrast T1: this sequence helps to distinguish T1 "bright" fat within the skull base

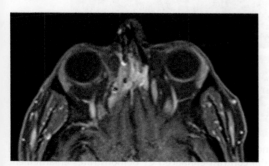

Fig. 11. Axial T1 postcontrast fat-saturated MRI of PNS along the right nasociliary nerve (*red arrow*) in a 53-year-old man with ethmoidal sarcoma. (*Courtesy of* Dinesh Rao, MD, Jacksonville, FL.)

foramina and from the CNs, which have lower signal intensity. A decrease in the amount of fat within a neural foramen or distortion of fat around a nerve suggests tumor involvement (see **Fig. 7**). Chronic muscular denervation can be detected in this sequence by depicting atrophy and fat infiltration of affected muscles.

- Postcontrast T1: the use of gadolinium allows PNS to be more visible, and this sequence is less likely to be degraded by artifacts.[7] In practice, it can be challenging to distinguish enhancing PNS from the surrounding bright fat without fat suppression.
- Postcontrast T1 with fat suppression: this sequence improves contrast resolution between PNS and fat by suppressing the normal bright T1 fat signal rendering it dark. This sequence can pose challenges because chemical-shift fat suppression techniques may be inhomogeneous particularly at areas of air-bone interface and near metallic implants and dental fillings, which can lead to false-positive diagnoses, as such areas can mimic pathologic enhancement.

T2 Sequences

- T2 without and with fat suppression: T2 sequences help identify denervation edema.

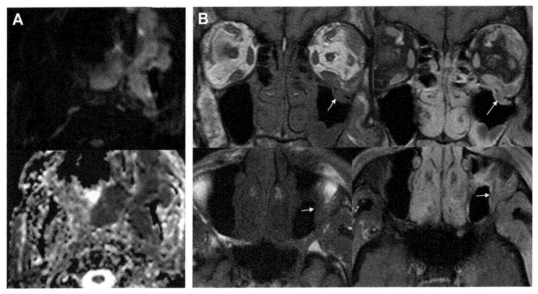

Fig. 12. Patient with human immunodeficiency virus (HIV) and lymphoma. (*A*) Axial diffusion-weighted imaging demonstrates left transpatial mass with restricted diffusion commonly seen with lymphoma. (*B*) Coronal and axial T1 precontrast and postcontrast images demonstrate V2 PNS (*arrows*).

The fat suppression makes neurogenic edema from muscular denervation more conspicuous by rendering the adjacent fat dark.

- Specialized T2 sequences CISS, FIESTA: these high-resolution T2-weighted sequences are useful in evaluating the cisternal segments of cranial nerves, which are surrounded by cerebrospinal fluid.

Short tau inversion recovery sequence can be used in conjunction with or as an alternative to T2 sequence with fat suppression to identify muscle denervation edema, as it provides more uniform fat suppression.[34]

Emerging Imaging Techniques

- 3D magnetic resonance neurography: this technique may provide more detailed assessment of the extracranial and peripheral branches of CNs due to higher image resolution and less artifacts.[24,35]
- CN diffusion tensor imaging tractography: this technique may be useful in depicting cranial

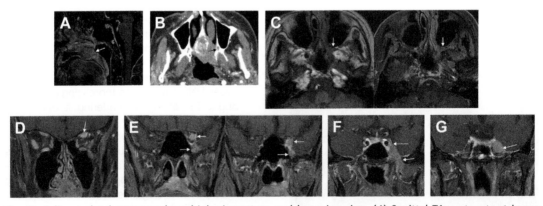

Fig. 13. Salivary gland type neoplasm biphasic pattern and bone invasion. (*A*) Sagittal T1 postcontrast image demonstrates primary mass in hard palate (*arrow*). (*B*) Axial contrast-enhanced CT demonstrates enlargement of the left greater palatine canal (*arrow*). (*C*) Axial T1 precontrast and postcontrast fat-saturated images demonstrate PNS in left PPF (*arrows*). (*D*) Coronal T1 fat-saturated postcontrast images demonstrate antegrade PNS along V1 (*arrow*). (*E*) PNS in superior orbital fissure (*upper arrow*) and foramen rotundum (*inferior arrow*), (*F*) cavernous sinus (*upper arrow*), foramen ovale (*inferior arrow*) and (*G*) Meckel's cave (*arrow*).

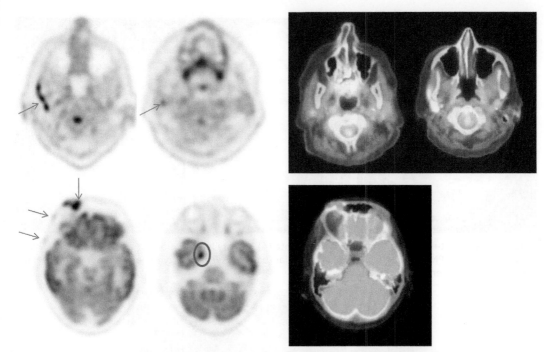

Fig. 14. Axial PET-CT images demonstrating FDG avid primary right supraorbital SCC (*blue arrow*) with retrograde PNS along right facial nerve branches to parotid gland (*blue arrows*) and along auriculotemporal nerve posterior to mandibular ramus/condylar head to V3 and intracranial to cavernous sinus (*blue circle*).

nerve trajectories especially when anatomy is distorted due to tumor.[36]

Imaging Scan Planes

Axial and coronal planes are the most commonly used for assessment of PNS especially for CN V and CN VII.[7] Coronal image reformats are essential for assessing vertical oriented nerves such as the mandibular nerve through foramen ovale and the mastoid segment of the facial nerve (see **Fig. 6**).[37]

DIFFERENTIAL DIAGNOSIS AND PITFALLS

Two main differential diagnostic considerations to PNS include benign nerve tumors and neuritis. Schwannomas and neurofibromas can affect any portion of a cranial nerve and manifest as bulky enlargement mimicking PNS.[7,13] Skull base meningiomas can also mimic PNS, especially those of cavernous sinus or Meckel's cave origin (**Fig. 17**).[13] Neuritis typically manifests as enhancement of the nerve without significant enlargement with various infectious causes including different viruses, fungi (mucormycosis), Lyme disease, poliomyelitis, and syphilis (**Fig. 18**). Other causes include trauma, autoimmune conditions such as sarcoidosis, amyloidosis, or immunoglobulin G disease, and postradiation changes.[7,13,24] Patients who have undergone maxillectomy may have long-term enhancement within the PPF, which can seem similar to PNS.[13] In equivocal cases, short-term (6–8 weeks) imaging follow-up and/or biopsy may be helpful in establishing the correct diagnosis. PNS tends to progress, whereas neuritis

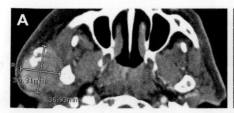
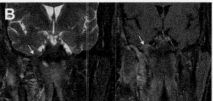

Fig. 15. High-grade salivary duct carcinoma. (*A*) Axial postcontrast CT image demonstrates primary tumor in right parotid gland. (*B*) Coronal T2 and T1 postcontrast fat-saturated images demonstrate right foramen ovale PNS (*arrows*) likely via auriculotemporal nerve given primary tumor location.

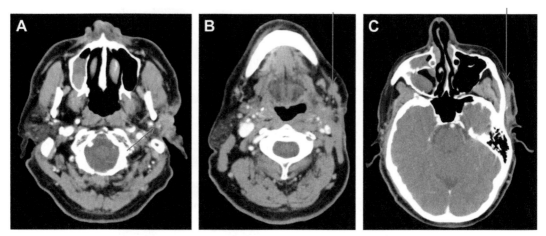

Fig. 16. Axial contrast-enhanced CT images demonstrate (*A*) primary left preauricular and infraauricular skin SCC (*blue arrow*) with (*B*) PNS involving marginal mandibular (*blue arrow*) and (*C*) zygomatic temporal branches (*blue arrow*) of the facial nerve.

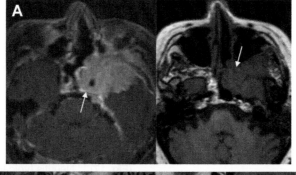

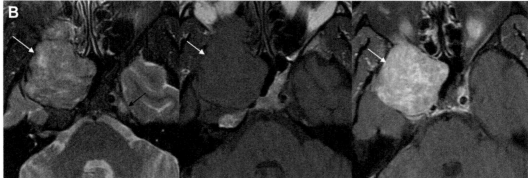

Fig. 17. (*A*) Axial T1 postcontrast fat-saturated and axial T1 noncontrast images demonstrate left skull base meningioma involving left cavernous sinus and PPF (*arrows*). (*B*) Axial T2 fat-saturated and T1 precontrast and postcontrast fat-saturated images demonstrate right trigeminal schwannoma (*white arrows*) and normal left Meckel's cave (*black arrow*).

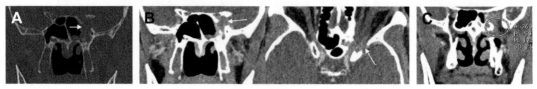

Fig. 18. (*A*) Coronal bone kernel image demonstrates erosion of lateral wall of left sphenoid sinus (*arrow*). (*B*) Coronal and axial contrast-enhanced CT images demonstrate tissue in superior orbital fissure and (*C*) inferior orbital fissure (*circle*). Endoscopic sinonasal surgery and biopsy demonstrated Aspergillus.

improves, and benign tumors are relatively stable overtime/demonstrate slow growth.[7,24]

Another potential pitfall is that the facial nerve typically demonstrates physiologic enhancement within the geniculate ganglion and tympanic segment. Enhancement of the facial nerve within the labyrinthine, mastoid, or canalicular segments is more likely to represent pathologic enhancement.[38] Anatomic variants such as variation of the venous pterygoid plexus can lead to asymmetric enhancement in the infratemporal fossa and parapharyngeal space and can be mistaken for PNS. Noting flow voids on T2-weighted sequence can avoid this pitfall.[7]

SUMMARY

PNS in head and neck cancers must be identified, as it carries important prognostic and therapeutic implications. Understanding the anatomy of the neural pathways of the head and neck, using appropriate imaging protocols and techniques, and scrutinizing important checkpoints can aid in accurately defining tumor extent and staging to offer the patient appropriate therapy and the best possible chance of disease control or cure.

CLINICS CARE POINTS

- Clinical symptoms of PNS include pain, paresthesia, dysesthesia, weakness, or paralysis; however, up to 40% of patients with PNS are asymptomatic.

- Trigeminal and facial nerves and their connections are most commonly involved.

- MRI is the most sensitive modality for detection of PNS, and imaging features include nerve enhancement, nerve thickening/enlargement and loss of fat around the nerve, and muscle denervation. Imaging should include the entire course of the suspected CN with a small FOV, no more than 18 cm, and slice thickness of 3 mm or less. Postcontrast imaging with fat suppression makes it easier to identify PNS by making previously bright fat dark so that enhancing PNS is more visible.

- CT is less sensitive in detecting PNS relying on indirect/secondary features such as neural foramen enlargement and erosions, thus detecting PNS at later stages.

- PET/CT can detect PNS; however, it generally has low sensitivity and appears as linear or curvilinear FDG uptake along the course of the CN.

ACKNOWLEDGMENTS

The author thanks medical illustrator Dominique Garcia for providing the digital illustrations.

REFERENCES

1. Cruveilheri J. Maladies des nerfs anatomie pathologique du corps Humain. 2nd edition. Paria: JB Bailiere; 1835.

2. Neumann E. Secundäre Cancroidinfiltration des Nervus mentalis bei einem Fall von Lippencancroid. Archiv für pathologische Anatomie und Physiologie und für klinische Medizin 1862; 24(102):201–2.

3. Ballantyne AJ, McCarten AB, Ivanez ML. The extension of cancer of the head and neck through peripheral nerves. Am J Surg 1963; 106(4):651–67.

4. Liebig C, Ayala G, Wilks J, et al. Perineural invasion in cancer: a review of the literature. Cancer 2009; 115(15):3379–470.

5. Moonis G, Cunnane MB, Emerick K, et al. Patterns of perineural tumor spread in head and neck cancer Magn Reson Imaging. Clin N Am 2012 Aug;20(3): 435–46.

6. Barrett AW, Speight PM. Perineural invasion in adenoid cystic carcinoma of the salivary glands: a valid prognostic indicator? Oral Oncol 2009 Nov; 45(11):936–40.

7. Kirsch CFE, Schmalfuss IM. Practical Tips for MR Imaging of Perineural Tumor Spread. Magn Reson Imaging Clin N Am 2018 Feb;26(1):85–100.

8. Maroldi R, Farina D, Borghesi A, et al. Perineural tumor spread. Neuroimaging Clin N Am 2008;18(2): 413–29, xi.

9. Stambuk HE. Perineural tumor spread involving the central skull base region. Semin Ultrasound CT MR 2013;34(5):445–58.

10. Marchesi F, Piemonti L, Mantovani A, et al. Molecular mechanisms of perineural invasion, a forgotten pathway of dissemination and metastasis. Cytokine Growth Factor Rev 2010;21(1):77–82.

11. Nemzek WR, Hecht S, Gandour-Edwards R, et al. Perineural spread of head and neck tumors: how accurate is MR imaging? AJNR Am J Neuroradiol 1998;19(4):701–6.

12. Badger D, Aygun N. Imaging of Perineural Spread in Head and Neck Cancer. Radiol Clin North Am 2017; 55(1):139–49.

13. Ginsberg LE. Imaging of perineural tumor spread in head and neck cancer. Semin Ultrasound CT MR 1999;20(3):175–86.

14. Woodruff WW Jr, Yeates AE, McLendon RE. Perineural tumor extension to the cavernous sinus from superficial facial carcinoma: CT manifestations. Radiology 1986;161(2):395–9.

15. Banerjee TK, Gottschalk PG. Unusual manifestations of multiple cranial nerve palsies and mandibular metastasis in a patient with squamous cell carcinoma of the lip. Cancer 1984;53(2):346–8.

16. Williams LS, Mancuso AA, Mendenhall WM. Perineural spread of cutaneous squamous and basal cell carcinoma: CT and MR detection and its impact on patient management and prognosis. Int J Radiat Oncol Biol Phys 2001;49(4):1061–9.

17. Solares CA, Mason E, Panizza BJ. Surgical Management of Perineural Spread of Head and Neck Cancers. J Neurol Surg B Skull Base 2016;77(2):140–9.

18. Bakst RL, Glastonbury CM, Parvathaneni U, et al. Perineural Invasion and Perineural Tumor Spread in Head and Neck Cancer. Int J Radiat Oncol Biol Phys 2019;103(5):1109–24.

19. Johnston M, Yu E, Kim J. Perineural invasion and spread in head and neck cancer. Expert Rev Anticancer Ther 2012;12(3):359–71.

20. Caldemeyer KS, Mathews VP, Righi PD, et al. Imaging features and clinical significance of perineural spread or extension of head and neck tumors. Radiographics 1998;18(1):97–110.

21. Lian K, Barlett E, Yu E. Perineural tumor spread along the sixth cranial nerve: CT and MR imaging. AJNR Am J Neuroradiol 2011;32(9):E178.

22. Ginsberg L, Eicher S. Great auricular nerve: anatomy and imaging in a case of perineural tumor spread. ANJR Am J Neuroradiol 2000;21(3):58–639.

23. Hanna E, Vural E, Prokopakis E, et al. The sensitivity and specificity of high-resolution imaging in evaluating perineural spread of adenoid cystic carcinoma to the skull base. Arch Otolaryngol Head Neck Surg 2007;133(6):541–5.

24. Medvedev O, Hedesiu M, Ciurea A, et al. Perineural spread in head and neck malignancies: imaging findings - an updated literature review. Bosn J Basic Med Sci 2022;22(1):22–38.

25. Lee H, Lazor JW, Assadsangabi R, et al. An Imager's Guide to Perineural Tumor Spread in Head and Neck Cancers: Radiologic Footprints on 18F-FDG PET, with CT and MRI Correlates. J Nucl Med 2019;60(3):304–11.

26. Raslan OA, Muzaffar R, Shetty V, et al. Image findings of cranial nerve pathology on [18F]-2- deoxy-D-glucose (FDG) positron emission tomography with computerized tomography (PET/CT): a pictorial essay. Cancer Imaging 2015;15:20.

27. Carter RL, Foster CS, Dinsdale EA, et al. Perineural spread by squamous carcinomas of the head and neck: a morphological study using antiaxonal and antimyelin monoclonal antibodies. J Clin Pathol 1983;36(3):269–75.

28. Shah K, Esmaeli B, Ginsberg LE. Perineural tumor spread along the nasociliary branch of the ophthalmic nerve: imaging findings. J Comput Assist Tomogr 2013;37(2):282–5.

29. Ginsberg LE. MR imaging of perineural tumor spread. Neuroimaging Clin N Am 2004;14(4):663–77.

30. Carlson KC, Roenigk RK. Know your anatomy: perineural involvement of basal and squamous cell carcinoma on the face. J Dermatol Surg Oncol 1990;16(9):827–33.

31. Gandhi MR, Panizza B, Kennedy D. Detecting and defining the anatomic extent of large nerve perineural spread of malignancy: comparing "targeted" MRI with the histologic findings following surgery. Head Neck 2011;33(4):469–75.

32. Fischbach F, Müller M, Bruhn H. Magnetic resonance imaging of the cranial nerves in the posterior fossa: a comparative study of t2-weighted spin-echo sequences at 1.5 and 3.0 tesla. Acta Radiol 2008;49(3):358–63.

33. Kirsch CF. Advances in magnetic resonance imaging of the skull base. Int Arch Otorhinolaryngol 2014;18(Suppl 2):S127–35.

34. Malhotra A, Tu L, Kalra VB, et al. Neuroimaging of Meckel's cave in normal and disease conditions. Insights Imaging 2018;9(4):499–510.

35. Khalilzadeh O, Fayad LM, Ahlawat S. 3D MR Neurography. Semin Musculoskelet Radiol 2021;25(3):409–17.

36. Jacquesson T, Cotton F, Attyé A, et al. Probabilistic Tractography to Predict the Position of Cranial Nerves Displaced by Skull Base Tumors: Value for Surgical Strategy Through a Case Series of 62 Patients. Neurosurgery 2019;85(1):E125–36.

37. Ong CK, Chong VF. Imaging of perineural spread in head and neck tumours. Cancer Imaging 2010;(1A):S92–8, 10 Spec no A.

38. Martin-Duverneuil N, Sola-Martínez MT, Miaux Y, et al. Contrast enhancement of the facial nerve on MRI: normal or pathological? Neuroradiology 1997;39(3):207–12.

Anatomy and Pathology of the Skull Base
Malignant and Nonmalignant Lesions

Emilio P. Supsupin Jr, MD[a],*, Noelani S. Gonzales, MS-IV[b],
James Matthew Debnam, MD[c]

KEYWORDS

- Skull base anatomy • Sphenoid bone • Central skull base • Cephalocele
- Caroticoclinoid foramen (ring) • Pituitary macroadenoma • Gradenigo syndrome
- Endoscopic endonasal approaches

KEY POINTS

- The skull base (SB) is the osseous foundation of the cranial vault containing many openings that allow communication between the extracranial and intracranial structures.
- The sphenoid is a complex bony structure that is likened to a bird with unfurled wings.
- Ossification of the dural fold that stretches between the anterior and middle clinoid processes may form a caroticoclinoid foramen (ring).
- Pituitary macroadenomas are by far the most frequently encountered intrasellar pathology, followed by meningiomas and craniopharyngiomas.
- The most common cerebellopontine angle lesions include vestibular schwannomas, meningiomas, and epidermoid cysts.

 Video content accompanies this article at http://www.oralmaxsurgery.theclinics.com.

INTRODUCTION

The skull base (SB) is the osseous foundation of the cranial vault that separates the intracranial and extracranial structures. It contains many openings and apertures that transmit critical neurovascular structures and allow communication between intracranial and extracranial contents. This communication is crucial for normal physiologic processes, however, may also allow spread of disease between the extracranial and intracranial environments. Knowledge of imaging anatomy is important in narrowing the differential diagnosis of SB lesions, staging, and in surgical planning. In this chapter, we provide a comprehensive review of SB imaging anatomy including important landmarks and anatomic variants of clinical relevance to endoscopic endonasal and open transbasal approaches to the SB. In addition, we illustrate the diverse array of pathologies affecting the SB using cases from our clinical practices.

Skull Base Anatomy

The SB is comprised of five bones: two paired frontal and temporal bones and unpaired sphenoid, ethmoid, and occipital bones[1] (**Fig. 1**A). The SB has two surfaces: endocranial and exocranial

[a] Radiology/Neuroradiology, Radiology Residency Program, University of Florida College of Medicine, 655 West 8th. Street, Jacksonville, FL 32209, USA; [b] Nova Southeastern University, Dr. Kiran C. Patel College of Osteopathic Medicine, Fort Lauderdale, FL 33314, USA; [c] Neuroradiology, The University of Texas MD Anderson Cancer Center, Houston, TX 77030, USA
* Corresponding author. Department of Radiology, University of Florida College of Medicine, 655 West 8th Street, Jacksonville, FL 32209.
E-mail addresses: Emilio.Supsupin@jax.ufl.edu; Emilio.P.Supsupin@uth.tmc.edu

Oral Maxillofacial Surg Clin N Am 35 (2023) 413–433
https://doi.org/10.1016/j.coms.2023.03.001

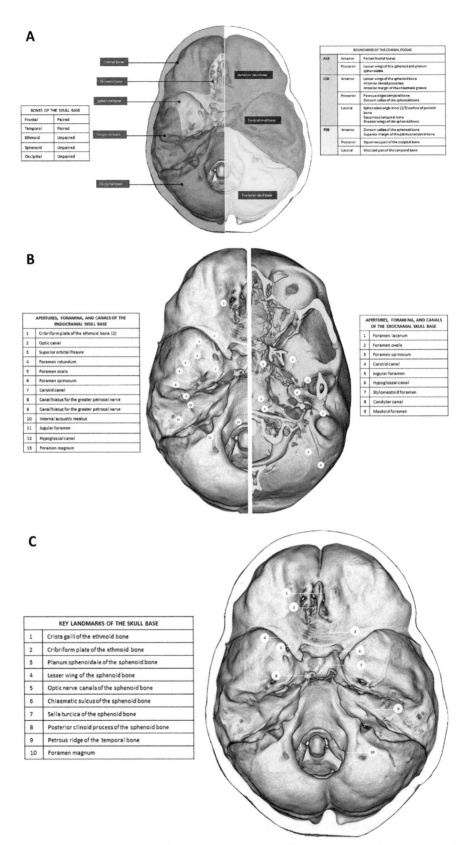

Fig. 1. (*A*) Bones, boundaries, contents of the ASB, CSB, and PSB. (*B*) Endocranial and exocranial surfaces of the SB. (*C*) Key landmarks of the SB.

(**Fig. 1**B). The endocranial surface serves as the floor of the cranium where the brain and neurovascular structures are seated. The exocranial surface is situated above multiple neck compartments. The anterior exocranial surface of the SB is superiorly related to the orbits and sinonasal structures.[1] The central exocranial surface of the SB lies above multiple compartments of the suprahyoid neck, including the roof of the pharyngeal mucosal and the parapharyngeal, masticator, and parotid spaces.[1] The posterior exocranial surface of the SB is rostral to the pharyngeal mucosal, the carotid, retropharyngeal, perivertebral spaces, and the craniocervical junction.[1]

When viewed from above, the endocranial surface may be divided into three compartments namely anterior skull base (ASB), central skull base (CSB), and posterior skull base (PSB). The designation of the boundaries (**Table 1**) between these compartments is arbitrary.[1] This approach may oversimplify the separation between compartments and may not perfectly incorporate the three-dimensional structures of the SB.[1] However, this comprehensively organizes the anatomy and pathologic conditions of the SB for practical discussion.

The ASB houses the frontal lobes and the olfactory bulbs and is bounded anteriorly and laterally by the paired frontal bones. The lesser wing of

the sphenoid and the planum sphenoidale define the posterior border of the ASB (**Fig. 1**C). The chiasmatic sulcus, a shallow shelf between the medial aspects of the optic nerve canals between the anterior border of the sella and planum sphenoidale is regarded by some authors as part of the ASB, while others consider it to be a CSB structure.[1] **Fig. 2**A–C summarizes the neurovascular structures of the SB.

The crista galli (**Fig. 3**A) is an important landmark in ASB surgery, particularly in endoscopic endonasal approaches. The falx cerebri attaches to the frontal ridge (see **Fig. 3**A) and crista galli. The cribriform plate is porous to allow for transmission of the olfactory nerves originating from the olfactory bulb and terminating in the nasal cavity. The Keros classification is used to ascertain the depth of the olfactory sulcus (**Fig. 3**B), which contains the anterior ethmoidal artery (**Fig. 3**C). The CSB is made up of the sphenoid and temporal bones (**Fig. 4**A–E). The posterior boundary of the CSB is defined by the dorsum sellae and posterior clinoid processes medially and the petrous ridges laterally.[1] The CSB contains the temporal lobes and many important neurovascular structures including the internal carotid arteries and cranial nerves. The CSB anatomy and pathology may be divided into the sella and parasellar structures. Important parasellar structures include the cavernous sinuses and their tributaries, the internal carotid arteries and accompanying venous plexus (ie, the venous plexus of Rectorzik), and multiple cranial nerves (see **Fig. 4**D).

The sphenoid is a complex bony structure that is likened to a bird with unfurled wings.[2] (see video 1 and **Fig. 4**A). The body of the sphenoid bone is at the center stage in the discussion of anatomy and pathology of the CSB. The lesser (LSW) and greater (GSW) sphenoid wings contain openings and apertures that transmit critical neurovascular structures (**Table 2**). The GSW forms the floor of the CSB. The LSW provides an important communication between the exocranial and intracranial environments through the orbital fissures that has important implications in the spread of disease. The parts of the sphenoid bone are summarized (see **Fig. 4**A–C).

The vidian and palatovaginal canals run along the floor of the sphenoid sinus (see **Fig. 4**B) and are important landmarks in endoscopic SB surgery. The temporal bone (see **Fig. 4**E) is another complex osseous structure in the SB which may be involved in various pathologic conditions.

The PSB is composed of the posterior temporal and occipital bones. The latter forms the posterior boundary of the PSB. The PSB houses the cerebellum and brainstem and contains the major dural venous sinuses including the jugular bulbs. The

Table 1 Boundaries of the cranial fossae		
ASB	Anterior	Paired frontal bones
	Posterior	Lesser wings of the sphenoid and planum sphenoidale
CSB	Anterior	Lesser wings of the sphenoid bone
		Anterior clinoid processes
		Anterior margin of the chiasmatic groove
	Posterior	Petrous ridges of the temporal bone
		Dorsum sellae of the sphenoid bone
	Lateral	Sphenoidal angle inner (two-thirds) surface of parietal bone
		Squamous temporal bone
		Greater wings of the sphenoid bone
PSB	Anterior	Dorsum sellae of the sphenoid bone
		Superior margin of the petrous temporal bone
	Posterior	Squamous part of the occipital bone
	Lateral	Mastoid part of the temporal bone

A

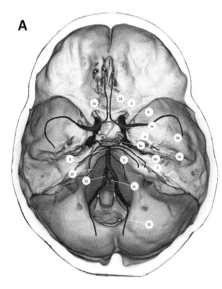

ARTERIES OF THE SKULL BASE	
1a	A1 segment of the anterior cerebral artery
1b	A2 segment of the anterior cerebral artery
2	Anterior communicating artery
3	Internal carotid artery
4	Ophthalmic artery
5a	M1 segment of the middle cerebral artery
5b	M2 segment of the middle cerebral artery
6a	P1 segment of the posterior cerebral artery with posterior communicating artery
6b	P2 segment of the posterior cerebral artery
7	Superior cerebellar artery
8	Basilar artery
9	Pontine artery
10	Anterior inferior cerebellar artery
11	Vertebral artery
12	Anterior spinal artery
13	Posterior inferior cerebellar artery
14	Middle meningeal artery

B

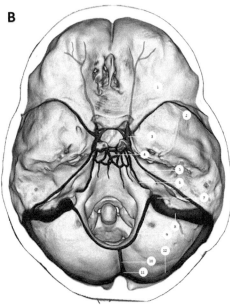

MAJOR DURAL VENOUS SINUSES AND TRIBUTARIES	
1	Ophthalmic vein
2	Sphenoparietal sinus
3	Cavernous sinus
4	Basilar venous plexus
5	Superior petrosal sinus
6	Inferior petrosal sinus
7	Jugular bulb
8	Sigmoid sinus
9	Marginal sinus
10	Straight sinus
11	Confluence of sinuses
12	Transverse sinus

C

CRANIAL NERVES OF THE SKULL BASE	
1	CN I Olfactory bulb
2	CN II Optic nerve
3	CN III Oculomotor nerve
4	CN IV Trochlear nerve
5a	CN V1 Ophthalmic division of the Trigeminal nerve
5b	CN V2 Maxillary division of the Trigeminal nerve
5c	CN V3 Mandibular division of the Trigeminal nerve
6	CN VI Abducens nerve
7	CN VII Facial nerve
8	CN VIII Vestibulocochlear nerve
9	CN IX Glossopharyngeal nerve
10	CN X Vagus nerve
11	CN XI Accessory nerve
12	CN XII Hypoglossal nerve

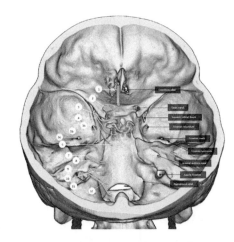

Fig. 2. (A) Endocranial surface–arteries of the SB. (B) Endocranial surface–veins of the SB. (C) Endocranial surface–cranial nerves and foramina of the SB.

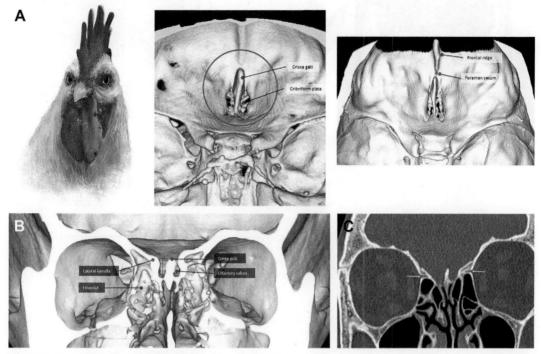

Fig. 3. (*A*) The crista galli and ASB landmarks. Crista galli is Latin for "crest of the rooster," or more simply, a chicken crown. The lateral lamellae that sit on both sides of the crista galli are important landmarks for SB surgery via endoscopic endonasal approach (EEA). The crista galli and frontal ridge serve as attachments of the falx cerebri, a dural membrane that separates the cerebral hemispheres. The *red circle* is showing the crista galli to point out its resemblance to the chicken crown. (*B*) Cribriform plate and lateral lamella. Depth of the olfactory sulcus (Keros classification) denoted by red line is used to assess risk of injury to the ASB during endoscopic endonasal surgery. The bottom of the red line is the cribriform plate. (*C*) The anterior ethmoidal artery foramina. Anterior ethmoidal artery foramina is seen as a bony notch at the medial orbital walls (*yellow arrows*).

internal auditory canal contains the canalicular segments of CN VII and CN VIII (**Fig. 5**A). The foramen magnum in the PSB is the largest opening in the SB that transmits the brainstem and cervicomedullary structures. The temporal and occipital bones form the jugular foramen. The jugular spine splits the jugular foramen into two compartments: the pars nervosa and pars vascularis. The pars nervosa is the anteromedial compartment that transmits the glossopharyngeal nerve and its tympanic branch (Jacobsen nerve). The pars vascularis, which is larger than its counterpart, contains CN X (vagus) and CN XI (spinal accessory) (**Fig. 5**B). The anterior condylar canal (AKA hypoglossal canal) (**Fig. 5**C and D) harbors CN XII and the anterior condylar vein.

The apertures of the skull allow for transmission of the cranial nerves and vessels (see **Table 2**).

The lesser sphenoid wing forms the optic canal that transmits the ophthalmic artery, traveling sympathetic fibers, and the optic nerve before joining the optic chiasm. This canal is a pathway from the orbit to the middle cranial fossa that allows spread of disease.

The superior orbital fissure (see **Fig. 4**C) is a cleft formed by the lesser and greater wings of the sphenoid bone. This transmits the superior and inferior ophthalmic veins, CN III (oculomotor nerve), CN IV (trochlear nerve), ophthalmic division (V1—lacrimal, frontal, and nasociliary branches) of the trigeminal nerve, CN VI (abducens nerve), orbital branch of the middle meningeal artery, recurrent branch of lacrimal artery, and the superior and inferior ophthalmic veins. The greater sphenoid wing, body of the maxillary bone at the orbital floor, and the palatine bones form the inferior orbital fissure (see **Fig. 4**C). This transmits the infraorbital and zygomatic branches of the maxillary division (V2) of the trigeminal nerve, the infraorbital artery and vein, inferior ophthalmic vein, and emissary veins to the pterygoid venous plexus.

The foramen rotundum (see **Fig. 2**C) is a circular aperture of the greater wing of the sphenoid beneath the anterior clinoid process. This contains the maxillary division (V2) of the trigeminal nerve. The foramen ovale (see **Fig. 2**C) is an oval-shaped opening within the greater wing of the

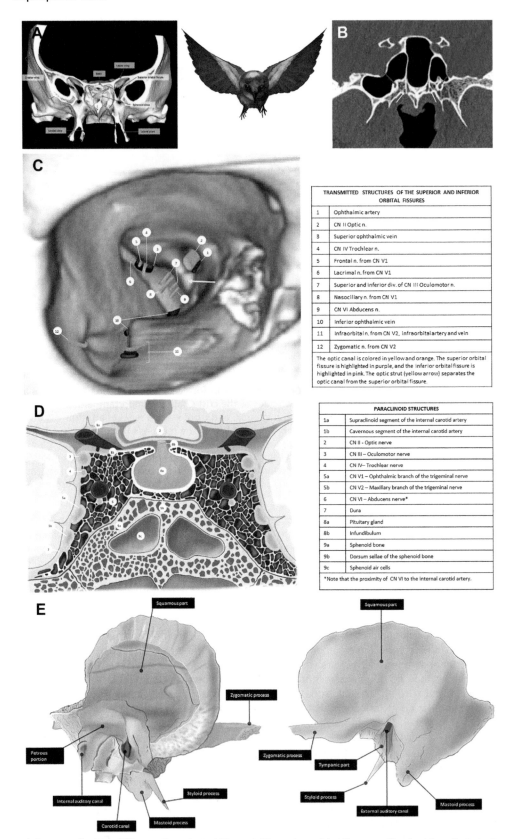

Fig. 4. (*A*) 3D CT of sphenoid bone. The sphenoid bone is likened to a bird (barn swallow) with unfurled wings. (*B*) Vidian and palatovaginal canals. Medial and inferior location of the palatovaginal canals (*yellow arrows*) relative to the vidian canals (*red arrows*). (*C*) Sphenoid bone–superior and inferior orbital fissures. (*D*) Paraclinoid structures. (*E*) Parts of the temporal bone.

Table 2
Skull base apertures and transmitted structures

Apertures/Foramen	Location	Transmitted Structure(s)
Cribriform plate	Anterior cranial fossa (Ethmoid bone)	CN I Olfactory n.
Optic canal	Anterior cranial fossa (Sphenoid bone)	CN II Optic n.
Superior orbital fissure	Middle cranial fossa (Sphenoid bone)	CN III Oculomotor n. CN IV Trochlear n. CN V1 Ophthalmic div. Trigeminal n. CN VI Abducens n.
Inferior orbital fissure	Orbit	CN V2 Maxillary div. Trigeminal n. Infraorbital a. and v.
Foramen rotundum	Middle cranial fossa (Sphenoid bone)	CN V2 Maxillary div. Trigeminal n.
Foramen ovale	Middle cranial fossa (Sphenoid bone)	CN V3 Mandibular div. Trigeminal n.
Foramen spinosum	Middle cranial fossa (Sphenoid bone)	Middle meningeal a.
Foramen lacerum	Middle cranial fossa (Sphenoid bone)	Internal carotid a.
Internal auditory meatus	Posterior cranial fossa (Petrous part of the Temporal bone)	CN VII Facial n. CN VIII Vestibulocochlear n.
Jugular foramen	Posterior cranial fossa (B/w Temporal and Occipital bones)	CN IX Glossopharyngeal n. CN X Vagus n. CN XI Accessory nerve Sigmoid sinus to inferior jugular v.
Hypoglossal canal	Posterior cranial fossa (Occipital bone)	CN XII Hypoglossal n. Anterior condylar vein

sphenoid, lateral to the dorsum sellae. This carries the mandibular division (V3) of the trigeminal nerve that innervates the muscles of mastication.

The foramen spinosum (see **Fig. 2**C) is located inferolateral to the foramen ovale and is also an opening created by the greater wing of the sphenoid. This foramen transmits the middle meningeal artery (MMA), a vessel that supplies the lateral dural surfaces of the brain. Because of its location beneath the articulation point of four skull bones called the pterion, skull fracture may cause a tear to this artery and result in epidural hematoma. The MMA may be embolized to treat chronic subdural hematomas.

Landmarks and Anatomic Variants of Clinical Importance and Relevance to Skull Base Surgery

Understanding the relationship of SB lesions to important anatomic landmarks and recognizing anatomic variants is crucial in planning the surgical approach. Knowledge of relevant anatomy and anatomic variants may help avoid complications.

ASB

The crista galli has important clinical implications in ASB surgery particularly in endoscopic transcribriform approaches.[3] Knowledge of dimensions of the crista galli is important in preoperative planning of access to the lesion and instrumentation.[4] The crista galli, being part of the ethmoid bone, may be pneumatized and accumulate fluid (**Fig. 6**) that can get infected and simulate rhinosinusitis.[5] Mucoceles may expand the crista galli and produce bone resorption and new bone formation.[6] Alterations in the morphology of bony landmarks (such as the foramen cecum and frontal ridge) (see **Fig. 3**A) may serve as important clues to the diagnosis and extent of disease. Lesions such as meningoencephalocele may produce expansion of the foramen cecum and erosion of the crista galli.[7]

The olfactory recess contains the olfactory bulb and anterior ethmoidal artery (see **Fig. 3**C). The depth of the olfactory fossa is defined by the height of the lateral lamella. The Keros classification is the most common criterion used to assess

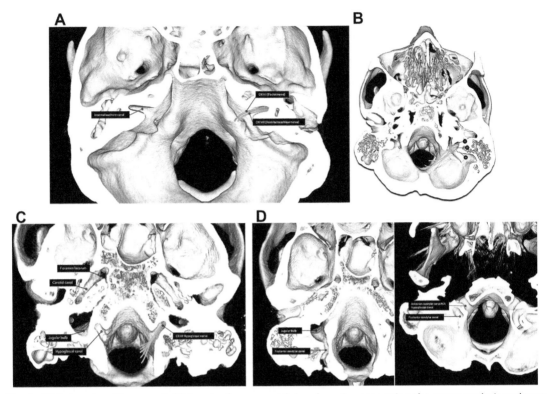

Fig. 5. (*A*) Internal auditory canal. (*B*) Jugular foramen with jugular spine separating the pars vascularis and pars nervosa. The jugular spine separates the jugular foramen (*dashed lines*) into the pars nervosa (anteromedial compartment in blue) and pars vascularis (posterolateral compartment in red). The pars nervosa houses CN IX, while CN X and XI travel into the pars vascularis. (*C*) Hypoglossal canal, jugular bulb, and carotid canal. (*D*) Posterior condylar canal.

the risk of injury to the anterior cranial base. It provides helpful information on the depth of the olfactory fossa in surgical planning and in avoiding iatrogenic injury to the cribriform plate and medial ethmoid roof.[8,9] Preoperative CT is necessary for identifying the anterior ethmoidal artery and avoiding injury to this vessel during endoscopic sinus surgery.[10]

CSB

The vidian canal (see **Fig. 4**B) is an important landmark for identification of the petrous segment of the internal carotid artery (ICA), particularly during extended endoscopic endonasal approaches to cranial base surgery. The vidian canal lies along the medial pterygoid plateau and harbors the vidian artery, vein, and nerve.[11] It has a critical

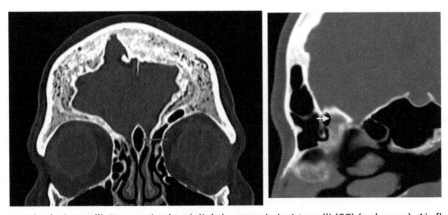

Fig. 6. Pneumatized crista galli. Pneumatized and slightly expanded crista galli (CG) (*red arrow*). Air-fluid level in the pneumatized CG (*yellow arrow*). The fluid filling the pneumatized CG may become infected.

role in planning endoscopic SB surgeries because of its relationship to the ICA. The vidian canal is found to be below the level of the anterior genu of the petrous (ICA) in most patients (89%), and less commonly at the same level or above the petrous ICA (7% and 4%, respectively).[11] This implies that a working room inferior and medial to the vidian canal might not always be safe because this could be located superior to the level of the anterior genu of the petrous ICA.[11] Because the vidian nerve lies immediately underneath the sphenoid sinus mucosa, bony dehiscence of the vidian canal may have implications regarding potential injury to the vidian nerve.[11]

The palatovaginal canal runs along the floor of the sphenoid sinus, medial to the vidian canal (see **Fig. 4**B).[12] The constant relationship of the external orifice of the vidian and palatovaginal canals and sphenopalatine artery can be used as an anatomic landmark when performing endoscopic vidian neurotomy.[12]

The intimate relationship of the anterior clinoid process (ACP) to the clinoid segment of the ICA makes treatment of vascular and neoplastic lesions related to the ACP challenging.[13] Preoperative CT is useful in detecting anatomic variations of the ACP. Appropriate modifications may be required when performing extradural anterior clinoidectomy to ensure a safe approach.[13] Pneumatization of the ACP should not be mistaken for flowvoids in the ICA (**Fig. 7**A).

The middle clinoid process is an inconsistent anatomic variant (**Fig. 7**B). Ossification of the dural fold that stretches between the anterior and middle clinoid processes may form a caroticoclinoid foramen (ring) (see **Fig. 7**B). Another anatomic variant is an interclinoid bridge (**Fig. 7**C), an osseous connection between the anterior and posterior clinoid processes. These anatomic variants must be recognized and properly managed to avoid injury to the cavernous carotid artery during expanded endoscopic endonasal surgery.[14]

Protrusions of the ICA into the sphenoid sinus are also important anatomic variants to recognize during transsphenoidal surgery (**Fig. 7**D and E). A radiological *teddy bear sign* (**Fig. 7**F) has been described as a useful preoperative tool for the identification of anatomy predisposing to a high risk of ICA injury.[15,16] Preoperative CT to evaluate the relationship of the intersphenoid septum to the ICA is crucial in avoiding arterial injury (see **Fig. 7**D).

Other anatomic variants in the central SB may be encountered in the routine imaging of craniofacial structures. SB defects such as persistent craniopharyngeal canal, canalis basilaris medianus, and fossa navicularis magna (**Fig. 7**G) incidentally found on brain imaging should not be mistaken for pathology. Other anatomic variants include canaliculus innominatus,[17] foramen of Vesalius[17] (**Fig. 7**H), among others.

PSB

The hypoglossal canal contains the anterior condylar vein and hypoglossal nerve. The posterior condylar canal (see **Fig. 5**D) houses the posterior condylar vein that connects the sigmoid sinus or jugular fossa into the suboccipital venous plexus, an important pathway for venous outflow in normal physiologic conditions and in high-flow vascular malformations/fistulas.[18] The hypoglossal canal and posterior condylar canal may harbor dural AV fistulas.[19–26]

An enlarged posterior condylar canal may provide access for treatment of dural AV fistulas. Recognizing an enlarged or prominent mastoid emissary vein (**Fig. 8**A) is important to avoid complications during retrosigmoid craniotomies and far lateral approaches.

An elongated and ossified styloid process of the temporal bone (**Fig. 8**B) may produce symptoms because of compression of soft tissues and neurovascular structures, termed Eagle syndrome.

Skull Base Pathology

Diverse pathologies of the SB may be encountered in clinical practice. These may be categorized into congenital, traumatic, infection, neoplastic and tumor-like lesions, and vascular.

Anterior Skull Base

Aggressive diseases such as infections and malignancies frequently breach the ASB.[27]

Congenital lesions in the ASB include meningoencephalocele (**Fig. 9**A), intracranial extension of midline frontonasal masses such as nasal glioma (**Fig. 9**B), and nasal dermoid cyst. With advances in imaging techniques, cephaloceles may be incidentally discovered protruding into the sphenoid sinuses when located in the ASB or in the temporal bones when situated in the CSB. Those in the ASB are often repaired prophylactically.[28] Spontaneous cerebrospinal fluid (CSF) leak commonly occurs in the cribriform plate. Thinner bones in the anterior and lateral SB are associated with spontaneous CSF leak.[29]

Cephaloceles may develop in traumatic SB fractures. The most common locations are in the orbital roof, ethmoid, and sphenoid regions.[30] Clinical presentations of cephaloceles may include CSF rhinorrhea, exophthalmos, and hearing loss.[30] Surgical treatment is often required for

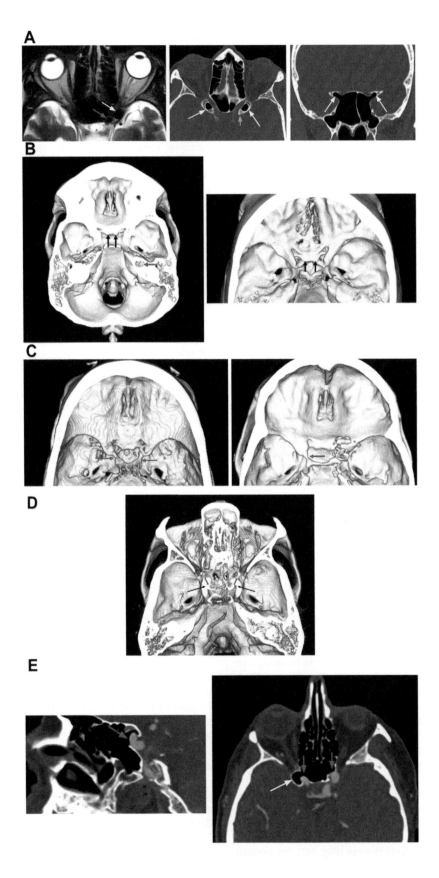

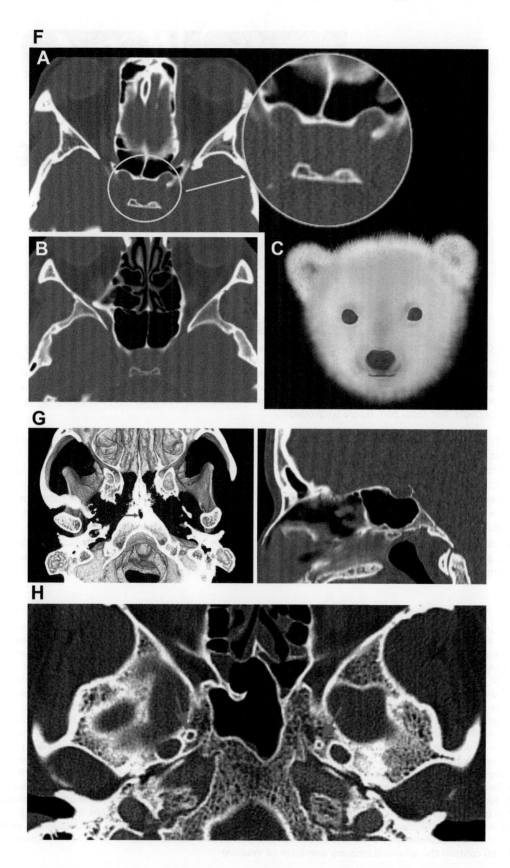

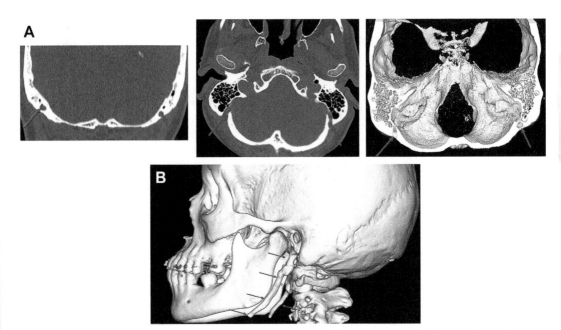

Fig. 8. (*A*) Prominent mastoid emissary veins. Prominent mastoid emissary veins (*red arrows*) are important venous outflow channels in physiologic and high-flow states (such as dural AV fistulas). Recognizing this anatomic variant may help avoid complications such as uncontrollable bleeding and air embolism during far lateral and retrosigmoid approach craniotomies. (*B*) Temporal bone-elongated and ossified styloid processes. Elongated, ossified styloid process (*red arrows*) may produce symptoms such as throat pain, foreign body sensation, dysphagia, and facial pain (Eagle syndrome).

definitive symptomatic improvement or resolution in most cases.[30]

Cephalocele associated with a metameric syndrome, CAMS (cerebrofacial arteriovenous metameric syndrome) has been described.[31] Traumatic iatrogenic meningocele in an infant following difficult intubation resulting in perforation of the cribriform plate has been reported.[32] The nasoseptal flap is an effective and safe technique for reconstructing SB defects.[33]

Olfactory groove and planum sphenoidale meningiomas (**Fig. 9**C) are common lesions in the ASB.[34] These lesions are unique as they remain clinically silent but may become large masses upon diagnosis.[35] Headache is the most common symptom prompting neuroradiological workup, followed by behavioral changes. Other symptoms include hyposmia/anosmia and visual impairment. These lesions are treated by open and endoscopic endonasal approaches.[36]

Fig. 7. (*A*) Pneumatized ACP. On axial T2 MRI, the dark signal of the pneumatized anterior clinoid process (ACP, *yellow arrows*) mimicking the flow-void (*red arrow*) of the adjacent ICA must not be confused for an aneurysm. CT confirms pneumatization of the ACP (*yellow arrows*), avoiding the need for additional imaging. The small triangular piece of bone (*blue arrows*) corresponds to the non-pneumatized, posteriorly directed part of the ACP. (*B*) Middle clinoid process and caroticoclinoid rings. Ossification of the middle clinoid processes (*black arrows*) or dural sheaths connecting them to the ACP forming caroticoclinoid rings (*red asterisks*). Pneumatized petrous apices (*red arrows*). (*C*) Interclinoid bridges (*red arrows*): osseous connections between the anterior and posterior clinoid processes. (*D*) Protrusions of the ICAs. The ICAs (*black arrows*) protrude into the sphenoid sinus (*red line*), increasing the risk of injury during endonasal endoscopic surgery. It is also important to know the location of the intersphenoid sinus septum (*red arrow*) relative to the ICA to avoid arterial injury. (*E*) Bony dehiscence with protrusion of the ICA into the sphenoid sinus (*red arrows*). On the right side, the ICA also protrudes into the sphenoid sinus through the pneumatized ACP (*yellow arrow*). (*F*) Teddy bear signprotrusions of the ICA into the sphenoid sinuses (*A* with inset) resembling a teddy bear (*C*). This radiologic sign may be used to assess high-risk injury to the ICAs during transsphenoidal SB surgery. Lack of protrusion of the ICAs into the sphenoid sinuses (*B*) indicates a low risk of injury to the ICAs. (*G*) Midline clival defect benign midline bony defect (*red arrows*) in the clivus. Differential considerations include persistent craniopharyngeal canal, canalis basilaris medianus, and fossa navicularis magna. (*H*) Foramen of Vesalius (*red arrows*) situated anterior to the foramen ovale (*red asterisks*) contains the sphenoid emissary vein (vein of Vesalius).

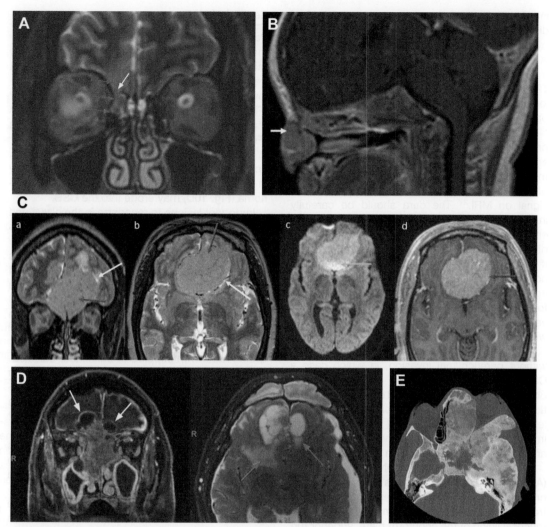

Fig. 9. (*A*) Meningoencephalocele. A 39-year-old woman with seizures. Coronal T2-weighted MRI shows protrusion of the right inferior frontal lobe (*red arrows*) through a bony defect in the fovea ethmoidalis, the lateral roof of the ethmoid bone (*yellow arrow*). (*B*) Midline frontonasal mass-nasal glioma. Evaluation for intracranial extension of nasal glioma (*yellow arrow*) before resection can be challenging. Intracranial extension may not be apparent on imaging. (*C*) Olfactory groove/planum sphenoidale meningioma. (a and b). Coronal and axial T2-weighted MRI showing a large extra-axial mass in the olfactory groove (*red arrows*) isointense to gray matter. CSF cleft (*yellow arrows*) consistent with extra-axial location of the mass. (c) MRI showing elevated DWI signal reflecting hypercellularity of the mass (*blue arrow*). (d) Avidly enhancing extra-axial mass in the olfactory groove, consistent with meningioma (*red arrow*). (*D*) Olfactory neuroblastoma (esthesioneuroblastoma) with intracranial extensionheterogeneously enhancing sinonasal mass with SB erosion and intracranial extension into the anterior cranial fossa. There are cystic changes (*yellow arrows*), mass effect, and vasogenic edema (*red arrows*) in the bilateral inferior frontal lobes. (*E*) Fibrous dysplasia (FD) - axial CT depicting extensive FD in the anterior and central SB with typical ground glass and sclerotic and lucent bony changes.

Following resection, olfactory groove meningiomas are often associated with loss of smell. However, smell preservation surgery in the lateral endoscopic endonasal approach has been described.[37] Ga 68 Tetraxetan, 1,4,7,10-tetraazacyclododecane-tetraacetic acid/Tyr^3-Octreotate - d-Phe1-Tyr^3-Octreotide (DOTA-TOC) PET/CT fused MRI in postoperative evaluation of olfactory groove meningioma millimetric remnants have been described.[38]

Most extracranial tumors that involve the ASB arise from the sinonasal cavities.[27] Aggressive sinonasal tumors such as the common squamous cell carcinoma and the rarer olfactory neuroblastoma (**Fig. 9**D) may erode into ASB. These lesions are amenable to biopsy and the primary role of imaging is to determine the intracranial extent of disease.[27] The cribriform plate is easily violated by sinonasal malignancies.[27] The cribriform plate is well evaluated on coronal CT, and on MRI shows a linear hypointense signal on T1-weighted and T2-weighted sequences.[27] The more laterally located orbital plates are thick and serve as strong barriers to intracranial spread of disease.[27]

Intracranial extension of disease includes breach of the SB with involvement of the dura and invasion of the brain parenchyma.[27] Compromise of SB integrity is suspected with dehiscence of the cribriform plate on CT and loss of its normal signal on MRI.[27] The dura should be carefully inspected for evidence of disease such as thickening and enhancement.[27] It can be difficult to differentiate reactive change from dural invasion. If the visualized dura is grossly thickened with nodular contour, dural invasion is assumed and aggressive resection of potentially involved dura followed by radiotherapy is undertaken.[27] Dural invasion is associated with a high recurrence rate with poor prognostic implications.[27]

The tumor may indent the base of the brain without parenchymal invasion, in which case a CSF cleft at the tumor–brain interface may be observed. The brain has normal signal characteristics. However, invasion of the brain by aggressive lesions such as squamous cell carcinoma results in loss of CSF cleft with presence of brain edema and abnormal enhancement on imaging.[27]

Olfactory neuroblastoma (ONB) (see **Fig. 9**D) (AKA esthesioneuroblastoma) is a rare neuroendocrine malignancy of neural crest origin. It arises from the neuroectodermal stem cells found in the mucosal lining of the cribriform plate, superior turbinates, anterior ethmoids, and nasal roof and septum.[39] ONBs may have a slow onset of symptoms. There is an emerging role of Ga 68 Dotatate PET MRI and PET/CT in the diagnosis, staging, and treatment response monitoring of ONBs.[40,41] The role of diffusion-weighted MRI in distinguishing ONBs from other sinonasal malignancies has been described.[42]

Fibrous dysplasia (FD) (**Fig. 9**E) is an uncommon bone disease that may be encountered in the ASB.[43] It is characterized by replacement of normal bone architecture by abnormal fibro-osseous connective tissue.[43] Patients may present with a wide range of symptoms such as facial pain, hypoesthesia, headaches, proptosis, diplopia, nasal obstruction, or facial deformity.[43,44] The diagnosis of FD is based on clinical and typical imaging features. CT is the imaging modality of choice, providing anatomic depiction of the extent of disease and morphologic bone changes of ground glass opacities, sclerosis, and cysts.

Central Skull Base

Pathologic conditions in the CSB may arise primarily from the sella or parasellar regions. Pituitary macroadenomas (**Fig. 10**A) are by far the most frequently encountered intrasellar pathology, followed by meningiomas and craniopharyngiomas[45] (**Fig. 10**B). A giant aneurysm of the cavernous ICA may compress the surrounding cranial nerves (**Fig. 10**C).

Pathologies in the CSB may arise from the sella, sphenoid sinus, and clivus. Extracranial pathology in the nasopharynx such as nasopharyngeal carcinoma (**Fig. 10**D) may erode into the CSB.

Important lesions to recognize in the clivus and petroclival regions include chondrosarcomas (**Fig. 10**E) and chordomas[45] (**Fig. 10**F and G).

Chondrosarcoma is a malignant cartilaginous tumor with 5% to 10% occurring in the head and neck.[46] The peak incidence is in the fourth to fifth decades, with male sex predominance.[47] SB chondrosarcomas arise off midline, most often occurring at the petro-occipital synchondrosis.[48] On CT, chondrosarcomas may contain a chondroid matrix with stippled or curvilinear calcifications in a "ring and arc" pattern.[47] Due to high water content, chondrosarcomas are T1 hypointense and T2 hyperintense. However, calcification of the chondroid matrix can cause T1 and T2 signal hypointensity.[49]

Chordomas are rare locally aggressive neoplasms arising from embryonic notochordal remnants in the axial skeleton. Approximately one-third arise in the midline of the clivus at the spheno-occipital junction.[50] Chordomas most commonly occur in the fourth decade with male sex predominance. On CT, chordomas are well-circumscribed, expansile, hyperdense mass with bone destruction and show moderate to marked enhancement.

Irregular calcifications may represent sequestra from bony destruction. On MRI, chordomas are T1 hypo to isointense and markedly T2 hyperintense and demonstrate moderate to marked enhancement.[50]

The parasellar region (see **Fig. 4**D) contains the cavernous sinuses and Meckel's caves and houses multiple neurovascular structures (including the ICA and cranial nerves III, IV, V1, V2, and VI). Therefore, a wide range of inflammatory, infectious, or neoplastic processes (including perineural spread of disease) may be encountered in the parasellar regions. Symptoms may arise from compression and/or infiltration of these cranial nerves.

CSB infection may develop in elderly people with diabetes and result from necrotizing otitis externa. Atypical SB osteomyelitis (ASBO) (**Fig. 10**H) is an important diagnostic

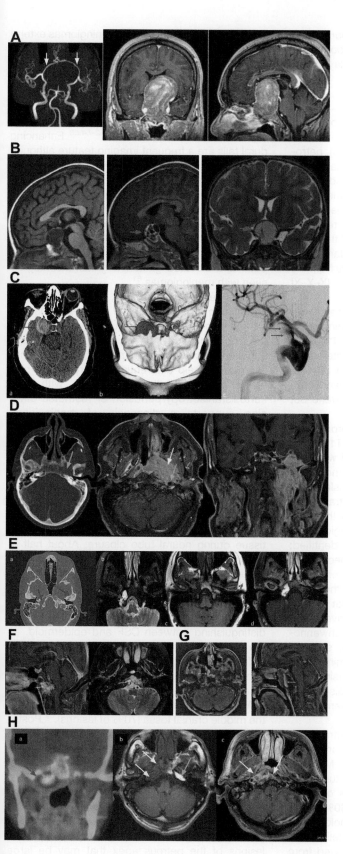

Fig. 10. (*A*) Pituitary macroadenoma. Pituitary macroadenoma with a very large sellar and suprasellar mass producing splaying of the bilateral ICA (*red arrows*) and circle of Willis. The A-1 segments of both anterior cerebral arteries are elevated and draped over the suprasellar component of the mass (*yellow arrows*). (*B*) A 19-month-old woman with cystic craniopharyngioma. Cystic sellar and suprasellar mass (*red arrows*) with enhancing components and internal septations. (*C*) Giant aneurysm of the right cavernous carotid artery. (a) Heterogeneous hyperattenuating lesion in the right parasellar/paraclinoid region (*red arrow*) (b) 3-D CTA demonstrating a giant aneurysm of the right cavernous carotid artery (*red arrow*). (c) Catheter angiogram showing a partially thrombosed aneurysm with incomplete filling of the aneurysm sac (*red arrows*). A giant aneurysm may produce symptomatic compression of multiple cranial nerves in the cavernous sinus (ie, CN III and VI palsies). (*D*) Nasopharyngeal carcinoma. NPCA with intracranial extension into the middle cranial fossa. CT shows bony erosion in the SB (*blue arrow*). The nasopharyngeal mass (*yellow arrow*) partially encased and displaced the carotid artery (*green arrow*) and extended in the middle cranial fossa with brain invasion (*red arrows*). (*E*) Petroclival chondrosarcoma. (a) Lytic lesion with pattern of rings and arcs in the petroclival region on CT. (b Hyperintense signal on T2-weighted MRI. (c) Hypointense on T1-weighted MRI. (d) Avid enhancement on postcontrast T1-weighted MRI. (*F*) Petroclival chordoma. A 61-year-old woman with petroclivcal chordoma (*yellow arrows*) who subsequently underwent resection via midline EEA. The lesion is heterogeneously enhancing and T2 hyperintense. (*G*) Petroclival chordoma s/p midline endoscopic endonasal resection postoperative MRI following endoscopic endonasal resection and nasoseptal flap reconstruction. The hyperintense signal (*yellow arrows*) corresponds to the fatty component of the nasoseptal flap. (*H*) ASBO. (a) Ceretec WBC scan demonstrates increased uptake of tagged white blood cells (*red arrow*). (b) Loss of normal fatty marrow signal in the SB and paraclival soft tissue infiltration (*yellow arrows*). Note bright T1 signal of normal fatty marrow in the clivus and petrous apex (*blue arrows*). (c) Heterogeneous soft tissue enhancement in the SB and adjacent soft tissues (*yellow arrows*).

consideration.[51] ASBO has a predilection to the CSB, and stroke can be a devastating complication when the diagnosis is missed or delayed.

Posterior Skull Base

Important anatomic structures in the posterior skull base (PSB) include the cerebellopontine angles (CPAs), internal auditory canals (IACs), petromastoid, jugular foramen, and hypoglossal canal.

The CPA is a triangular subarachnoid space within the PSB centered at the level of the IAC.[52] The apex of the space is medially positioned within the prepontine cistern.[52] The petrous temporal bone forms the anterolateral border and the cerebellum defines the posteromedial boundary of the CPA.[52] The space extends craniocaudally from the cranial nerve V to the cranial nerve IX–X–XI complex.[52–54]

The most common CPA lesions include vestibular schwannomas (VSs) (**Fig. 11**A), meningiomas (**Fig. 11**B), and epidermoid cysts[52] (**Fig. 11**C).

VSs are the most commonly encountered lesions in the CPA[52] comprising 70% to 80% of masses. Most develop from the Schwann cells within the internal auditory canal and extend out of the porus acousticus into the CPA.[52]

Bilateral VSs are diagnostic of neurofibromatosis type II.[54] VSs show isointense signal on T1 and intermediate to hyperintense signal on T2 with avid enhancement, although heterogeneity and cystic degeneration may be found with increasing size. The presence of susceptibility due to intratumoral microhemorrhage may help distinguish these lesions from other masses such as meningiomas.[52] Three enhancement patterns have been identified: homogeneous in most cases, heterogeneous, and central cystic change without enhancement.[52,53,55–57] T2 hyperintense signal in the dorsal brainstem is another imaging feature that may be seen with VSs and may reflect degenerative demyelination of the vestibular nucleus.[53,58] Schwannomas arising from other cranial nerves, such as cranial nerves V, VII, and IX–XI may mimic VSs with similar imaging features. Tumor arising from the facial nerves may be difficult to distinguish from VSs. However, the former may extend along the course of the facial nerve canal.[52]

Meningiomas are the most common intracranial extra-axial masses and are also the second most common mass in the CPA, after VSs. Meningiomas account for 10% to 50% of all tumors in the CPA,[52] and 10% of meningiomas occur in the CPA.[59] Facial pain is seen in up to 30% of patients with meningiomas.[59] Histopathologically, meningiomas arise from meningoepithelial cells and within the CPA are most often derived from

the posterior petrous dura.[52] Meningiomas extend into but do not expand the porus acousticus, unlike VSs.[52] Hyperostosis is more common than bony erosion.[53,59] CT exhibits a hyperattenuating mass in the CPA with occasional calcification, while MRI shows a dural-based extra-axial lesion that is isointense to cortex on T1-weighted imaging with intense enhancement.[52–54,59] Enhancing dural tails are a frequent imaging feature although they are nonspecific. Meningiomas and VSs may have a similar appearance on imaging, although cystic degeneration and intratumoral hemorrhage are typical of VSs while a "dural tail" sign and osteoproliferation favor CPA meningiomas. Relative tumor volume has been demonstrated to be higher in the meningiomas than VSs.[53,60] Alanine peak and elevated glutamine/glutamate may be seen with meningiomas.[61]

Advanced MRI techniques, including diffusion kurtosis imaging (DKI) and three-dimensional arterial spin labeling (3D-ASL), may complement the morphologic and physiologic information supplied by conventional imaging.[62] These techniques may help differentiate VS from CPA meningiomas.[62] A solid CPA tumor with high kurtosis/anisotropy/perfusion or restricted diffusion supports a diagnosis of meningioma. Conversely, low kurtosis/anisotropy/perfusion or facilitated diffusion is consistent with a diagnosis of schwannoma.[62]

Epidermoid cysts (ECs) are the third most common tumors in the CPA, accounting for 5% of all lesions in this location and 1% of intracranial tumors.[52,53,59,63,64] ECs are congenital lesions arising from the inclusion of ectodermal epithelial tissue during neural tube closure. About half of the intracranial ECs are in the CPA.[52,63,65] ECs are isoattenuating to CSF on CT and conventional MRI sequences show characteristic signal hyperintensity on diffusion-weighted imaging. Fluid-attenuated inversion recovery (FLAIR) is useful in distinguishing between CSF and epidermoid, as the signal is incompletely suppressed in an EC.[52] Diffusion weighted imaging (DWI) is also helpful in postoperative evaluation of residual tumor after resection.[52]

Arachnoid cysts (**Fig. 11**D) are typically found in the middle cranial fossa (70% of lesions).[52] Posterior fossa and CPA arachnoid cyst may cause compression of the brainstem and cerebellum. On imaging, they are seen as smooth lesions that follow the signal of CSF on all pulse sequences, including complete suppression on FLAIR. They can be differentiated from epidermoids by lack of diffusion restriction.[52]

Cholesterol granulomas (**Fig. 11**E) are expansile lesions of the petrous apex that may be large

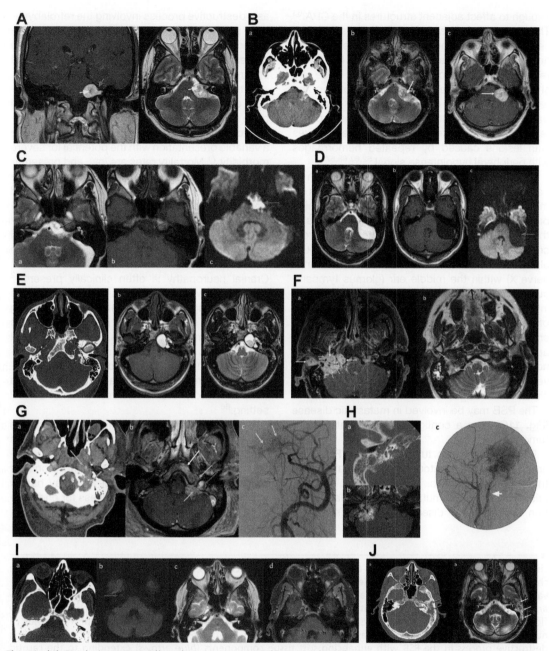

Fig. 11. (*A*) CPA lesion–VS. Avidly enhancing extra-axial mass in the left CPA with expansion of the porus acousticus (PA, *red arrows*). Dark signal on T2-weighted MRI with lack of enhancement reflects intratumoral hemorrhage (*yellow arrows*). Expansion of the PA and intratumoral hemorrhage and/or cystic degeneration favor VS over meningioma. (*B*) CPA lesion–meningioma. (a) Calcified mass in the left cerebellopontine angle (CPA) (*yellow arrow*). (b) Extra-axial mass with heterogeneous signal on T2-weighted MRI. Dark signal corresponds to the calcification on CT (*yellow arrow*). (c) Avidly enhancing extra-axial mass (*arrow*) in the left CPA consistent with meningioma (*yellow arrow*). Note the lack of expansion of the PA (*arrowhead*), unlike in VSs. (*C*) CPA lesion–epidermoid cyst. T2 hyperintense (a) and T1 hypointense (b) extra-axial mass (*red arrows*) with diffusion restriction on DWI (*red arrow*) (c). ECs may follow the signal of CSF but have a characteristic bright signal (*red arrow*) on diffusion-weighted MRI, a feature that is absent in arachnoid cysts. (*D*) Cerebellopontine angle lesion–arachnoid cyst. T2 hyperintense (a) and T1 hypointense (b) extra-axial mass in the left cerebellopontine angle (CPA). There is NO diffusion restriction on DWI (*red arrow*) (c), which differentiates this mass from an epidermoid cyst. (*E*) Petrous apex cholesterol granuloma. (a) Expansile lesion with soft tissue attenuation in the left petrous apex on CT. (b *and* c) Expansile lesion with hyperintense T1 and T2 signal with heterogeneity on T2, consistent with

enough to affect adjacent structures in the CPA.[63] They result from obstruction of petrous apex air cells and with consequent repeated hemorrhage and inflammation lead to expansion of bone with remodeling and resorption.[66] On CT, these are sharply marginated lesions with remodeling of the temporal bone and density similar to the brain parenchyma. MRI shows heterogeneous hyperintensity on T1-weighted and T2-weighted images with lesions caused by repeated hemorrhages with peripheral hypointense signal.[52,63,66,67]

The jugular foramen may harbor lesions such as paragangliomas that are also known as glomus tumors (**Fig. 11**F). These are highly vascular, benign but locally aggressive neuroendocrine tumors in the head and neck. In the CPA, these arise from cranial nerve X at the jugular foramen (glomus jugulare), Arnold nerve (auricular branch of cranial nerve X) within the middle ear (glomus tympanicum), or from cranial nerve IX.[63,67–69] CT shows infiltrative osseous changes with loss of the cortex of the jugular foramen and temporal bone with avid enhancement after contrast. A salt and pepper appearance on MRI represents linear and serpiginous flow voids often with prominent draining veins and regions of T1 hyperintensity from intralesional hemorrhage.[63,67–69]

The PSB may be involved in metastatic disease (**Fig. 11**G) from a contiguous or distant primary tumor.

Endolymphatic sac tumors (ELSTs) (**Fig. 11**H) are papillary adenomatous tumors that arise from the endolymphatic sac. Twenty percent of cases arise from sporadic mutations unassociated with Von Hippel-Lindau disease. The ELSTs appear as a destructive process involving the retrolabyrinthine petrous temporal bone.[70] They show heterogeneous signal intensity on MRI because of the presence of intratumoral hemorrhage and avid enhancement.[52,66,67,70]

Petrous apicitis (**Fig. 11**I) is an inflammatory process centered in the petrous apex of the temporal bone resulting as a sequela of otitis media and otomastoiditis[52] (**Fig. 11**J). Petrous apicitis may have a variable presentation with the potential for severe morbidity.[71] Mortality rates are low, and presentation with Gradenigo's triad is uncommon.[71] Gradenigo syndrome refers to the presence of fever and CN VI neuropathies in the setting of petrous apicitis.[66,71] Prompt diagnosis and appropriate medical management with surgical drainage can avoid serious complications such as meningitis, brain abscess, and dural venous sinus thrombosis.[71] Cranial neuropathy is often clinically present.[52] CT may show destructive changes in the petrous apex with imaging features of otitis media including mastoid air cell effusion.[52] MRI demonstrates edema, inflammatory changes, and enhancement in the petrous apex which may or may not be pneumatized.[52] The cavernous sinus should be evaluated for thrombosis and enhancement along the fifth and sixth cranial nerves in this clinical setting.[66]

Dural arteriovenous fistulas (DAVFs) around the hypoglossal canal[19–21] and in the marginal sinus (venous sinus associated with the foramen magnum) are well described. The posterior condylar canal is an inconstant channel that may harbor DAVFs[22–26] and may provide access for endovascular treatment of these lesions when enlarged.

---

cholesterol granuloma. The expansile appearance, signal characteristics, and location in the petrous apex are characteristic imaging features of cholesterol granuloma. (*F*) Paraganglioma-glomus jugulotympanicum. Hypervascular mass in the right jugular fossa extending to the middle ear cavity and external auditory canal (*yellow arrows* in a) exhibiting the classic "salt and pepper" appearance. The bright areas ("salt") correspond to slow flow and blood products (*blue arrows* in *a* and *b*). The dark areas (pepper) correspond to the flow-voids of numerous small vessels within the mass (*red arrows* in *a* and *b*). (*G*) Posterior SB metastasis. (a) CT showing destructive process in the PSB with enhancing soft tissue components (*blue arrows*) extending to the carotid space. (b) MRI depicting bony infiltration with abnormal marrow signal (*yellow arrow*) and mass-like enhancement in the cerebellomedullary angle and hypoglossal canal (*green arrows*). Tumor thrombus in the left jugular bulb (*red arrow*). (c) Catheter angiogram demonstrating tumor blush (*orange arrows*) mainly from the ascending pharyngeal artery (*purple arrow*). (*H*) Endolymphatic sac tumor. (a) Destructive lesion in the right mastoid and SB. (b) Avidly enhancing mass in the mastoid extending into the right CPA corresponding to destructive lesion on CT. (c) Tumor blush with the mass fed by multiple branches of the external carotid artery—predominantly by a recanalized otic artery (*arrow*). (*I*) Petrous apicitis (apical petrositis). (a) Abnormal soft tissue attenuation within the right petrous apex (PA) on CT (*red arrow*) (b) MRI showing focal abnormal DWI signal elevation in the right PA corresponding to the CT finding (*red arrow*) (c) Elevated T2-signal in the right PA on T2-weighted MRI sequence (*red arrow*) (d) Peripheral enhancement surrounding the described abnormality in the right PA (*red arrow*). Imaging findings and the clinical presentation of right facial pain in this patient are consistent with petrous apicitis. (*J*) Coalescent mastoiditis. (a) CT showing opacification of the left mastoid air cells and middle ear cavity with bony erosions and loss of normal septations in the mastoid air cells (*red arrows*). (b) Mastoid effusion on T2-weighted MRI (*yellow arrows*).

CLINICS CARE POINTS

- The crista galli has important clinical implications in anterior SB surgery, particularly in endoscopic transcribriform approaches.

- The Keros classification is the most common criteria used to assess the risk of injury to the anterior cranial base in functional endoscopic sinus surgery.

- Protrusions of the ICA into the sphenoid sinus are important anatomic variants to recognize during transsphenoidal surgery.

- The constant relationship of the external orifice of the vidian and palatovaginal canals and sphenopalatine artery can be used as an anatomic landmark when performing endoscopic vidian neurotomy.

- Advanced MRI techniques such as DKI and 3D-ASL may help differentiate VSs from CPA meningiomas.

DISCLOSURE

The authors have nothing to disclose.

REFERENCES

1. Chapman PR. Head and neck. Philadephia, PA: Elsevier; 2019.
2. Hallinan JTPD, Sia DSY, Yong C, et al. The sphenoid bone. In: Skull base imaging. St. Louis, MO: Elsevier; 2018. p. 39–64.
3. Ucar H, Bahsi I, Orhan M, et al. The Radiological Evaluation of the Crista Galli and Its Clinical Implications for Anterior Skull Base Surgery. J Craniofac Surg 2021;32(5):1928–30.
4. Lee JM, Ransom E, Lee JY, et al. Endoscopic anterior skull base surgery: intraoperative considerations of the crista galli. Skull Base 2011;21(2):83–6.
5. Socher JA, Santos PG, Correa VC, et al. Endoscopic surgery in the treatment of crista galli pneumatization evolving with localized frontal headaches. Int Arch Otorhinolaryngol 2013;17(3):246–50.
6. Shidanshid M, Taghi AS, Kuchai R, et al. Endoscopic resection of a mucocele of the crista galli. Ear Nose Throat J 2015;94(9):E23–5.
7. Barkovich AJ, Vandermarck P, Edwards MS, et al. Congenital nasal masses: CT and MR imaging features in 16 cases. AJNR Am J Neuroradiol 1991; 12(1):105–16.
8. Nair S, Ibrahim A. The Importance of Cribriform-Lamella Angle in Endoscopic Sinus Surgery. Indian J Otolaryngol Head Neck Surg 2021;73(1):66–71.
9. Babu AC, Nair M, Kuriakose AM. Olfactory fossa depth: CT analysis of 1200 patients. Indian J Radiol Imaging 2018;28(4):395–400.
10. Gupta A, Ghosh S, Roychoudhury A. Radiological and clinical correlations of the anterior ethmoidal artery in functional endoscopic sinus surgery. J Laryngol Otol 2022;136(2):154–7.
11. Adin ME, Ozmen CA, Aygun N. Utility of the Vidian Canal in Endoscopic Skull Base Surgery: Detailed Anatomy and Relationship to the Internal Carotid Artery. World Neurosurg 2019;121:e140–6.
12. Liu T, Li P, Meng Q, et al. [The role of palatovaginal canal and sphenopalatine artery in the localization of vidian canal during vidian neurotomy]. Lin Chung Er Bi Yan Hou Tou Jing Wai Ke Za Zhi 2020;34(7):606–9.
13. Baidya NB, Tang CT, Ammirati M. Intradural endoscope-assisted anterior clinoidectomy: a cadaveric study. Clin Neurol Neurosurg 2013;115(2):170–4.
14. Zhao X, Labib MA, Avci E, et al. Navigating a Carotico-Clinoid Foramen and an Interclinoidal Bridge in the Endonasal Endoscopic Approach: An Anatomical and Technical Note. J Neurol Surg B Skull Base 2021;82(5):534–9.
15. Twigg V, Carr SD, Balakumar R, et al. Radiological features for the approach in trans-sphenoidal pituitary surgery. Pituitary 2017;20(4):395–402.
16. Yeung W, Twigg V, Carr S, et al. Radiological "Teddy Bear" Sign on CT Imaging to Aid Internal Carotid Artery Localization in Transsphenoidal Pituitary and Anterior Skull Base Surgery. J Neurol Surg B Skull Base 2018;79(4):401–6.
17. Ginsberg LE, Pruett SW, Chen MY, et al. Skull-base foramina of the middle cranial fossa: reassessment of normal variation with high-resolution CT. AJNR Am J Neuroradiol 1994;15(2):283–91.
18. Ginsberg LE. The posterior condylar canal. AJNR Am J Neuroradiol 1994;15(5):969–72.
19. Spittau B, Millan DS, El-Sherifi S, et al. Dural arteriovenous fistulas of the hypoglossal canal: systematic review on imaging anatomy, clinical findings, and endovascular management. J Neurosurg 2015; 122(4):883–903.
20. Cyril C, Ofelia M, Herve D. Dural arteriovenous fistula involving the anterior condylar canal. J Neuroimaging 2013;23(3):425–8.
21. Liu JK, Mahaney K, Barnwell SL, et al. Dural arteriovenous fistula of the anterior condylar confluence and hypoglossal canal mimicking a jugular foramen tumor. J Neurosurg 2008;109(2):335–40.
22. Miyachi S, Ohshima T, Izumi T, et al. Dural arteriovenous fistula at the anterior condylar confluence. Interv Neuroradiol 2008;14(3):303–11.
23. Okahara M, Kiyosue H, Tanoue S, et al. Selective transvenous embolization of dural arteriovenous fistulas involving the hypoglossal canal. Interv Neuroradiol 2007;13(1):59–66.

24. Suyama K, Nakahara I, Matsumoto S, et al. Posterior condylar canal dural arteriovenous fistula treated with transvenous embolization through the deep cervical vein. J Stroke Cerebrovasc Dis 2022;31(12): 106808.

25. Kim JH, Lee CY. Posterior condylar canal dural arteriovenous fistula as a rare cause of glossopharyngeal neuralgia: A case report. Headache 2021; 61(8):1281–5.

26. Kiyosue H, Okahara M, Sagara Y, et al. Dural arteriovenous fistula involving the posterior condylar canal. AJNR Am J Neuroradiol 2007;28(8):1599–601.

27. Sia DSY, Yong C, Hallinan JTPD, et al. Anterior Skull Base. In: *Skull base imaging*. St. Louis, MO: Elsevier; 2018. p. 1–19.

28. Arnaout MM, Hanz SZ, Heier LA, et al. Prevalence and Outcome of Anterior and Middle Cranial Fossae Encephaloceles without Cerebrospinal Fluid Leak or Meningitis. World Neurosurg 2021;149:e828–35.

29. Ganjaei KG, Soler ZM, Mappus ED, et al. Novel Radiographic Assessment of the Cribriform Plate. Am J Rhinol Allergy 2018;32(3):175–80.

30. Langman M, Stopa BM, Cuoco JA, et al. Natural History of Traumatic Encephaloceles: A Systematic Literature Review. J Craniofac Surg 2022;34(1): 120–5.

31. Fernandez-Gajardo R, Almeida JP, Suppiah S, et al. Ethmoid Meningoencephalocele in a Patient with Cerebrofacial Arteriovenous Metameric Syndrome. World Neurosurg 2018;114:1–3.

32. Renaud M, Fath L, Cheptou M, et al. Iatrogenic meningoencephalocele after traumatic perforation of the cribriform plate during nasal intubation of a preterm infant. Int J Pediatr Otorhinolaryngol 2019;118: 120–3.

33. Shah N, Deopujari C, Bommakanti V. The reconstruction of skull base defects in infants using pedicled nasoseptal flap-a review of four cases. Childs Nerv Syst 2019;35(11):2157–62.

34. DeMonte F, Raza SM. Olfactory groove and planum meningiomas. Handb Clin Neurol 2020;170:3–12.

35. Fountas KN, Hadjigeorgiou GF, Kapsalaki EZ, et al. Surgical and functional outcome of olfactory groove meningiomas: Lessons from the past experience and strategy development. Clin Neurol Neurosurg 2018;171:46–52.

36. Zenga F, Penner F, Cofano F, et al. Trans-Frontal Sinus Approach for Olfactory Groove Meningiomas: A 19year Experience. Clin Neurol Neurosurg 2020; 196:106041.

37. Orgain CA, Kuan EC, Alvarado R, et al. Smell Preservation following Unilateral Endoscopic Transnasal Approach to Resection of Olfactory Groove Meningioma: A Multi-institutional Experience. J Neurol Surg B Skull Base 2020;81(3):263–7.

38. Salgues B, Graillon T, Guedj E. [(68)Ga]Ga-DOTA-TOC PET/CT fused to MRI in post-operative evaluation of olfactory groove meningioma: a case on millimetric remnants. Eur J Nucl Med Mol Imaging 2021;48(1):316–7.

39. Lufkin RB, Borges A, Villablanca P. Teaching atlas of head and neck imaging. New York: Thieme; 2000.

40. Roytman M, Tassler AB, Kacker A, et al. [68Ga]-DOTATATE PET/CT and PET/MRI in the diagnosis and management of esthesioneuroblastoma: illustrative cases. J Neurosurg Case Lessons 2021;1(2): CASE2058.

41. Verma P, Singh BK, Singh I, et al. Ga-68 DOTATATE Positron Emission Tomography/Computed Tomography in a Rare Case of Esthesioneuroblastoma. Indian J Nucl Med 2021;36(2):217–9.

42. Xiao Z, Tang Z, Qiang J, et al. Differentiation of olfactory neuroblastomas from nasal squamous cell carcinomas using MR diffusion kurtosis imaging and dynamic contrast-enhanced MRI. J Magn Reson Imaging 2018;47(2):354–61.

43. Hussaini AS, Swanson DD, Nguy PL, et al. Malignant Sarcomatous Degeneration of Craniofacial Fibrous Dysplasia. J Craniofac Surg 2022;33(6):1787–90.

44. Grover M, Gupta A, Samdhani S, et al. Anterior and Central Skull Base Fibrous Dysplasia: A 12 Years' Experience. Indian J Otolaryngol Head Neck Surg 2022;74(Suppl 2):1462–7.

45. Quirk B, Connor S. Skull base imaging, anatomy, pathology and protocols. Pract Neurol 2020;20(1): 39–49.

46. Banks KP, Ly JQ, Thompson LDR, et al. Mesenchymal chondrosarcoma of sinonasal cavity: a case report and brief literature review. Eur J Radiol Extra 2004;49(2):47–51.

47. Mahalingam HV, Mani SE, Patel B, et al. Imaging Spectrum of Cavernous Sinus Lesions with Histopathologic Correlation. Radiographics 2019;39(3): 795–819.

48. Korten AG, ter Berg HJ, Spincemaille GH, et al. Intracranial chondrosarcoma: review of the literature and report of 15 cases. J Neurol Neurosurg Psychiatry 1998;65(1):88–92.

49. Eller R, Sillers M. Common fibro-osseous lesions of the paranasal sinuses. Otolaryngol Clin North Am 2006;39(3):585–600, x.

50. Erdem E, Angtuaco EC, Van Hemert R, et al. Comprehensive review of intracranial chordoma. Radiographics 2003;23(4):995–1009.

51. Chapman PR, Choudhary G, Singhal A. Skull Base Osteomyelitis: A Comprehensive Imaging Review. AJNR Am J Neuroradiol 2021;42(3):404–13.

52. Chapman MN, Sakai O. In: Imaging of the Cerebellopontine Angle, In: *Skull base imaging*. St. Louis, MO: Elsevier; 2018. p. 247–68.

53. Bonneville F, Savatovsky J, Chiras J. Imaging of cerebellopontine angle lesions: an update. Part 1: enhancing extra-axial lesions. Eur Radiol 2007; 17(10):2472–82.

54. Smirniotopoulos JG, Yue NC, Rushing EJ. Cerebellopontine angle masses: radiologic-pathologic correlation. Radiographics 1993;13(5):1131–47.

55. Charabi S, Tos M, Thomsen J, et al. Cystic vestibular schwannoma–clinical and experimental studies. Acta Otolaryngol Suppl 2000;543:11–3.

56. Gomez-Brouchet A, Delisle MB, Cognard C, et al. Vestibular schwannomas: correlations between magnetic resonance imaging and histopathologic appearance. Otol Neurotol 2001;22(1):79–86.

57. Delsanti C, Regis J. [Cystic vestibular schwannomas]. Neurochirurgie 2004;50(2–3 Pt 2):401–6.

58. Okamoto K, Furusawa T, Ishikawa K, et al. Focal T2 hyperintensity in the dorsal brain stem in patients with vestibular schwannoma. AJNR Am J Neuroradiol 2006;27(6):1307–11.

59. Friedmann DR, Grobelny B, Golfinos JG, et al. Nonschwannoma tumors of the cerebellopontine angle. Otolaryngol Clin North Am 2015;48(3):461–75.

60. Hakyemez B, Erdogan C, Bolca N, et al. Evaluation of different cerebral mass lesions by perfusion-weighted MR imaging. J Magn Reson Imaging 2006;24(4):817–24.

61. Cho YD, Choi GH, Lee SP, et al. (1)H-MRS metabolic patterns for distinguishing between meningiomas and other brain tumors. Magn Reson Imaging 2003;21(6):663–72.

62. Lin L, Chen X, Jiang R, et al. Differentiation between vestibular schwannomas and meningiomas with atypical appearance using diffusion kurtosis imaging and three-dimensional arterial spin labeling imaging. Eur J Radiol 2018;109:13–8.

63. Bonneville F, Savatovsky J, Chiras J. Imaging of cerebellopontine angle lesions: an update. Part 2: intra-axial lesions, skull base lesions that may invade the CPA region, and non-enhancing extra-axial lesions. Eur Radiol 2007;17(11):2908–20.

64. Hasegawa M, Nouri M, Nagahisa S, et al. Cerebellopontine angle epidermoid cysts: clinical presentations and surgical outcome. Neurosurg Rev 2016;39(2):259–66. discussion: 266-257.

65. Hasegawa T, Wakamatsu K, Fujii T, et al. [Cerebellopontine angle epidermoid showing a positive enhancement upon metrizamide CT cisternography]. Rinsho Hoshasen 1985;30(4):497–500.

66. Chapman PR, Shah R, Cure JK, et al. Petrous apex lesions: pictorial review. AJR Am J Roentgenol 2011;196(3 Suppl):WS26–37. quiz: S40-23.

67. Bonneville F, Sarrazin JL, Marsot-Dupuch K, et al. Unusual lesions of the cerebellopontine angle: a segmental approach. Radiographics 2001;21(2):419–38.

68. Fernandez-de Thomas RJ, De Jesus O. Glomus Jugulare. In: StatPearls. FL: Treasure Island; 2022.

69. Ikram A, Rehman A. Paraganglioma. In: StatPearls. FL: Treasure Island; 2022.

70. Geng Y, Gu X, Lin M, et al. Endolymphatic sac tumour: exploring the role of CT and MRI features in the diagnosis of 22 cases. Clin Radiol 2022;77(8):e592–8.

71. Talmor G, Vakil M, Tseng C, et al. Petrous Apicitis: A Systematic Review and Case Presentation. Otol Neurotol 2022;43(7):753–65.

SUPPLEMENTARY DATA

Supplementary data related to this article can be found online at https://doi.org/10.1016/j.coms.2023.03.001.

Imaging of Major Salivary Gland Lesions and Disease

Elliott Friedman, MD[a],*, Yu Cai, MD, MS[b], Bo Chen, MD[c]

KEYWORDS

- Salivary gland • Sialoadenitis • Sialolithiasis • Salivary gland neoplasm • CT • MRI

KEY POINTS

- Computed tomography with contrast provides excellent anatomic resolution for the diagnosis of sialolithiasis and infectious or inflammatory disorders.
- MRI with contrast is needed to distinguish cystic from solid T2 hyperintense masses.
- Although some neoplasms have distinctive imaging features, imaging is not usually reliable to provide a specific histopathologic diagnosis of salivary gland tumors, and biopsy is usually required.
- Certain imaging features may be useful to suggest a mass is more likely benign or low-grade malignant versus a high-grade malignancy.

INTRODUCTION

Salivary glands are exocrine glands in the head and neck that produce saliva, which play a significant role in normal digestive function. A variety of pathologies can affect the salivary glands including infection, autoimmune disease, trauma, obstruction and inflammation, and neoplasia, as well as iatrogenic causes. Imaging of salivary glands plays a key role in diagnosing salivary gland disorders. Contrast-enhanced CT (CECT) is the most common initial diagnostic modality for salivary pathology in adults and is the imaging modality of choice for inflammatory and obstructive etiologies which represent the most commonly encountered pathologies. MRI has better soft-tissue resolution compared with CT and is the preferred imaging modality when a salivary mass is present. Ultrasound (US) is often the initial imaging modality of choice in children and can also complement CT and MRI in certain cases.[1]

SALIVARY GLAND ANATOMY

Parotid Glands

The parotid glands are the largest of the salivary glands and are located in the parotid space, which is enclosed by fascia from the superficial layer of the deep cervical fascia and situated anterior to the mastoid tip and external auditory canal (EAC), posterior to the masticator space, anterolateral to the carotid space and lateral to the parapharyngeal space. The anterior superficial aspect of the gland overlies the masseter muscle and mandible. The main parotid duct (Stensen's duct) drains into the oral cavity through the buccal mucosa opposite the upper second molar after coursing over the masseter and piercing the buccinator muscle.[1,2] Although classically divided into superficial and deep lobes based on the plane of the facial nerve, there is no actual anatomic division within the gland. As the facial nerve branches within the parotid gland are not well depicted on routine imaging, the retromandibular vein can be used to infer its location.[3] The parotid tail is the tissue at the inferior aspect of the superficial lobe, located between the platysma and posterior belly of the digastric muscle and anterolateral to the sternocleidomastoid muscle.[2] The deep lobe reflects a smaller portion of the gland that extends through the stylomandibular tunnel into the prestyloid parapharyngeal space. Pathology in this location is less accessible for clinical assessment.[3,4]

[a] Department of Radiology, Houston Methodist Hospital, 6565 Fannin Street, Houston, TX 77030, USA; [b] Ascension Seton Medical Center Austin, 1201 West 38th Street, Austin, TX 78705, USA; [c] Department of Diagnostic and Interventional Radiology, McGovern Medical School at the University of Texas HSC Houston, 6431 Fannin Street, MSB 2.130B, Houston, TX 77030, USA
* Corresponding author.
E-mail address: erfriedman@houstonmethodist.org

Oral Maxillofacial Surg Clin N Am 35 (2023) 435–449
https://doi.org/10.1016/j.coms.2023.02.007
1042-3699/23/© 2023 Elsevier Inc. All rights reserved.

Location of a mass within superficial or deep lobes of the parotid gland has surgical implications. Tumors limited to the superficial lobe can usually be treated by partial parotidectomy whereas total parotidectomy is often needed for deep lobe lesions. The goals of parotid tumor surgery are ideally complete tumor removal and facial nerve preservation, and imaging is crucial for accurate preoperative localization and staging.[1,5]

It is estimated that more than 20% of the normal population has accessory parotid glands(APGs), which are situated superficial to the masseter muscles. APGs are distinct from the main parotid gland and are located 6 mm anterior to it, as opposed to a facial process of the parotid which is a contiguous extension of tissue anteriorly over the masseter. APGs drain by a single accessory duct into Stensen's duct. APGs are susceptible to pathologies such as neoplasia and inflammation that occur in the parotid gland, however, sometimes the anterior location may be clinically confusing for a salivary pathology.[6]

A unique feature of parotid glands compared with other major salivary glands is that they contain lymph nodes, due to the parotid gland's relatively late encapsulation. The majority of lymph nodes are in the superficial lobe. The parotid nodes receive drainage from superficial soft tissues of the face and scalp and external ear, with efferent drainage into IIA and IIB nodes.[1] The presence of intraparotid lymph nodes explains the unique occurrence of Warthin tumor (WT) in the parotid gland as well as harboring regional and distant metastatic disease.[6,7]

Parotid glands tend to be mildly hypoattenuating with respect to muscle on non-contrast CT (NCCT) in adults and iso attenuating in children, due to differences in intraglandular fat. On MRI, normal parotid glands tend to be mildly hyperintense on T1-weighted imaging and T2-weighted imaging (T1WI and T2WI) with respect to muscle in adults and isointense in children. Parotid glands demonstrate diffuse enhancement after contrast administration.[2] Fat content of the parotids tends to increase with age and also tends to be higher in men[8] (**Fig. 1**).

Submandibular Glands

The submandibular gland forms a C shape, wrapping around the posterior free edge of the mylohyoid muscle which divides the gland into the larger superficial lobe in the submandibular space (SMS) and the deep lobe which projects into the posterior aspect of the sublingual space (SLS). The submandibular gland is located inferior to the mandible with the superficial lobe inferolateral to the mylohyoid and bounded by the anterior and posterior bellies of the digastric. The submandibular gland is separated from the parotid gland by the stylomandibular ligament. The SMS also contains lymph nodes, the facial artery and vein, and branches of the hypoglossal nerve.[1,3] If a mass is separated from the submandibular gland by the facial vein then it must be a lymph node or other extraglandular mass.[9] The main duct (Wharton's duct) exits the anteromedial aspect of the gland and courses anterior superiorly between the sublingual gland and genioglossus muscle to terminate at the sublingual papilla in the anterior floor of the mouth. The duct is larger in width than the papilla so sialoliths commonly become lodged at the junction.[1] A normal variant is a Stafne cyst, which is a well-defined radiographically lucent lesion in the posterior mandibular body from the intraosseous extension of submandibular tissue.[10]

On CT, the normal submandibular glands tend to be symmetric in size and with a density between muscle and the parotid glands. On MRI, submandibular glands are slightly T1 hypo and T2 hyperintense compared with parotid gland, with diffuse enhancement[2] (**Figs. 2 and 3**).

Sublingual Glands

The sublingual glands are the smallest of the major salivary glands, lying deep to the body of the mandible and lateral to the root of the tongue musculature within the SLS. The sublingual gland is not truly encapsulated and drains by numerous small ducts into the floor of the mouth, although sometimes some of the ducts fuse to form Bartholin's duct which drains into the main submandibular duct. The mylohyoid muscle sling separates the SLS and floor of the mouth from the submandibular and submental spaces. Posteriorly, there is free communication between the SMS and SLS, and the majority of people have a defect in the mylohyoid (boutonniere), which may contain herniated sublingual gland and provides another potential route of spread of disease between the SLS and SMS. The SLS also contains the lingual artery, nerve, and vein, part of the hyoglossus muscle, and the submandibular duct and deep lobe (**Fig. 2**).[11]

Minor Salivary Glands

The minor salivary glands are small aggregations of glandular tissue (~800–1000) scattered throughout the submucosa of the oral cavity, paranasal sinuses, pharynx, larynx, trachea, and bronchi.[1] The minor salivary glands are beyond the scope of this article. Large case reviews of intraoral minor salivary gland neoplasms yield a 40% to 50% malignancy rate, with the junction

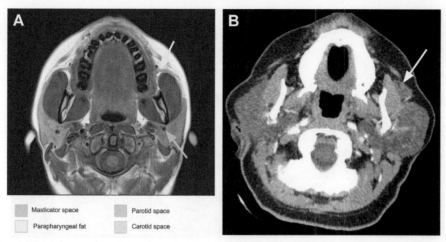

Fig. 1. (*A*) Axial T1WI image shows the parotid gland (*red shading*) in relation to adjacent spaces. Retromandibular vein (*green arrow*) and insertion of Stensen's duct (*yellow arrow*). (*B*) Axial NCCT shows APG anterior to the masseter (*white arrow*).

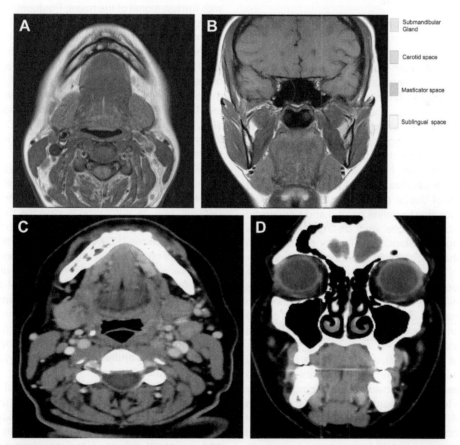

Fig. 2. (*A, B*) Axial (*A*) and coronal (*B*) T1WI show the normal appearance of the submandibular gland and its association with adjacent structures. (*C, D*) Axial (*C*) and coronal (*D*) CT show the normal appearance of the SLS and floor-of-mouth.

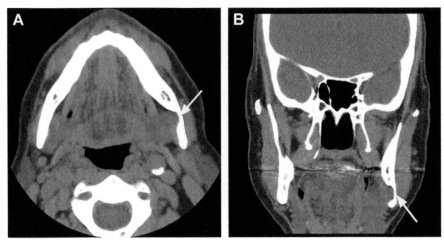

Fig. 3. (*A*, *B*) Axial (*A*) and coronal (*B*) NCCT images show a concave defect (*arrows*) in the left mandible with protrusion of submandibular tissue, a Stafne cyst.

of the hard and soft palate being a relatively common location.[12]

IMAGING TECHNIQUE

CT is the most common initial imaging modality performed for suspected salivary gland pathology. It is widely available and easily interpreted, provides excellent cross-sectional anatomic resolution, and evaluates for cervical lymphadenopathy. CT is also superior to MRI in assessing osseous changes such as bone destruction and foraminal enlargement. CECT is the preferred imaging modality for inflammatory disease and suspected calcifications. Contrast does not generally interfere with the ability to detect ductal calcifications yet provides excellent delineation of ductal dilatation and has excellent spatial resolution to define parotid and periparotid inflammatory changes and distinguish abscess from phlegmon. Standard CT neck protocol with venous phase acquisition is preferred. A face protocol can also be used but will not screen the whole neck for lymphadenopathy. In patients with significant beam hardening artifacts from dental amalgam or facial hardware, angled gantry acquisition may be needed to provide adequate image quality.[2]

CECT is also sensitive for detection of salivary gland masses, however, MRI with its improved soft-tissue contrast provides the imaging modality of choice for assessment of salivary gland tumors (SGTs). MRI adequately defines local extension of tumor, including extraglandular extension and perineural spread.[13] MRI techniques vary by institution but generally include axial and coronal noncontrast T1WI without fat saturation (FS) and

T1FS + C as well as some combination of axial and coronal T2WI without and with FS. T1 precontrast images are performed without FS because the bright signal of the fat provides good contrast with the low signal of the mass. Postcontrast imaging is necessary to distinguish whether a T2 hyperintense mass is cystic or solid, and to delineate perineural disease. Diffusion-weighted imaging (DWI) is also recommended to allow apparent diffusion coefficient (ADC) analysis of salivary masses.[14] Advanced imaging techniques, such as MRI perfusion and spectroscopy imaging, are also being used in combination with DWI/ADC analysis to help distinguish benign from malignant salivary neoplasms.[15,16]

US is able to distinguish solid from cystic salivary masses, detect sialolithiasis, diagnose and follow-up acute and chronic inflammatory disorders as well as autoimmune disease (Sjogren's syndrome) of the major salivary glands, and evaluate lymph nodes.[17] Given its lack of ionizing radiation, US is often the first imaging study performed for salivary disorders in children. US is useful to guide fine needle aspiration biopsies of salivary gland masses and cervical lymphadenopathy. US is limited compared with CT and MRI in assessing deeper spaces of the neck, skull base, and floor of the mouth. Additionally, US is operator-dependent, and artifacts may obscure evaluation or confuse the diagnosis.[18]

Fluorodeoxyglucose (FDG)-PET detects areas of increased metabolic activity and is used for staging and restaging many types of cancers and monitoring response to therapy. As both benign and malignant salivary gland neoplasms as well as non-neoplastic entities such as inflammatory diseases may be FDG avid, FDG-PET has limited value in the initial diagnosis of SGTs. FDG-PET can however be extremely useful for evaluating metastatic disease and in post-treatment cases, both for defining the extent of residual or recurrent disease and providing prognostic information.[19]

Sialography is generally not a first-line imaging study. MR sialography, obtained with heavily T2-weighted sequences provides a noninvasive alternative to conventional or digital subtraction sialography in the detection of sialolithiasis, ductal stenoses, and ectasia, which helps evaluate disorders such as chronic recurrent sialoadenitis, Sjogren syndrome (SjS), juvenile recurrent parotitis, and post-trauma.[20]

SALIVARY GLAND PATHOLOGY
Non-neoplastic Etiologies

Sialadenitis
Inflammatory pathologies are the most common disorders to affect the salivary glands. The choice of imaging modality varies with the suspected cause and location but generally CT or US is employed initially for suspected obstructive or inflammatory disease.[21]

Sialolithiasis
The majority of salivary gland stones occur in the submandibular gland and are most commonly solitary. Most submandibular calculi are located in the main duct, most commonly at the ostium or along the bend at the posterior margin of the mylohyoid. The opening of Wharton's duct is narrower than the caliber of the duct, resulting in stone impaction at this point. Submandibular duct stones are more likely to be chronic than parotid duct stones and may present with intermittent symptoms. Chronic sialolithiasis may demonstrate glandular atrophy. Tiny asymptomatic calculi within the parotid glands are sometimes present on CT scans.[1]

CT has increased sensitivity over plain films for detecting focal calcifications. It has been estimated that 20% of submandibular stones and 40% of parotid stones may not be detected on plain films.[1] Suspected cases of uncomplicated sialolithiasis have traditionally been imaged with NCCT due to concerns that contrast might interfere with the ability to detect calcified stones. CECT, however, has not been shown to have significantly decreased sensitivity compared with NCCT for the detection of obstructive sialolithiasis and allows for evaluation of potential complications like glandular inflammation or abscess or alternative diagnosis, such as tumor.[22] NCCT images are not indicated due to unnecessary radiation. Dual-energy CT techniques allow for virtual unenhanced CT images.[23] US is effective at diagnosing sialolithiasis, especially stones > 2 mm, and is often the first-line modality in children. MRI is less sensitive than CT at detecting calcifications but MR sialography can identify radiolucent stones as hypointense foci in a dilated duct[24] (**Fig. 4**).

Infectious sialadenitis
Acute suppurative (bacterial) sialadenitis most commonly presents as acute painful unilateral salivary gland swelling, more commonly affecting the parotid than the submandibular glands. Acutely on CT and MRI, there is unilateral glandular enlargement with increased enhancement, ductal dilatation, edema in the adjacent fat, reactive lymphadenopathy, and potential spread of infectious/inflammatory changes into adjacent muscles and soft tissues. T2 signal can be high or low depending on whether more edema or cellular infiltrate is present. US most commonly shows an enlarged, hypoechoic gland. Imaging is helpful to detect findings such as a drainable abscess or large obstructing calculus that indicate the process is unlikely to respond to conservative treatment alone (**Fig. 5**).

Viral sialadenitis worldwide is most commonly due to the mumps virus, although it is a much less common cause in the United States. Different from bacterial sialadenitis, viral infection may begin with a prodromal period. On imaging, there

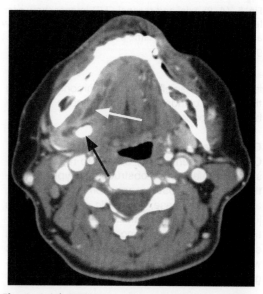

Fig. 4. Axial CECT image in a patient with "submandibular swelling." Dilated Wharton's duct (*white arrow*) with large calcified stone at the submandibular gland hilum (*blue arrow*). Note that intravenous contrast does not interfere with delineation of the calcified stone.

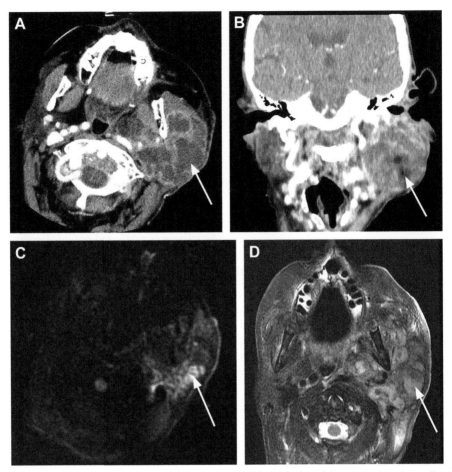

Fig. 5. (*A, B*) Axial and coronal CECT images show a large multiloculated peripherally enhancing collection in the left parotid gland (*arrows*) and adjacent soft tissues which were confirmed to be an abscess. (*C, D*) DWI (*C*) and axial T2FSWI (*D*) in the same patient show areas of restricted diffusion and T2 hyperintensity (*arrows*) in the pyogenic abscess.

is edema and swelling most commonly affecting the parotid glands bilaterally, although this may be asynchronous[24] (**Figs. 6 and 7**).

Chronic sialadenitis

Chronic sialadenitis may be due to repeated episodes of infection or obstruction, atypical infections, HIV sialopathy, granulomatous disease, autoimmune disease, idiopathic entities such as juvenile recurrent parotitis, and chronic post-treatment sequela among other causes. With chronic sialadenitis, imaging appearance varies with the underlying pathology, as well as the degree and duration of inflammation.[1,24]

Human immunodeficiency virus sialopathy

An uncommon manifestation of human immunodeficiency virus (HIV) is painless bilateral parotid gland enlargement with cystic, partially cystic, and/or solid lesions (benign lymphoepithelial

lesions) and lymphadenopathy.[24] On US, the cysts may not be purely anechoic and may demonstrate internal septa.[25] The imaging appearance can mimic SjS and sarcoidosis, but in addition to a different clinical profile, the presence of cervical lymphadenopathy and adenotonsillar hyperplasia helps to distinguish HIV-related parotid disease from SjS.[24] Glandular calcifications are not expected with HIV-related parotid disease (**Fig. 8**).

Autoimmune disease

SjS causes autoimmune-mediated inflammation of the salivary glands. The imaging appearance varies with the stage of the disease. Early on, the glands may appear normal, with subsequent gland enlargement and a miliary pattern of tiny bilateral cyst formation. Over time, there is development of larger cysts and mixed cystic and solid lesions as well as solid lymphocytic aggregates, with premature fat deposition, punctate calcifications, and

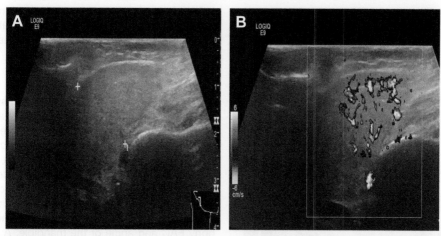

Fig. 6. (*A*, *B*) Grayscale (*A*) and color Doppler (*B*) US images show an enlarged parotid gland with increased vascularity in a patient with viral parotitis.

eventual atrophy and micronodularity. On CT, the gland initially develops hyperattenuation followed by a honeycomb appearance.[26] A characteristic "salt and pepper" appearance has been described on MRI.[27] MR sialography has been found to be sufficiently accurate compared with conventional sialography in staging the disease. Initial punctate peripheral ductal sialectasis progresses to larger globular and ultimately cavitary and destructive lesions, as well as areas of stenosis and dilatation in the parotid duct and truncated intraglandular branches.[28] Any dominant solid parotid mass in SjS should be concerning for development of lymphoma[1] (**Fig. 9**).

Sarcoidosis

Salivary manifestations of sarcoidosis affect a minority of patients, and may affect multiple glands simultaneously, most commonly bilateral. Imaging findings are nonspecific and may mimic other inflammatory or neoplastic conditions. Most commonly multiple noncavitary salivary masses are present with an appearance sometimes described as "foamy" on cross-sectional imaging. Heerfordt's syndrome, an association with facial nerve paralysis, can confuse for a malignant diagnosis. The panda sign on Gallium-67 citrate scintigraphy (bilateral lacrimal and parotid gland and nasopharyngeal tracer uptake) is characteristic of sarcoidosis.[1,29]

Post-radiation sialadenitis

Radiation-induced sialadenitis may occur after conventional 2D radiotherapy for oral cavity or pharyngeal cancers, most commonly affecting the parotid gland which may be within or in

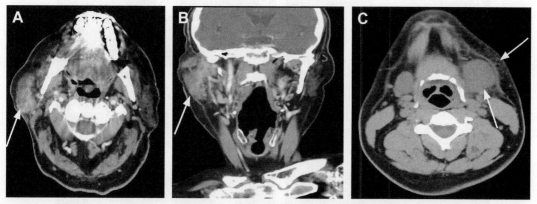

Fig. 7. (*A*, *B*) Axial (*A*) and coronal (*B*) CECT shows an enlarged, heterogeneously enhancing right parotid gland (*arrows*) and mild subcutaneous edema in a patient with parotitis. (*C*) Axial CECT in a patient with submandibular sialadenitis shows an enlarged left submandibular gland (*white arrow*) with overlying edema (*yellow arrow*) and mild platysma thickening.

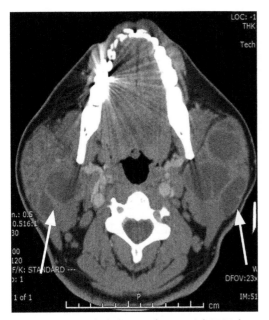

Fig. 8. Benign epithelial cysts of HIV. Axial CECT shows bilateral parotid enlargement with circumscribed cysts demonstrating rim enhancement (*arrows*).

proximity to the radiated field. Radiation injury is less severe with modern conformal techniques. Chronic changes on imaging include decreased gland size with diffuse enhancement, low T1 and T2 signal on MRI, and hyperattenuation on CT. US shows heterogeneous echotexture with hypoechogenic foci and echogenic lines.[30]

Radioactive iodine used to treat thyroid cancers accumulates in the saliva and results in dose-dependent injury to the salivary glands.[31] There is a decrease in salivary gland size and increased parotid attenuation on NCCT. MR sialography shows ductal stenosis and sialectasis as well as nonvisualized ducts.[24]

Cystic lesions

Cystic lesions can be seen with HIV-associated salivary disease, SjS, and sarcoidosis as previously discussed. Sialoceles may form after trauma or surgery. A number of developmental cysts can occur within or adjacent to the major salivary glands. Among these, first branchial cleft cysts appear on imaging as a cyst in or around the parotid gland, near the pinna or EAC, or along a tract between the junction of the membranous and bony EAC and angle of the mandible. A fistulous connection to the EAC can be present. There is usually no or minimal peripheral enhancement unless the cyst is infected[32] (**Figs. 10 and 11**).

Simple ranulas are mucosal retention cysts arising from the sublingual gland or minor salivary glands of the SLS and appear on imaging as a simple cyst confined to the floor of the mouth. Diving or plunging ranulas are pseudocysts resulting from rupture of a simple ranula and classically have a tail in the SLS and body of the cyst below the mylohyoid in the SMS. The collapsed fluid-filled SLS component referred to as the tail sign is considered pathognomonic and can be detected by US, CT, or MRI. Ranulas can become infected which will show thicker peripheral enhancement and may alter the internal T1 and T2 signals.[33] The differential diagnosis for cystic lesions in this region includes floor-of-mouth dermoid or epidermoid, lymphatic malformation, abscess, suppurative lymph nodes, cystic salivary

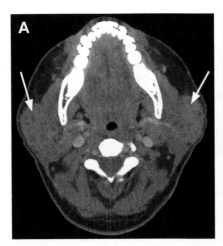

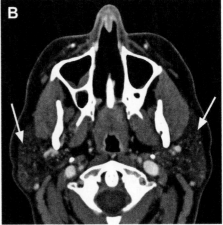

Fig. 9. (*A*) Axial CECT in a patient with SjS shows enlargement of the parotid glands bilaterally with numerous tiny hypodense cysts (*arrows*). (*B*) Axial CECT in a patient with late-stage SjS shows liposubstitution (fatty replacement) and punctate calcifications of the parotid glands bilaterally (*arrows*).

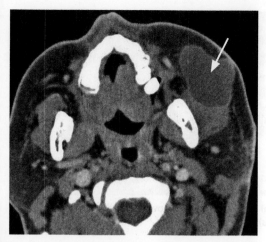

Fig. 10. Axial CECT shows a well-demarcated, low-density cystic lesion in the left masticator space compressing against the anterior aspect of the masseter in the region of Stensen's duct, a posttraumatic sialocele (*arrow*).

neoplasm, and submandibular gland mucocele (**Fig. 12**).

Tumors and Tumor-Like Conditions

SGTs are a histologically diverse group of neoplasms, consisting of benign and malignant epithelial and nonepithelial tumors. The proportion of benign to malignant neoplasms varies by the gland involved, with the risk of malignancy in adults increasing as gland size decreases for the major salivary glands. The majority of parotid gland tumors in adults are benign, submandibular gland tumors are more evenly split between benign and malignant, and the majority of sublingual gland tumors are malignant, such that regardless of appearance, sublingual masses should be considered malignant until proven otherwise. SGTs in children are more likely to be malignant.[34]

CT has good spatial resolution but is limited for soft-tissue characterization compared with MRI. Although some SGTs have characteristic imaging features by MRI, many imaging findings are nonspecific or demonstrate considerable overlap between benign and malignant tumors as well as some non-neoplastic entities such as inflammatory diseases. Ultimately, biopsy is usually needed to establish a definitive histopathologic diagnosis.

Certain imaging features can be useful in predicting that a SGT is more likely to be malignant, although not infallible. Irregular tumor margins, extraglandular extension, low T2 signal, low ADC value, rapid growth, perineural spread, and nodal metastasis are all features that may suggest a mass is more likely to be malignant. Infectious or inflammatory processes can mimic these characteristics with some processes having poorly defined margins, extraglandular spread, facial nerve enhancement, low T2 signal, lymphadenopathy, and rapid growth. Benign tumors may be complicated by sialadenitis. Some low-grade malignancies, such as mucoepidermoid carcinoma, can have well-defined margins. Slow growth rate cannot be used to assume benignity because some malignant SGTs such as adenoid cystic carcinoma are notoriously slow growing.[34] WT can rarely present with cervical nodal involvement[35] (**Fig. 13**).

Solid malignancies in the neck are more likely to have lower ADC values than benign lesions,

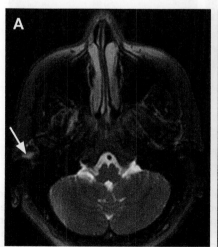
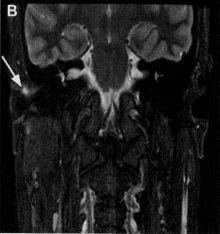

Fig. 11. (*A, B*) T2FSWI axial (*A*) and coronal (*B*) images show a small T2 hyperintense cyst (*white arrows*) adjacent to the right EAC, a first branchial cleft cyst.

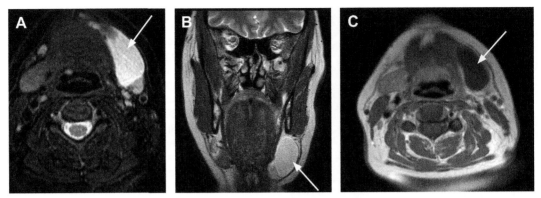

Fig. 12. (*A–C*) Axial T2FSWI (*A*), coronal T2WI (*B*), and axial T1+C (*C*) images show a well-demarcated T2 hyperintense cyst with rim enhancement in the left SMS (*arrows*), a diving ranula.

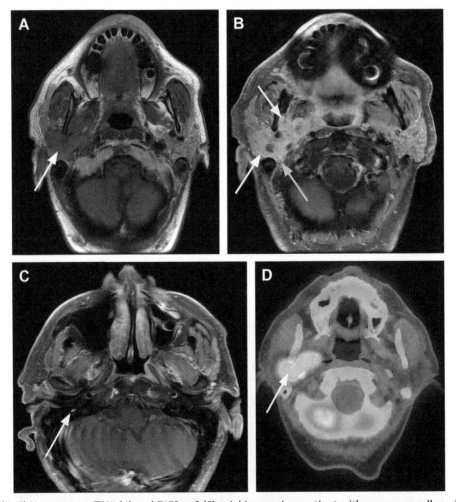

Fig. 13. (*A, B*) Non-contrast TIWI (*A*) and T1FS + C (*B*) axial images in a patient with squamous cell carcinoma of the parotid gland show an enhancing soft-tissue mass involving the superficial and deep lobes of the right parotid gland (*white arrows*). Margins are poorly defined particularly along the deep aspect. Perineural spread with enhancement of the inferior alveolar nerve (V3) at the mandibular foramen (*yellow arrow, B*) and tumor extending to the stylomastoid foramen (*green arrow, B*). (*C*) T1FS + C image at a higher level than image *B* shows enhancement of the mastoid segment of the right facial nerve (*arrow*) from retrograde perineural tumor spread. (*D*) PET/CT image shows intense FDG avidity in the tumor (*arrow*).

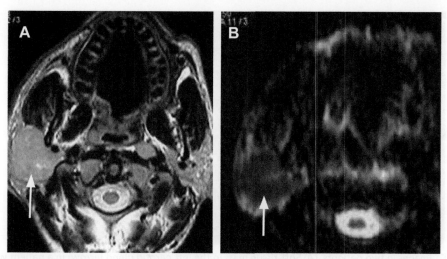

Fig. 14. (A) Axial T2WI shows a hyperintense mass in right parotid gland (*white arrow*). (B) ADC map shows low ADC values in the mass (*white arrow*). Pathology-proven mucoepidermoid carcinoma.

however, there is overlap in ADC values between benign and malignant SGTs. Only pleomorphic adenoma (PA) was significantly distinguishable from other SGT due to its facilitated diffusion (high ADC).[14] DWI can also be used for post-treatment follow-up with low ADC soft tissue more concerning for recurrent tumor[36] (**Fig. 14**).

There is a wide overlap in the imaging appearance of salivary gland malignancies. Mucoepidermoid carcinoma, the most common malignant SGT, can have a wide variety of imaging appearances, which tend to vary with tumor grade.[37] Adenoid cystic carcinoma has the highest tendency for perineural spread.[38] Multiple solid masses in the parotid glands may reflect lymphoma, metastatic or another lymphadenopathy,

multifocal WT, oncocytoma, recurrent PA, or granulomatous disease (**Figs. 15 and 16**).

Some benign SGTs have characteristic imaging findings. PA, the most common SGT, is most frequently a solitary T2 hyperintense, enhancing mass, with high ADC values in the superficial lobe of the parotid gland. Larger masses may have a heterogeneous appearance and dystrophic calcifications may be present. T2 signal higher than cerebrospinal fluid is specific for PA.[1,14,39] Rapid growth, development of irregular margins or areas of low T2 or ADC signal, and pathologic lymphadenopathy is concerning for malignant degeneration into carcinoma ex-PA[40] (**Figs. 17 and 18**).

WT, the second most common benign SGT, is a smoking-induced tumor in older adults. It occurs

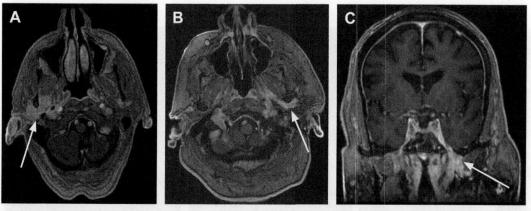

Fig. 15. Perineural spread in two patients. Axial T1FS + C image (A) shows thickened enhancement along the right auriculotemporal nerve (*arrow*). Axial (B) and coronal (C) T1FS + C in another patient shows perineural spread along the left auriculotemporal nerve (*arrow, B*) and extending retrograde along V3 branches to foramen ovale (*arrow, C*).

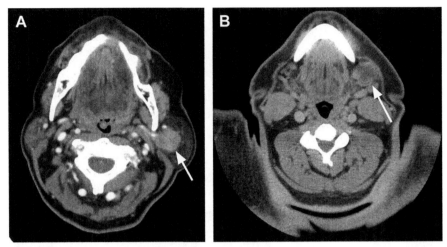

Fig. 16. CECT images in two patients. (*A*) Soft-tissue mass in the left parotid gland (*arrow*) in a patient with renal cell carcinoma. Pathology-proven nodal metastasis. (*B*) Patient with left buccal space squamous cell carcinoma shows a heterogenous metastatic SMS lymph node (*arrow*). Unlike the parotid glands, the submandibular glands do not contain lymph nodes within the gland substance.

almost exclusively in the parotid glands, characteristically at the parotid tail, and may be multifocal and bilateral. Although benign, low ADC values are characteristic, similar to low ADC values seen in malignancies.[41] Oncocytomas are rare benign tumors worth mentioning because they have a characteristic inconspicuous appearance within the parotid gland on T2FSWI and T1FS + C and are therefore known as "vanishing tumors."[42] Certain mesenchymal tumors may also have characteristic appearances. Lipomas obviously consist of diffuse fat signal. Nerve sheath tumors in the salivary glands are rare but may sometimes demonstrate a target sign of hypointense central and hyperintense peripheral T2 signal.[43] Vascular malformations and hemangiomas uncommonly occur in the salivary glands with imaging appearances as demonstrated elsewhere in the head and neck (**Figs. 19 and 20**).

Imaging plays a key role in staging of salivary gland cancers. Locoregional tumor, nodes, metastasis staging is largely a function of the size of the mass and involvement of adjacent structures, size and laterality of nodal disease and whether more than one node is involved, and the presence of extraglandular or extranodal extension.[44] Postcontrast imaging is crucial to delineate perineural spread, primarily involving the facial nerve or the auriculotemporal nerve, or trigeminal nerve branches.[45]

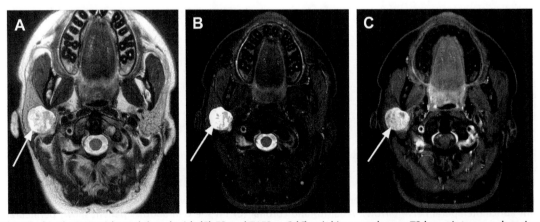

Fig. 17. (*A–C*) T2WI without (*A*) and with (*B*) FS and T1FS + C (*C*) axial images show a T2 hyperintense enhancing mass in the right parotid gland (*arrows*) spanning the stylomandibular tunnel. Pathology-proven PA.

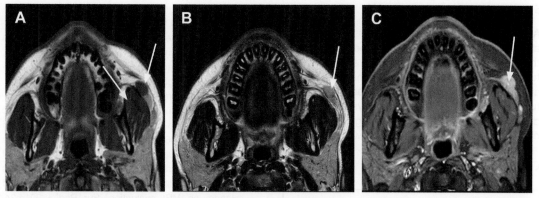

Fig. 18. (*A–C*) MRI axial T1WI (*A*), T2WI (*B*), and T1FS + C (*C*) images show a small enhancing mass (*white arrows*), overlying the masseter muscle (*yellow arrow*, *A*). Pathology-proven PA of the APG.

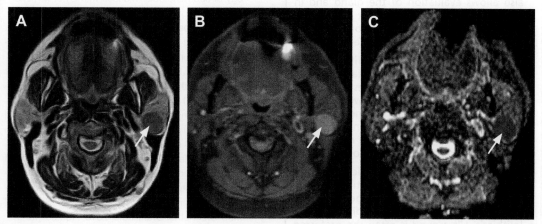

Fig. 19. (*A–C*) Axial T2WI (*A*), T1FS + C (*B*), and ADC map (*C*) of an older male patient with a pathologically-proven WT show a sharply demarcated homogenous low T2 signal enhancing mass with characteristic low ADC values in the left parotid tail (*arrows*). Some WT may have cystic components.

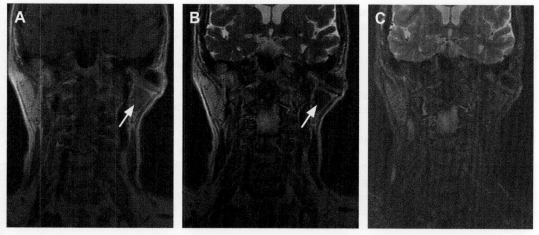

Fig. 20. (*A–C*) Coronal T1WI (*A*), T2WI (*B*), and T2FSWI (*C*) images in a patient with pathologically-proven oncocytoma show a low T1 and T2 signal left parotid mass (*arrows*), which becomes inconspicuous with FS (*C*).

SUMMARY

An incredible variety of pathology occurs within and around the salivary glands including sialolithiasis, a wide range of infectious and inflammatory disorders as well as autoimmune diseases, and a range of benign and malignant tumors and tumor-like conditions. Imaging plays a key role in diagnosis and treatment planning, and in the case of SGTs, post-treatment follow-up.

CLINICS CARE POINTS

- Noncontrast CT is unnecessary for sialolithiasis evaluation, as vessels and calculi are different densities. Contrast-enhanced CT also allows evaluation of the gland and in the case of submandibular duct obstruction for a potential obstructing floor of mouth mass, in addition to calculus detection.

- MRI is the best imaging modality to assess salivary gland tumors, and certain imaging features can be used to suggest a mass is more likely to be malignant. However, given the overlap in imaging appearance of malignant SGTs as well as some benign tumors, biopsy is often necessary to establish a definitive histopathologic diagnosis.

- Ultrasound can distinguish cystic from solid masses and provides another option for evaluation of submandibular or superficial lobe parotid masses or inflammatory disease or sialolithiasis. Ultrasound is often the preferred initial imaging modality for evaluation of major salivary gland disease in children.

DISCLOSURE

None of the authors have any relevant disclosures related to the content of this article.

REFERENCES

1. Som PM, Brandwein-Gensler M. In: Chapter 40: Anatomy and pathology of the salivary glands, In: *Head and neck imaging.* St Louis, MO: Mosby Elsevier; 2011. p. 2449–609.
2. Atkinson C, Fuller J, Huang B. Cross-sectional Imaging Techniques and Normal Anatomy of the Salivary Glands. Neuroimaging Cl N Am 2018;28(2):137–58.
3. Kessler AT, Bhatt AA. Review of the Major and Minor Salivary Glands, Part 1: Anatomy, Infectious, and Inflammatory Processes. J Clin Imaging Sci 2018;8:47.
4. Bag AK, Curé JK, Chapman PR, et al. Practical imaging of the parotid gland. Curr Probl Diagn Radiol 2015;44:167–92.
5. Guntinas-Lichius O, Silver CE, Thielker J, et al. Management of the facial nerve in parotid cancer: preservation or resection and reconstruction. Eur Arch Oto-Rhino-Laryngol 2018;275:2615–26.
6. Rosa MA, Łazarz DP, Pękala JR, et al. The accessory parotid gland and its clinical significance. J Craniofac Surg 2020;31:856–60.
7. Nuyens M, Schüpbach J, Stauffer E, et al. Metastatic disease to the parotid gland. Otolaryngol Head Neck Surg 2006 Dec;135:844–8.
8. Chang HC, Juan CJ, Chiu HC, et al. Effects of gender, age, and body mass index on fat contents and apparent diffusion coefficients in healthy parotid glands: an MRI evaluation. Eur Radiol 2014;24:2069–76.
9. Weissman JL, Carrau RL. Anterior facial vein and submandibular gland together: predicting the histology of submandibular masses with CT or MR imaging. Radiology 1998;208:441–6.
10. Aps JKM, Koelmeyer N, Yaqub C. Stafne's bone cyst revisited and renamed: the benign mandibular concavity. Dentomaxillofac Radiol 2020;49:20190475.
11. La'porte SJ, Juttla JK, Lingam RK. Imaging the floor of the mouth and the sublingual space. Radiographics 2011;31:1215–30.
12. Pires FR, Pringle GA, de Almeida OP, et al. Intra-oral minor salivary gland tumors: a clinicopathological study of 546 cases. Oral Oncol 2007;43:463–70.
13. Liu Y, Li J, Tan YR, et al. Accuracy of diagnosis of salivary gland tumors with the use of ultrasonography, computed tomography, and magnetic resonance imaging: a meta-analysis. Oral Surg Oral Med Oral Pathol Oral Radiol 2015;119:238–45.
14. Habermann CR, Arndt C, Graessner J, et al. Diffusion-weighted echo-planar MR Imaging of primary parotid gland tumors: Is a prediction of different histologic subtypes possible? AJNR Am J Neuroradiol 2009;30:591–6.
15. Razek AA, Samir S, Ashmalla GA. Characterization of parotid tumors with dynamic susceptibility contrast perfusion-weighted Magnetic Resonance Imaging and diffusion-weighted imaging. J Comput Assist Tomogr 2017;41:131–6.
16. King AD, Yeung DK, Ahuja AT, et al. Salivary gland tumors at in vivo Proton MR Spectroscopy. Radiol 2005;237:563–9.
17. Katz P, Hartl DM, Guerre A. Clinical ultrasound of the salivary glands. Otolaryngol Clin North Am 2009;42:973–1000.
18. Białek EJ, Jakubowski W. Mistakes in ultrasound examination of salivary glands. J Ultrason 2016;16:191–203.
19. Larson CR, Wiggins RH. FDG-PET Imaging of Salivary Gland Tumors. Semin Ultrasound CT MR 2019;40:391–9.
20. Kalinowski M, Heverhagen JT, Rehberg E, et al. Comparative study of MR sialography and digital

subtraction sialography for benign salivary gland disorders. AJNR Am J Neuroradiol 2002 Oct;23:1485–92.

21. Madani G, Beale T. Inflammatory conditions of the salivary glands. Semin Ultrasound CT MR 2006 Dec;27:440–51.

22. Purcell YM, Kavanagh RG, Cahalane AM, et al. The Diagnostic Accuracy of Contrast-Enhanced CT of the Neck for the Investigation of Sialolithiasis. AJNR Am J Neuroradiol 2017;38:2161–6.

23. Pulickal GG, Singh D, Lohan R, et al. Dual-Source Dual-Energy CT in Submandibular Sialolithiasis: Reliability and Radiation Burden. AJR Am J Roentgenol 2019;213:1291–6.

24. Abdel Razek AAK, Mukherji S. Imaging of sialadenitis. NeuroRadiol J 2017;30:205–15.

25. Martinoli C, Pretolesi F, Del Bono V, et al. Benign lymphoepithelial parotid lesions in HIV-positive patients: spectrum of findings at gray-scale and Doppler sonography. AJR Am J Roentgenol 1995;165:975–9.

26. Sun Z, Zhang Z, Fu K, et al. Diagnostic accuracy of parotid CT for identifying Sjögren's syndrome. Eur J Radiol 2012;81:2702–9.

27. Takashima S, Takeuchi N, Morimoto S, et al. MR Imaging of Sjögren Syndrome: Correlation with Sialography and Pathology. J Comput Assist Tomogr 1991; 15:393–400.

28. Cho A, Lee YR, Jeon YT, et al. Correlations of MR Sialographic Gradings with the Clinical Measures of Sjögren's Syndrome. Laryngoscope 2022. https://doi.org/10.1002/lary.30150.

29. Chapman MN, Fujita A, Sung EK, et al. Sarcoidosis in the Head and Neck: An Illustrative Review of Clinical Presentations and Imaging Findings. AJR Am J Roentgenol 2017;208:66–75.

30. Cheng SC, Wu VW, Kwong DL, et al. Assessment of post-radiotherapy salivary glands. Br J Radiol 2011; 84:393–402.

31. Mandel S, Mandel L. Radioactive iodine and the salivary glands. Thyroid 2003;13:265–71.

32. Friedman E, Patiño MO, Udayasankar U. Imaging of Pediatric Salivary Glands. Neuroimaging Clin N Am 2018;28:209–26.

33. Kurabayashi T, Ida M, Yasumoto M, et al. MRI of ranulas. Neuroradiology 2000;42:917–22.

34. Friedman E, Patino MO, Abdel Razek AAK. MR Imaging of Salivary Gland Tumors. Magn Reson Imaging Clin N Am 2022;30:135–49.

35. Rimmer RA, Cottrill EE. Multifocal Warthin's Tumor: An Uncommon Presentation of Bilateral Cervical Lymphadenopathy. Case Rep Otolaryngol 2018; 2018:3791825.

36. Razek AA, Mukherji SK. Imaging of posttreatment salivary gland tumors. Neuroimag Clin N Am 2018; 28:199–208.

37. Kashiwagi N, Dote K, Kawano K, et al. MRI findings of mucoepidermoid carcinoma of the parotid gland: Correlation with pathologic features. Br J Radiol 2012;85:709–13.

38. Hanna E, Vural E, Prokopakis E, et al. The sensitivity and specificity of high-resolution imaging in evaluating perineural spread of adenoid cystic carcinoma to the skull base. Arch Otolaryngol Head Neck Surg 2007;133:541–5.

39. Tsushima Y, Matsumoto M, Endo K, et al. Characteristic bright signal of parotid pleomorphic adenomas on T2-weighted MR images with pathologic correlation. Clin Radiol 1994;49:485–9.

40. Kato H, Kanematsu M, Mizuta K, et al. Carcinoma ex pleomorphic adenoma of the parotid gland: Radiologic-pathologic correlation with MR imaging including diffusion-weighted imaging. AJNR Am J Neuroradiol 2008;29:865–7.

41. Ikeda M, Motoori K, Hanazawa T, et al. Warthin tumor of the parotid gland: Diagnostic Value of MR Imaging with histopathologic correlation. AJNR Am J Neuroradiol 2004;25:1256–62.

42. Patel ND, Zante AV, Eisele DW, et al. Oncocytoma: The vanishing parotid mass. AJNR Am J Neuroradiol 2011;32:1703–6.

43. Shimizu K, Iwai H, Ikeda K, et al. Intraparotid facial nerve schwannoma: a report of five cases and an analysis of MR imaging results. AJNR Am J Neuroradiol 2005;26:1328–30.

44. Amin MB, Edge SB, Greene FL, et al, editors. AJCC cancer staging manual. 8th edition. Chicago: Springer; 2017.

45. Schmalfuss IM, Tart RP, Mukherji S, et al. Perineural tumor spread along the auriculotemporal nerve. AJNR Am J Neuroradiol 2002;23:303–11.

Image-Guided Biopsies of Superficial and Deep Head and Neck and Skull-Base Lesions

Amit Agarwal, MD[a],*, John Murray, MD[a], S. Johnny Sandhu, MD[a]

KEYWORDS

• Neoplasm • Image-guided • Core • FNA • Biopsy • Procedure

KEY POINTS

- Excellent anatomical knowledge is required for head and neck biopsies given the critical structures in the region, including vital nerves and vessels.
- Core needle biopsies provide larger tissue samples with higher diagnostic accuracy as compared with fine-needle aspirations.
- Ultrasound should be the preferred modality for most superficial lesions, whereas computed tomography is generally the choice for deep neck lesions.
- Meticulous planning, and good pre- and post-procedural care are essential parts of a successful procedure.
- Although minor complications are occasionally seen, major complications with image-guided head and neck biopsies are extremely rare.

INTRODUCTION

Image-guided biopsies have largely replaced open surgical techniques as the preferred method for establishing a histologic diagnosis for most of head and neck (H&N) pathologies and add tremendous value in terms of accuracy, safety, efficacy, lower cost, and overall better patient care. Dedicated H&N radiologists or neuroradiologists with expertise in H&N disease, now form an essential part of the multidisciplinary ear nose throat (ENT) team. They can best provide high-quality care, both in the diagnostic and interventional realm, given the critical anatomy in the region of the biopsies, including major nerves and vessels. Over the past decade, there has been increasing subspecialization in the field of neuroradiology with many large centers having dedicated H&N radiologists or a small set of neuroradiologists with subspecialty expertise.[1,2] As the number of requisitions for percutaneous image-guided biopsies has increased tremendously, so has interest among radiologists.

H&N intervention is still an evolving field, and this service line is managed differently at different centers by interventional radiologists, abdominal radiologists, musculoskeletal radiologists, neurointerventional surgeons, and neuroradiologists. We believe that diagnostic H&N neuroradiologists who regularly interpret these scans, participate in ENT tumor boards, and gradually develop a high level of anatomical knowledge provide optimal care.

Image-guided biopsies can be either fine-needle aspiration (FNA) or core needle biopsy (CNB) and can be performed under computed tomography (CT) or ultrasound (US) guidance. In general, if a lesion is palpable or superficial in location, it should be amenable to US guidance. On the contrary, CT is the modality of choice for deep neck lesions. MRI-guided H&N interventions have failed to garner much support and widespread acceptability, despite the advancement in open high-field magnets and are generally felt to be unnecessary given the wider availability and ease of

a Department of Radiology, Mayo Clinic, 4500 San Pablo Road, Jacksonville, FL 32224, USA
* Corresponding author.
E-mail addresses: amitmamc@gmail.com; agarwal.amit@mayo.edu

Oral Maxillofacial Surg Clin N Am 35 (2023) 451–468
https://doi.org/10.1016/j.coms.2023.02.006

CT-guided procedures. Thyroid and parotid biopsies are usually FNAs, almost always done under US, and a detailed discussion of these is beyond the scope of this article.[3,4] In this review article, we focus primarily on the anatomical approaches and biopsy techniques for deep-seated neck lesions with an emphasis on CT-guided procedures. Suprahyoid neck biopsies, including skull-base biopsies, are more challenging than infrahyoid neck lesions, given the complex bony structures and narrow windows. Although SCCa forms the most common indication for image-guided biopsies, the range of lesions is diverse, including other benign and malignant neoplasms, infectious conditions like skull-base osteomyelitis, and inflammatory conditions such as immunoglobulin G4 (IgG4) disease. As with any other interventions, a comprehensive knowledge of anatomy and proper planning are critical. The anatomic approach is one of the most important factors in H&N biopsies, given the vital anatomic arrangement in this region. Despite the complexity, major complications with H&N biopsies are rare, with few minor complications reported in the literature, like small hematomas and minor infections.[5] Surgical biopsies are usually reserved for mucosal lesions easily accessible on endoscopic exams or for cases where image-guided biopsy is inconclusive.

PROTOCOL, REVIEW, AND SCHEDULING

The importance of thorough pre-biopsy planning cannot be overstated, and often requires more time and effort than performing the actual procedure. **Fig. 1** outlines the algorithm used at our institution before scheduling the patient for image-guided biopsy. This includes review of the case at the ENT tumor board, obtaining all current and prior imaging, and ordering additional imaging if needed. Input from the radiation oncologist is crucial for both previously treated cases and for post-biopsy management. A significant number of biopsy requests that arise from outside the multidisciplinary team are either felt to be unnecessary or can be delayed in lieu of serial imaging. The list of indications for H&N biopsies is extensive, with a primary diagnosis or follow-up of SCCa (primary lesion or nodal) being the most common. However, there is a list of "do not touch" lesions, which includes anatomic variants, "pseudo-masses," venolymphatic malformations (**Fig. 2**), and benign neurogenic tumors, which should be identified and completely avoided, especially if near the skull base or critical anatomic structures.[6] Apart from imaging, the team needs to review serological markers, including the levels of circulating tumor DNA (liquid biopsy), which has

gained prominence recently for the surveillance of cancer recurrence in human papillomavirus (HPV)-associated squamous cell carcinoma (SCCa) (**Fig. 3**).[7] Each H&N biopsy is protocolled at our institution by a member of the H&N biopsy group and scheduled on a day when a member of the H&N biopsy team is scheduled for procedures. Any need for the patient to be nothing per oral (NPO) should also be outlined in the protocol and communicated with the patient before the procedure.

PRE-PROCEDURAL WORKUP

Pre-procedural workup for H&N biopsies is like that of any interventional case. This includes withholding any anticoagulants such as aspirin, Plavix, warfarin, or medication that can alter platelets, prothrombin time (PT), and international normalized ratio (INR). Although lab evaluation for most H&N biopsies are not as stringent as spinal or vascular procedures, we do routinely check the INR (<1.5) for patients with a history of warfarin use.[8] The patient usually checks in 2 h before the procedure in the "Prep and Recovery" room followed by routine clinical evaluation by the nursing staff. Informed consent is usually standard, with a brief discussion about the procedure, indication, alternatives, risks, benefits, and common side effects. For parotid and deep H&N biopsies, we inform the patient about the risk of transient facial weakness and numbness.[9] Apart from general allergies documented in the electronic medical record, it is prudent to rule out allergies to lidocaine and latex, as these frequently go undocumented. The decision regarding no sedation, or mild or moderate sedation is made on a case-to-case basis with general anesthesia rarely necessary. We perform most of our deep H&N biopsies under mild sedation (Fentanyl: 25 to 50 µg) with continuous nursing support and vital monitoring during the procedure. Moderate sedation is preferred for skull base and osseous lesions, the latter requiring bone-cutting needles, such as osteo-site.[3,4] No sedation or nursing support is needed for most parotid and superficial biopsies. However, informing the patients regarding the high sensitivity of facial structures helps in set realistic expectations, as despite sedation, H&N biopsies are usually associated with some element of pain and discomfort.[10]

MODALITY SELECTION: ULTRASOUND VERSUS COMPUTED TOMOGRAPHY

The decision regarding US versus CT guidance for H&N biopsies is usually straightforward.

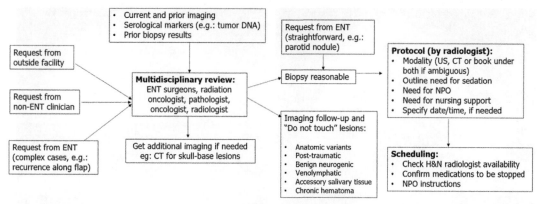

Fig. 1. The review process used at our program before scheduling biopsies, with multidisciplinary review forming the core of the process. All H&N biopsies are protocolled by a small group of neuroradiologists who perform these procedures.

Superficial (within 3 cm of the skin surface) and palpable lesions and generally easily accessible by US. Thyroid and superficial parotid lesions are almost always done under US. US is cost-effective and safe with the benefit of real-time visualization and needle localization along with instant maneuvering of the needle trajectory for accurate tissue sampling. US requires minimal procedural time and is easier to schedule in comparison to CT; the latter being used by other interventional teams with limited time slots. If there is ambiguity regarding the modality, we usually double book under CT and US and make every attempt to use US guidance (**Fig. 4**). Optimizing US parameters for proper lesion delineation is very important. This includes adjusting the depth and focus to the region of interest with the added advantage of a Doppler to evaluate the vascularity of a lesion and avoid any vessels along the tract. Linear high-frequency transducers are best suited for large skin surfaces, whereas compact high-frequency transducers (17 to 5 MHz; "hockey stick") are better for narrow windows like the parotid angle. The curved-array small footprint transducers (8 to 5 MHz) are ideal for lesions in a narrow window with a steep angle (**Fig. 5**). Although more straightforward than CT-guided procedures, US is not without its limitations. First, US procedures require more technical experience and are highly operator dependent. This is further accentuated by the fact that most neuroradiologists do not read US scans, leading to abdominal radiologists performing these at most centers. Second, lesions deep to osseous structures, calcifications, or metallic hardware are obscured on US.[11,12]

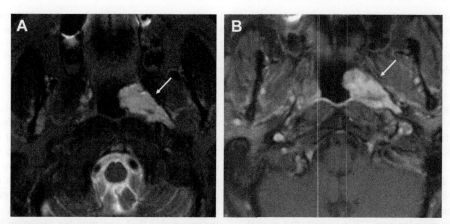

Fig. 2. Venolymphatic malformation of the left parapharyngeal space, an example of "do not biopsy" lesion. The lesion shows marked T2 hyperintensity on the axial T2 image (*A, arrow*) with patchy heterogenous enhancement (*B, arrow*) and fine internal septations. Imaging findings are characteristic of venolymphatic lesion and, at most can be followed up on imaging, to document stability.

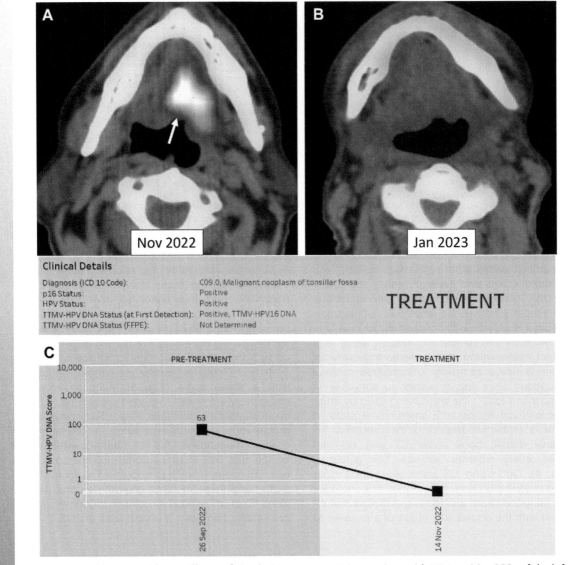

Fig. 3. "Liquid biopsy" with surveillance of circulating tumor DNA in a patient with HPV-positive SCCa of the left oropharynx. Post-treatment PET in November 2022 showed a hypermetabolic focus in the left tongue base (*A*, *arrow*) concerning tumor recurrence, which was amenable to CT-guided biopsy. However, the tumor DNA values were very low and were declining (*C*); therefore, the biopsy was deferred. Follow-up PET scan from Jan 2023 (*B*) shows resolution of uptake suggesting inflammatory changes.

Furthermore, US becomes even more challenging in the post-treated neck secondary to many factors, including lymphedema, chemoradiation-related fibrosis, and metallic hardware. There have been many instances where a large superficial lesion on CT was obscured on US due to dermal thickening and scarring associated with acoustic impedance. Apart from deep lesions, CT is usually the modality of choice for lesions at or near the skull base. CT provides excellent soft-tissue and osseous details and does not have the drawbacks of US. Near real-time CT fluoroscopy systems are available, with newer systems that feature a unique tablet-based mobile workflow for intuitive scanner operation. These systems also support users with innovative planning software. These newer scanners offer reduced radiation dose to protect the patient and the interventionist, whereas the tablet interface displays a dose thermometer that can monitor radiation levels in real-time. These also feature artifact reduction for the needle tip and intuitive touchscreen

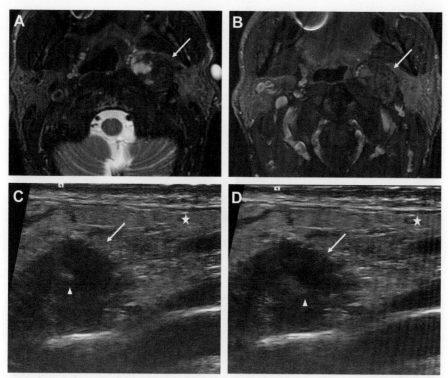

Fig. 4. Ultrasound-guided FNA of deep left parotid mass (mucoepidermoid carcinoma). The well-circumscribed lesion with low T2 signal (*A, arrow*) and poor enhancement (*B, arrow*) was seen clearly on ultrasound (*C* and *D, arrows*) with easy access. Multiple FNAs were obtained using a hypodermic 25-gauge needle. Normal overlying parotid tissue (*star*) and the needle-tip (*arrowhead*) can be seen on ultrasound.

functions that help in finding the proper position for the needle while measuring relevant distances.[13]

Fine-Needle Aspiration versus Core

FNAs and CNBs are the two most common tissue sampling techniques, each with pros and cons (**Table 1**). The preferred method of tissue sampling should be decided upon before the procedure; however, the flexibility to switch from FNA to CNB always exists. By convention, FNA is defined as a gauge (G) of ≤ 22 and CNB is performed with thicker needles ranging from 14 to 20 G.[14] In general, FNA is less traumatic but provides smaller tissue samples than core biopsies. FNA is usually sufficient for most parotid and thyroid lesions with few exceptions (like lymphoma) and offers a high diagnostic yield. FNA is also preferred for most nodal biopsies and lesions near neurovascular structures. For nodules with an initial nondiagnostic FNA, repeat FNA is futile and nondiagnostic in 28% to 53% of cases, whereas CNB provides a diagnostic sample in more than 95% of cases. In many cases, it is appropriate to perform FNA first with a cytopathologist present and then to proceed with core needle sampling if the cytologic samples are inadequate. The complication rates of CNB, such as infection, bleeding, and nerve injury, are not significantly higher than FNA if carried out under US guidance. The concern for seeding along the biopsy track is unfounded as the incidence is very low and usually related to the diameter of the needle, rather than the technique.[15,16] After inserting the needle into the lesion, applying suction to the syringe, and moving the needle back and forth (around 5 to 10 times) results in a better and more cellular sample (**Fig. 6**). Suction should be released when withdrawing the needle and should also be discontinued immediately if the blood becomes visible in the needle hub. If infection is on the differential and a discrete pocket of fluid or abscess is seen, it is better to use suction to aspirate. Frequent and rapid changes in the direction of the needle is painful for the patient and with poor results. The first pass usually yields the most diagnostic material; however, the diagnostic yield can be improved by using up to three passes. More than three passes are usually unnecessary and do not increase the yield. Suction should be avoided for thyroid

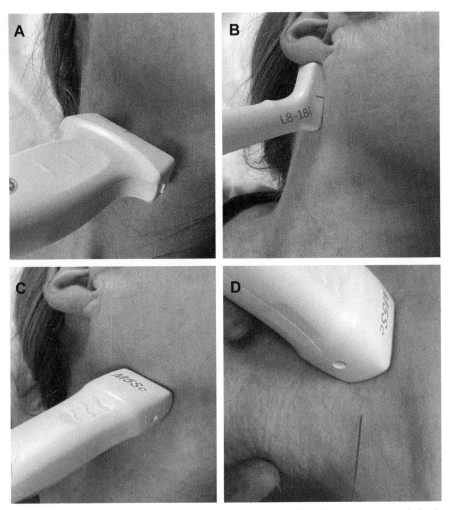

Fig. 5. High-frequency (12 to 8 MHz) linear transducers (*A*) is best suited for large areas of the lateral neck, whereas compact ("hockey-stick," 17 to 5 MHz) transducers (*B*) are ideal for narrow windows like the parotid angle. Small curved-array (*C*) transducers (8 to 5 MHz) are ideal for narrow window with a steep angle like the submandibular region. The needle should be parallel to the probe surface (*D*), angled at around 45° to the skin surface, and adjusted according to the depth of the lesion.

Table 1
Advantages and drawbacks of fine-needle aspiration and core needle biopsy

FNA	CNB
Rapid, less traumatic, lower complication rate	Higher sensitivity and diagnostic accuracy
Less expensive, rapid pathology turnaround	Provides larger tissue sample, larger intact tissue with preserved architecture
Preferred collection method for flow cytometry of lymphoid lesions	Preferred collection method for immunohistochemistry and most molecular markers
Standard for superficial parotid and thyroid lesions	Preferred for most deep neck and skull-base lesions
Limited tissue architecture characterization	More painful for the patient with need for sedation
Poor yield for fibrotic and cohesive lesions	Longer tissue-fixation and processing time
Poses limitation for immunohistochemistry and molecular testing	Higher complication rate including bleeding, tumor seeding etc.

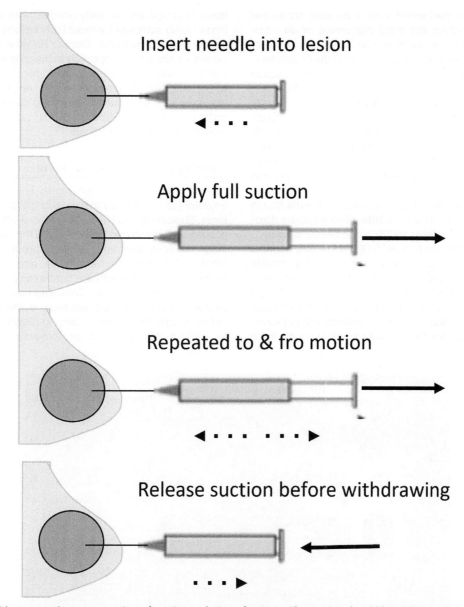

Insert needle into lesion

Apply full suction

Repeated to & fro motion

Release suction before withdrawing

Fig. 6. Diagrammatic representation of suction technique for FNAs. The suction should be maintained during the "to and fro" repeated motion; however, it is important to release suction before withdrawing the needle. Suction should be discontinued immediately if blood becomes visible in the needle hub.

and vascular lesions to minimize bleeding. For cystic neoplasms, FNA is frequently superior to CNB as the latter does not allow for content aspiration.[17,18]

INSTRUMENTATION

Lidocaine (1%) is generally used for local anesthesia, even in sedated patients, with a 25-G needle used to create a good skin wheal. A deeper neck lesion requires deep anesthetic injection, using a variable length (3.5 to 7 inches) 22-G spinal needle. If the lesion is transosseous, a spinal needle can be used to inject anesthetic beneath the periosteum. For superficial FNAs, including parotid and thyroid lesions, a simple hypodermic needle (22 to 25 G) is usually sufficient with no need for coaxial technique. Approximately 3 to 5 passes are obtained depending upon sample adequacy as assessed by the cytopathologist. Echogenic needles can be used for US-guided procedures, providing a clearer, more defined image from any angle with reduced acoustic shadowing. Core biopsies (and occasional deep neck

FNAs) are performed with a co-axial technique which involves the initial placement of an introducer thin-wall guide needle close to the target lesion followed by advancement of the biopsy needle through this needle to obtain multiple tissue samples with a single needle pass.[16,17] The coaxial needle size (length and thickness) is usually decided on a case-by-case basis. We usually use a 17 to 19 G introducer coaxial system with an 18 to 20 G biopsy needle, which has been shown to be safe with no adverse effects (**Fig. 7**A). Although thicker bore needles provide more tissue, there is increased trauma to tissue and risk of hemorrhage. Moreover, needle gauge has been shown to have little effect on tissue diagnosis when at least an 18-gauge needle is used.[19] Small caliber (as thin as 25 G) core biopsy needles are now available, which can consistently provide high-quality specimens with very low complication rates. Most biopsy needles have a "throw" length of 1 or 1 and 2 cm (**Fig. 7**B), with ultra-short throw needles available for smaller lesions. A 2-cm throw will provide the best tissue sample but with more

tissue damage, and is rarely needed, with a 1 cm throw being sufficient for most H&N lesions. Blunt needle (**Fig. 7**C) systems, such as Hawkins-Akins, permit an atraumatic approach to the target structure and allow for the deflection of vascular structures, which can be used for lesions very close to major vessels. Alternatively, the sharp diamond tip stylet can be replaced by a blunt tip needle after crossing a particular landmark.[16]

Planning the Tumor Biopsy Route

The most crucial part of H&N biopsy is planning a trajectory to avoid injury to critical anatomic structures. Suprahyoid neck lesions are more difficult to access than infrahyoid lesions, given the complex facial osseous anatomy. A good proportion of infrahyoid lesions are superficial and can be accessed using US, with the best example being lower neck nodal biopsies. Simulation software is available which uses segmentation, tracking, and virtual needle placement to help in planning with or without the utilization of three-dimensional

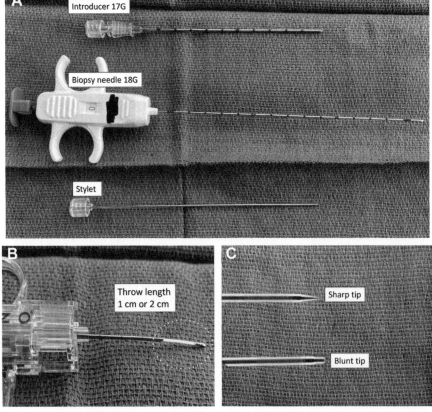

Fig. 7. Co-axial needles are used for core needles biopsies with a 17 to 19 G introducer system and 18 to 20 G biopsy needle (*A*) with "throw" length of 1 and 2 cm (*B*). Blunt "Hawkins-Akins" needle (*C*) permits an atraumatic approach to the target structure and allows for the deflection off vascular structures.

printing. The tables below outline the biopsy approach according to lesion localization and the anatomical structures to avoid in the trajectory. There is significant overlap in the anatomic approach and the same lesion can be approached through multiple routes depending upon the anatomic variance, operator experience, and preference.[2,5] For example, a prestyloid parapharyngeal lesion can be accessed using retromandibular, paramaxillary, and subzygomatic approaches (**Fig. 8**). Neck positioning plays an important part and can open access windows to the lesion, which might seem inaccessible on a standard axial image.

Subzygomatic approach

The subzygomatic approach is also known as the transcondylar, infratemporal, or sigmoid notch approach, with anatomic and technical considerations outlined in **Table 2**. This is ideal for lesions in masticator space and can also be used for parapharyngeal and retropharyngeal spaces as well as skull base (**Fig. 9**) lesions. The major anatomic structures of concern in the pathway of this approach are the internal maxillary artery and the mandibular division of the trigeminal nerve. The internal maxillary artery's origin is posterior to the neck of the mandible, embedded in the substance of the parotid gland, and then traverses either superficial or deep to the lateral pterygoid muscle.[2,5,20]

Retromandibular approach

This approach is also known as the transparotid approach, with anatomic and technical considerations outlined in **Table 3**. This is useful for deep parotid lesions (**Fig. 10**), lateral parapharyngeal, and carotid space lesions. The external carotid artery and the retromandibular vein run just posterior to the ramus and should be avoided. The facial nerve runs just lateral to the retromandibular vein. The styloid process serves as a very important landmark and keeping the trajectory anterior

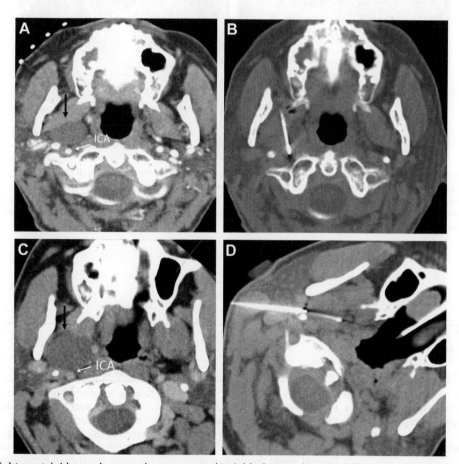

Fig. 8. Right prestyloid parapharyngeal space masses (*A, C, black arrows*) in two different patients, biopsied using paramaxillary (*B*) and retromandibular (*D*) approaches. Contrast-enhanced scan was performed during planning for better delineation of lesion and anatomic structures, including the ICA (*A, C, white arrows*).

Table 2
Subzygomatic approach

Target Lesions	Anatomical Concerns	Technique
• Masticator space (ideal approach) • Parapharyngeal space • Prevertebral region • Skull base	Risk of injury to the: • Mandibular branch of Vth nerve • Internal maxillary artery • Pterygoid venous plexus	Needle is inserted below the zygomatic arch and advanced through the intercondylar notch Wide-target as needle can be angulated cranially or caudally

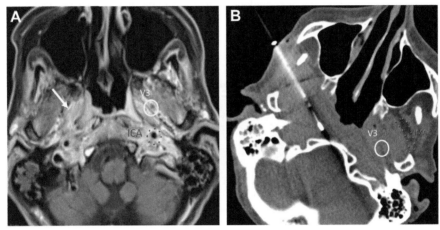

Fig. 9. Right subzygomatic approach for core needle biopsy of a poorly defined region of prevertebral soft tissue and skull-base enhancement (osteomyelitis) (*A, arrow*). The needle is advanced through the intercondylar notch (*B*) between the coronoid and condylar process with the IMA and mandibular (V3) division of the trigeminal nerve along the course. The ICA is usually posterior to the trajectory, however, should also be defined before needle insertion.

Table 3
Retromandibular approach

Target Lesions	Anatomical Concerns	Technique
• Deep parotid space • Parapharyngeal space • Pharyngeal mucosal space • Carotid sheath space	Risk of injury to the: • External carotid artery (medial vessel, immediately posterior to the ramus) • Retromandibular vein (lateral vessel, immediately posterior to the ramus) • Facial nerve (lateral to the vein)	Needle is inserted posterior to the mandible and anterior to the mastoid (transparotid) Potential risk to the facial nerve so thinner needle should be used No room for cranial angulation given the neurovascular anatomy

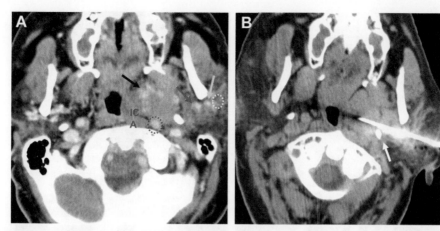

Fig. 10. Left retromandibular (transparotid) approach to a deep parotid space lesion (A, *black arrow*). Two vessels are identified just posterior to mandibular ramus with the medial vessel (A, *red arrow*) corresponding to ECA and the lateral vessel (A, *blue arrow*) corresponding to retromandibular vein. The yellow circle (A), corresponds to the expected location of the facial nerve, just lateral to the retromandibular vein. The styloid process (B, *white arrow*) serves as an important landmark and keeping the trajectory anterior to this avoids the ICA, as the artery runs posterior to the styloid.

to this avoids the internal carotid artery (ICA), as the artery runs posterior to the styloid.[2,5]

Paramaxillary approach

This is also known as the transfacial, transmalar, or retromaxillary approach with anatomic and technical considerations outlined in **Table 4**. This approach provides easy access to the lateral retropharyngeal space, the infrazygomatic masticator space, the posterior parapharyngeal, and the carotid sheath space (**Fig. 11**). This approach can also be used for skull-based lesions using cranial angulation and hyperextension of the neck. The access window can be narrow due to bony structures, including the maxillary antrum, the alveolar ridge, and the lateral pterygoid plate.[2,5,21]

Submastoid approach

Also known as the retroparotid approach, this trajectory is ideal for carotid space lesions, when the vessels are displaced medially, with details outlined in **Table 5**. The trajectory starts beneath the mastoid tip and courses posterior to the parotid gland with no risk to facial nerve or vessels within the parotid gland (**Fig. 12**).[2,5]

Transoral approach

This approach is used for open procedures by ENT surgeons, usually for pharyngeal mucosal lesions such as oropharyngeal SCCa or infectious lesions or drainage of peritonsillar and retropharyngeal abscesses (**Fig. 13**). Rarely, this approach can be used for image-guided procedures to biopsy retropharyngeal and prevertebral lesions.

Table 4
Paramaxillary approach

Target Lesions	Anatomical Concerns	Technique
• Lateral part of the retro-pharyngeal space • Infrazygomatic masticator space • Posterior parapharyngeal • Carotid sheath space.	Risk of injury to the: • Facial artery, coursing in the buccal space (easily identifiable)	Needle is inserted through the buccal space below the zygomatic coursing between the maxilla and mandible Narrow window limited by maxillary antrum, the alveolar ridge, the lateral pterygoid plate

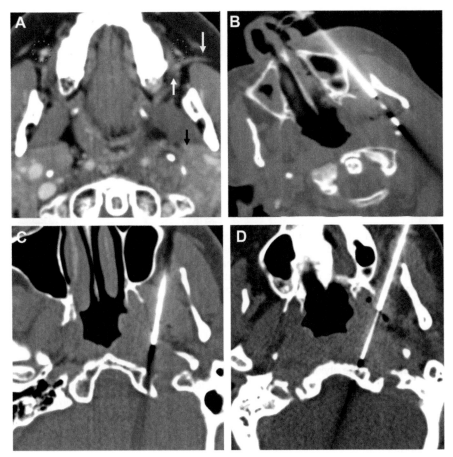

Fig. 11. Left paramaxillary approach for biopsy of deep parotid lesion (*A, B*; irradiation-induced sialadenitis on pathology) through the buccinator (*A, white arrow*). Facial artery and vein are identified in the buccal space (*A, B, red circle*) anterior to buccinator, adjacent to the parotid duct (*A, yellow arrow*). In two different patients, this approach is used to biopsy a posterior parapharyngeal (*C*) and retropharyngeal (*D*) lesion.

However, this requires an extensive set-up, including the need for general anesthesia. Although this approach is relatively safe, given the absence of critical neurovascular structures in the median or paramedian location, the small intraoral window makes it very challenging for the radiologist. The added risk of bleeding into the oropharyngeal airway and the inability to maintain sterility makes it even more complicated. This approach is rarely used by the radiologist, and should be considered only if no other route is available for access.[5,22]

Infrahyoid neck approach
Compared with suprahyoid, the infrahyoid neck lesions have much easier access. Nodal biopsies form the most common request for infrahyoid biopsies with the vast majority performed under US

Table 5
Submastoid approach

Target Lesions	Anatomical Concerns	Technique
• Lateral part of the perivertebral space • Carotid sheath space • Posterior parapharyngeal	Risk of injury to the: • Vertebral artery near the lateral mass of C2ICA for deep parapharyngeal access	Trajectory starts beneath the mastoid tip through the sternocleidomastoid muscle Path is posterior to the parotid gland with no risk to facial nerve or vessels within the parotid gland.

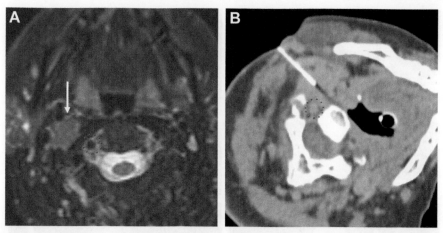

Fig. 12. Submastoid approach for biopsy of carotid sheath lesion (*A, B*; metastatic papillary thyroid carcinoma) through the sternocleidomastoid and posterior to the parotid gland. Lesion is displacing the ICA anteriorly. Although, the facial nerve is not at risk through this approach, the vertebral artery (*A, B, red circle*) lies in the trajectory.

guidance. However, like the suprahyoid neck, deep lesions in this compartment also require CT and more extensive workup and planning. The infrahyoid neck can be approached using anterolateral, posterolateral (**Fig. 14**), and posterior approaches which are outlined in detail in **Table 6**.[2,5]

SAMPLE COLLECTION AND CYTOPATHOLOGY

Currently, on-site evaluation of the adequacy of tissue samples has become standard and is usually provided by a cytotechnologist. The demand for on-site evaluation of tissue sample adequacy has increased, outpacing the capacity of available cytopathologists. Moreover, cytotechnologists

have been shown to be capable of providing this service with equivalent accuracy. In the absence of on-site evaluation, approximately 20% to 40% of FNAs can be nondiagnostic due to scant cellularity and poor smear preparation.[23] The onus for correct sample collection and labeling lies upon the radiologist as much as upon the pathologist/cytotechnologist. The specimen label must include the patient's name, date of birth, date and time of collection, and specimen source. The tissue sample is labeled as a "surgical pathology" specimen when a core biopsy has been obtained, even if slides are made. On the contrary, the tissue sample is ordered as a "cytology" for aspirates and FNA, when no core has been obtained.[24] FNA samples are placed on a glass slide which

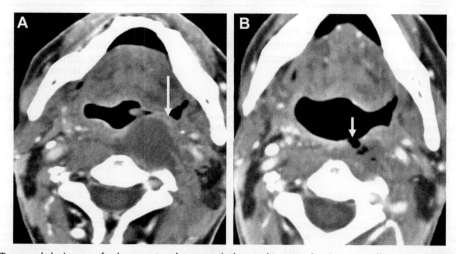

Fig. 13. Transoral drainage of a large retropharyngeal abscess (*A, arrow*) using a small incision by ENT surgeon and placement of radiolucent drainage tube (*B, arrow*). Though commonly used for open-surgical procedures, this approach is rarely used for image-guided biopsies.

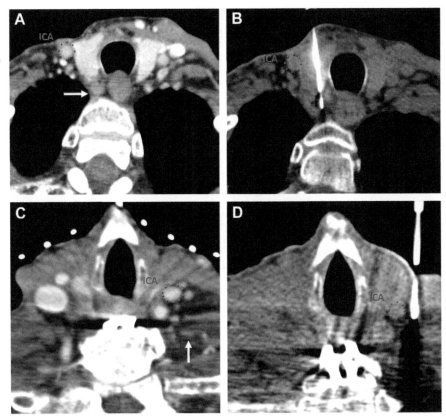

Fig. 14. Anterolateral (*A, B*) and posterolateral (*C, D*) approach biopsies in two different patients with nodal (*white arrows*) metastatic SCCa (showed high uptake on FDG PET). In the anterolateral approach, the needle traverses the thyroid gland and lies medial to the carotid sheath vessels (*red circle*) whereas in posterolateral approach it lies lateral to the carotid.

Table 6
Infrahyoid neck approaches

Target Lesions	Anatomical Concerns	Technique
Anterolateral(between carotid and airways) • Retrotracheal • Paraesophageal • Anterior perivertebral	Risk of injury to the: • Hypopharynx • Pyriform fossa • Carotid vessels	Trajectory starts anterior to the sternocleidomastoid muscle between the visceral space (containing thyroid gland, larynx, trachea, upper esophagus, hypopharynx) and carotid space
Posterolateral(lateral and posterior to carotids) • Retrotracheal • Lateral perivertebral • Posterior cervical space	Risk of injury to the: • Vertebral artery • Carotid vessels	Trajectory starts anterior to the sternocleidomastoid muscle between the visceral space (containing thyroid gland, larynx, trachea, upper esophagus, hypopharynx) and carotid space
Posterior • Vertebrae • Posterior perivertebral	No significant neurovascular risk, only muscles penetrated	Prone or lateral decubitus position. Keep checking on fluoroscopy to avoid penetration of thecal sac

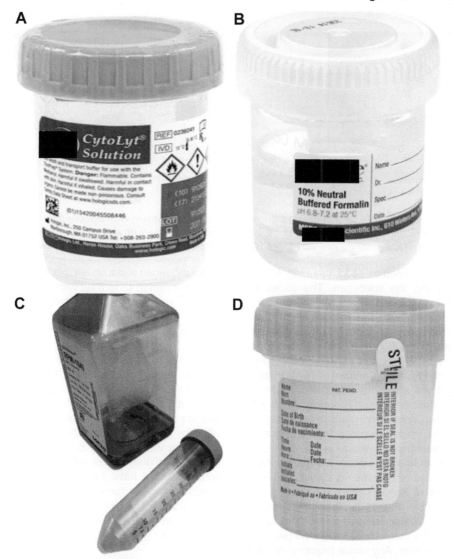

Fig. 15. Commonly used containers for head and neck tissue samples. FNA samples are placed in into a jar of preservative (CytoLyt) solution (*A*) whereas container with 10% neutral buffered formalin (*B*) is used for most core biopsies. If there is a clinical concern for hematopoietic malignancy (lymphoma/leukemia) the tissue is submitted in sterile container without formalin, with addition of RPMI (*C*). Microbiology samples for cultures are placed in sterile jar (*D*), with or without normal saline.

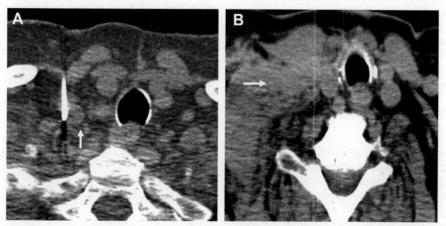

Fig. 16. Core biopsy of right supraclavicular node (*A*, *arrow*) complicated by lower neck hematoma, seen as amorphous high-density collection (*B*, *arrow*). The hematoma was self-resolving with no significant discomfort and no significant mass effect on the airways.

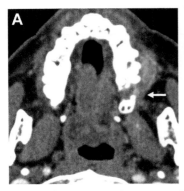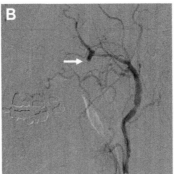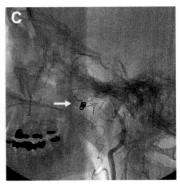

Fig. 17. Infiltrative mass (SCCa on pathology) along the left maxilla (*A, arrow*) with osseous destruction noted on CT. This was complicated by pseudoaneurysm of the internal maxillary artery (*B, arrow*) post-biopsy, seen on catheter angiogram. The pseudoaneurysm was coiled (*C*) given the high risk for rupture and bleeding.

is smeared with another slide resulting in two slides containing the specimen. The slides for wet fixation are placed immediately in alcohol (95%) for staining with the Papanicolaou stain. The rest of the specimen is put into a jar of preservative (CytoLyt) solution (**Fig. 15**A). Core biopsy samples are usually placed in 10% neutral buffered formalin (**Fig. 15**B). Multiple cores can go in a single jar if one site is being biopsied; however, if multiple sites are being biopsied, each site must be placed in its own individual jar. If there is a clinical concern for hematopoietic malignancy (lymphoma/leukemia) the tissue needs to be submitted fresh (sterile container) without formalin, with the addition of Roswell Park Memorial Institute (RPMI) (pink tissue culture media), for flow cytometric studies (**Fig. 15**C). Nodal core samples for disease processes other than lymphoma/leukemia (eg, SCCa metastasis) should be placed in a formalin container. Any tissue requiring cultures (microbiology) should be sent fresh (sterile jar, with or without normal saline) and not be placed in formalin (**Fig. 15**D). This includes submission of fluid aspirates from abscesses. Frequently, both microbiology and histology need to be performed and specimen pieces should be obtained in formalin and in sterile containers with normal saline.[25] Molecular and genetic tests are increasingly being performed on samples and should be placed in specific containers (eg, Affirma Gene Expression classifier for thyroid FNAs).[26]

POST-PROCEDURE CARE AND COMPLICATIONS

Many biopsies, primarily FNAs (like thyroid) can be performed in an outpatient office setting. However, core biopsies are usually done in a hospital-based setting. Routine post-procedure care with monitoring in the "Prep and recovery" area for around 1 h is sufficient for most patients. Patients

under moderate sedation are monitored for a more extended period (2 to 3 h), with the nursing team ensuring normal vitals before discharge. Image-guided H&N procedures are safe with very low complication rates. Immediate complications include hypotensive/vasovagal episodes, pain, hematoma formation, and facial weakness. These patients are monitored for a longer (2 to 3 h) period. Analgesics may be given post-procedure if the patient is in pain. Hematomas are uncommon and are usually small and self-resolving (**Fig. 16**). With the small-caliber needles used, the risk for significant vascular injury in H&N biopsies is very low with a slightly higher risk in post-radiated patients.[27] There have been few case reports of pseudoaneurysm formation (**Fig. 17**) and nerve injury post H&N biopsies; however, these are very uncommon, and generally, H&N procedures are low risk.[28]

SUMMARY

Despite the complex H&N anatomy, image-guided procedures are increasingly being used for superficial and deep neck lesions as an alternative to open biopsy. Image-guided techniques are relatively more straightforward, diagnostically expeditious, and very safe. However, this requires detailed anatomical knowledge along with expertise and experience. Dedicated H&N radiologists or radiologists with expertise in H&N anatomy and pathology can best contribute to the multidisciplinary teams caring for these patients. With the ever-growing demand for molecular markers and genetic testing, a large increase in the number of these procedures is expected over the next decade.

FUNDING INFORMATION

None.

CLINICS CARE POINTS

- Head and neck lesions can be safely biopsied using an image-guided approach.

- CT is the modality of choice for deep lesions and ultrasound is the modality of choice for superficial lesions.

- Excellent anatomical knowledge and pre-procedure trajectory planning are of utmost impotant for head and neck biopsies.

DISCLOSURES

No commercial or financial conflicts of interest for any authors.

REFERENCES

1. Curtin HD, Brogle N, Caruso P. Imaging-guided biopsy. Oral Maxillofacial Surg Clin N Am 2005; 13(1):51–62.

2. Loevner LA. Image-guided procedures of the head and neck: the radiologist's arsenal. Otolaryngol Clin North Am 2008;41(1):231–50.

3. McKnight CD, Glastonbury CM, Ibrahim M, et al. Techniques and approaches for safe, high-yield CT-Guided suprahyoid head and neck biopsies. AJR Am J Roentgenol 2017;208(1):76–83.

4. Hutchins T. Image guided head and neck biopsies: from superficial to deep. Tech Vasc Interv Radiol 2021;24(3):100769.

5. Gupta S, Henningsen JA, Wallace MJ, et al. Percutaneous biopsy of head and neck lesions with CT guidance: various approaches and relevant anatomic and technical considerations. Radiographics 2007;27(2):371–90.

6. Gopal N, Bhatt AA. Ten must know pseudolesions of the head and neck. Emerg Radiol 2021;28(1): 119–26.

7. Kong L, Birkeland AC. Liquid biopsies in head and neck cancer: current state and future challenges. Cancers 2021;13(8):1874.

8. Matsumoto M, Altman A, Jothishankar B, et al. Low utility of screening hematologic testing for image-guided biopsies in patients without bleeding risks. AJR Am J Roentgenol 2020;215(5):1279–85.

9. Olsson P, Ekblad F, Hassler A, et al. Complications after minor salivary gland biopsy: a retrospective study of 630 patients from two Swedish centres. Scand J Rheumatol 2023;52(2):208–16.

10. Lo WC, Cheng PW, Wang CT, et al. Pain levels associated with ultrasound-guided fine-needle aspiration biopsy for neck masses. Head Neck 2014;36(2): 252–6.

11. Learned KO, Lev-Toaff AS, Brake BJ, et al. US-guided biopsy of neck lesions: the head and neck neuroradiologist's perspective. Radiographics 2016;36(1):226–43.

12. Lorenzo G, Saindane AM. Pitfalls in image guided tissue sampling in the head and neck. Neuroimaging Clin N Am 2013;23(1):167–78.

13. Ernst RD, Kim HS, Kawashima A, et al. Near real-time CT fluoroscopy using computer automated scan technology in nonvascular interventional procedures. AJR Am J Roentgenol 2000;174(2): 319–21.

14. VanderLaan PA. Fine-needle aspiration and core needle biopsy: an update on 2 common minimally invasive tissue sampling modalities. Cancer Cytopathol 2016;124(12):862–70.

15. Eom HJ, Lee JH, Ko MS, et al. Comparison of fine-needle aspiration and core needle biopsy under ultrasonographic guidance for detecting malignancy and for the tissue-specific diagnosis of salivary gland tumors. AJNR Am J Neuroradiol 2015;36: 1188–93.

16. Aiken AH. Image-guided biopsies in the head and neck: practical value and approach. AJNR Am J Neuroradiol 2020;41(11):2123–5.

17. Hillen TJ, Baker JC, Long JR, et al. Percutaneous CT-guided core needle biopsies of head and neck masses: technique, histopathologic yield, and safety at a single academic institution. AJNR Am J Neuroradiol 2020;41(11):2117–22.

18. Oertel YC. Fine-needle aspiration and the diagnosis of thyroid cancer. Endocrinol Metab Clin North Am 1996;25:69–91.

19. Hong G, Koo JH. Evaluation of the gauge of needles used in the collection of specimens during endobronchial ultrasound-guided transbronchial needle aspiration. J Bras Pneumol 2019;45(1): e20180090.

20. Abrahams JJ. Mandibular sigmoid notch: a window for CT-guided biopsies of lesions in the peripharyngeal and skull base regions. Radiology 1998;208(3): 695–9.

21. Esposito MB, Arrington JA, Murtagh FR, et al. Anterior approach for CT-guided biopsy of skull base and parapharyngeal space lesions. J Comput Assist Tomogr 1996;20:739–41.

22. Mondal A, Raychoudhur BK. Peroral fine needle aspiration cytology of parapharyngeal lesions. Acta Cytol 1993;37:694–8.

23. Collins JA, Novak A, Ali SZ, et al. Cytotechnologists and on-site evaluation of adequacy. Korean J Pathol 2013;47(5):405–10.

24. Sehgal IS, Gupta N, Dhooria S, et al. Processing and reporting of cytology specimens from mediastinal lymph nodes collected using endobronchial

ultrasound-guided transbronchial needle aspiration: a state-of-the-art review. J Cytol 2020;37(2):72–81.

25. Keebler C, Somrak T. The manual of cytotechnology. Seventh Edition. Chicago: The American Society of Clinical Pathologists; 1993. p. 220.

26. Labourier E, Shifrin A, Busseniers AE, et al. Molecular testing for miRNA, mRNA, and DNA on fine-needle aspiration improves the preoperative diagnosis of thyroid nodules with indeterminate cytology. J Clin Endocrinol Metab 2015;100(7):2743–50.

27. Brown AP, Wendler DS, Camphausen K, et al. Performing nondiagnostic research biopsies in irradiated tissue: a review of scientific, clinical, and ethical considerations. J Clin Oncol 2008;26(24): 3987–94.

28. Walker AT, Chaloupka JC, Putman CM, et al. Sentinel transoral hemorrhage from a pseudoaneurysm of the internal maxillary artery: a complication of CT-guided biopsy of the masticator space. AJNR Am J Neuroradiol 1996;17(2):377–81.

Proton Radiotherapy for Skull-Base Malignancies
Imaging Considerations of Radiotherapy and Complications

Adam L. Holtzman, MD*, Roi Dagan, MD, MS, William M. Mendenhall, MD

KEYWORDS

- Proton • Radiotherapy • Skull-base • Cancer • Malignancy • Benign • Tumors • Complications

KEY POINTS

- Stereotactic, imaging-guided proton therapy (PT) is an effective and safe treatment of both benign and malignant skull-base tumors, which allows for improved normal tissue sparing
- Outcomes studies show the promising evidence of side-effect mitigation for skull-base tumors using PT.
- Reducing low and moderate radiation doses allows for the preservation of neurocognition and a reduction in second malignancies.
- High-dose conformity reduces the risk of central nervous system radionecrosis of sensitive neurovascular tissues immediately adjacent to the skull-base.
- Biologic optimization with dynamic arc delivery, relative biological effectiveness , ultrahigh dose rate delivery, and proton boron capture therapy, among others, may further improve the therapeutic ratio (defined as the probability of tumor control and the likelihood of normal tissue damage).

INTRODUCTION TO PROTON RADIOTHERAPY

With technological developments in mechanical and software engineering and computer processing speeds, the field of radiation oncology has embraced the widespread use of sophisticated and targeted forms of stereotactic, image-guided radiotherapy capable of highly conformal and precise treatment. External-beam radiotherapy (EBRT), the most common form of radiation delivered, is a noninvasive treatment delivery of ionizing radiation in the form of photons or particles.[1] Proton therapy (PT) has the physical advantages of a lower entry dose and limited distal fall-off compared with conventional photon radiotherapy. Clinically, this manifests as delivering equivalent therapeutic doses while reducing unnecessary low- and moderate-dose radiation to surrounding nontargeted normal tissue.[2,3] **Fig. 1** shows a comparison of proton and photon radiotherapy on CT planning studies for a skull-base meningioma.

In PT, two basic types of treatment delivery exist: double-scattered (DS) and pencil beam scanning (PBS). DS techniques use a brass aperture and Lucite compensator to physically shape the lateral and distal penumbra. In contrast, magnets are used to dose-paint a three-dimensional distribution with PBS. Both treatments rely on the physical property that protons have a reduced entry dose and stop shortly after maximal dose delivery. This is clinically delivered as the

Funding: None.
Department of Radiation Oncology, University of Florida College of Medicine, 2015 North Jefferson Street, Jacksonville, FL 32206, USA
* Corresponding author.
E-mail address: aholtzman@floridaproton.org

Oral Maxillofacial Surg Clin N Am 35 (2023) 469–484
https://doi.org/10.1016/j.coms.2023.02.003
1042-3699/23/

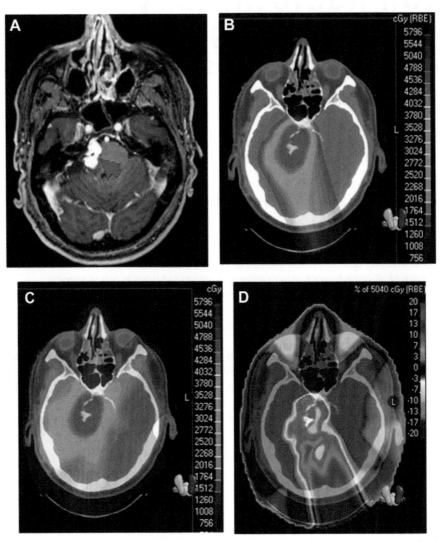

Fig. 1. Brain MRI of a right petrous apex World Health Organization (WHO) grade I meningioma (*red arrow*) (*A*). As noted on the enhanced Axial T1, there was extension to the prepontine cistern and brainstem compression at the time of radiation. A colorwash dose distribution comparison of two-field proton beam therapy (*B*), intensity-modulated radiotherapy (*C*), and a map depicting the differences between the two plans as measured by percent of the prescription dose of 50.4 GyRBE (*D*).

spread-out Bragg peak or the summation of multiple individual beams within a clinically therapeutic range.[2,3] **Fig. 2** shows the individual beamlets and the boost plan geometry for a petroclival chondrosarcoma using a single-field optimization technique. **Fig. 3** illustrates how the composite dosimetry compared with volumetric modulated arc therapy leads to reduced radiation within non-targeted normal tissues. Delivering a higher proportion of the treatment dose to the tumor relative to the surrounding normal tissues increases the therapeutic ratio, defined as the probability of tumor control and the likelihood of normal tissue damage.

Proton Therapy for Benign Base of Skull Tumors

The benefits of PT are documented for centrally located benign and low-grade extra-axial brain tumors. Given the excellent local control rates, favorable outcomes, and central location, the proton dosimetry allows a reduction in low- and moderate-dose bath to the frontal lobes, bilateral temporal lobes and hippocampi, circle of Willis, hypothalamic-pituitary axis, and the optic apparatus. These tumors include pituitary adenomas, craniopharyngiomas, and benign meningiomas.[4–10] Radiosurgical and fractionated proton

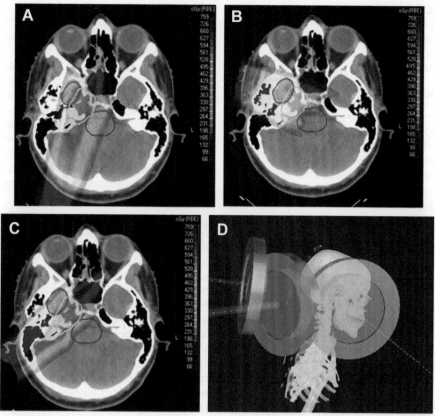

Fig. 2. Individual beamlets from a three-field boost plan of a right petroclival chondrosarcoma. Treatment is delivered by a single-field optimized right anterior (A) and posterior obliques (B, C) arrangement. The three-dimensional graphical representation of beam positioning on a digitally reconstructed radiographic (D). This illustration shows how each proton beam has a reduced entry dose with a limited exit dose in relation to the treatment target within the right petrous apex (demarcated in *lime green*).

schema have been documented with high local control rates and fewer toxicities.[7–9,11,12,13] Proton radiotherapy has demonstrated efficacy in lateralized base of skull (BOS) lesions (eg, vestibular schwannoma) with high control rates and low morbidity.[10,14] Other potential roles for PT include benign tumors involving both the brain and spine (eg, hemangioma and hemangioblastoma) when

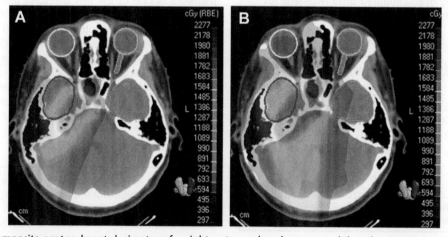

Fig. 3. Composite proton boost dosimetry of a right petrous chondrosarcoma (A) and comparison with a volumetric modulated arc technique comparison (B).

repeat or upfront surgery or other interventional procedures have high morbidity.[5,6] Conventional dose regimens range from 45 to 55.8 gray relative biological effectiveness (GyRBE) at 1.8 to 2 GyRBE (**Table 1**).

Pituitary Adenoma

Pituitary adenomas are common benign BOS tumors. Autopsy and radiographic series note that incidental, clinically insignificant findings may be present in as much as 20% of the population; however, they rarely cause issues related to hormone secretion or mass effect from tumor growth.[15] Radiotherapy is indicated for refractory secretory tumors and nonsecretory macroadenomas where medical management would imminently risk causing cranial neuropathy. Radiosurgery is preferred for secretory tumors as the biochemical response rate is more rapid, but it cannot be performed for a large tumor or those abutting the optic apparatus. In those situations, fractionated radiotherapy is indicated. PT is of particular interest as it has been shown to reduce the nontargeted low dose to the temporal lobes and hippocampi in these cases and thus may affect long-term neurocognition.[9,11]

Craniopharyngioma

Craniopharyngiomas are rare sellar tumors most commonly affecting children and adolescents. Radiation is used after subtotal resection, and disease control rates are equivalent to those obtained after macroscopic gross total resection when radiation is given adjuvantly. Given the good prognosis and the typical age at diagnosis

and location, several series document the efficacy of proton radiotherapy both in pediatric and adult populations, with local control rates nearing 90% with rare serious toxicity.[4,12,16–18]

Potential cyst expansion is particularly important during radiotherapy; clinical series have shown that up to 25% of patients can develop pseudoprogression in the form of cyst changes or expansion during treatment, necessitating treatment planning changes.[19] It is generally recommended that at least biweekly on-treatment MRI verification is performed to ensure that the prescription dose encompasses the target volume (**Fig. 4**).

Vestibular Schwannomas

Vestibular schwannomas are nerve sheath tumors affecting the vestibulocochlear nerve. Most are unilateral and sporadic, whereas a few are hereditary and bilateral (<5%). Observation is the primary management for newly diagnosed tumors, as approximately one-third will show growth within a time that precipitates therapeutic intervention. If treatment is indicated, surgery and radiation provide excellent control rates. Radiation has a lower rate of facial nerve injury and better hearing preservation than upfront surgery.[10,14,20] Pseudoprogression after treatment is a common feature of vestibular schwannoma. Thus, a transient, self-limited increase in the tumor size is a known phenomenon and should not be considered treatment progression (**Fig. 5**). Accordingly, it should be clinically observed, particularly in the absence of new or worsening neurologic symptoms.[18,21]

Meningioma

The diagnosis of an extra-axial tumor as meningioma can often be made radiographically and therefore is one of the few diseases that can be treated with radiation without tissue confirmation (85% are benign). Like other benign BOS tumors, 5-year local control rates are over 95% with PT.[7,8,13,22] Recent studies have shown that the utilization of gallium Ga 68-DOTATATE positron emission tomography improves target delineation for radiation treatment planning, particularly useful for difficult-to-interpret postsurgical skull-base cases (**Fig. 6**).[23]

Malignant Skull-Base Tumors

In addition to low- and moderate-dose reduction, PT provides a high-dose conformal radiotherapy for BOS malignancies. These tumors include bone sarcomas (eg, chordoma and chondrosarcoma), sinonasal tumors, soft tissue sarcomas (eg, rhabdomyosarcoma, hemangioblastoma,

Table 1
Summary of fractionated dose regimens for benign tumors of the skull-base

Histology	Conventional Fractionation Dose Regimens
Craniopharyngioma	54 GyRBE at 1.8–2 GyRBE
Hemangioma	45 GyRBE at 1.8 GyRBE
Meningioma (WHO grade I)	45–54 GyRBE at 1.8–2 GyRBE
Pituitary adenoma	Secretory 50.4–54 GyRBE at 1.8–2 GyRBE Nonfunctioning 45 GyRBE at 1.8 GyRBE
Vestibular schwannoma	50.4 GyRBE at 1.8 GyRBE

Abbreviation: GyRBE, gray relative biological effectiveness.

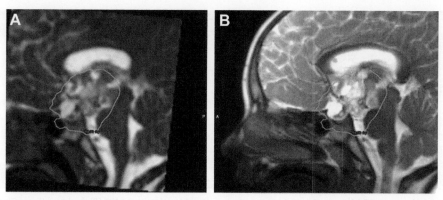

Fig. 4. Example of verification 0.23 T MRI simulation (*A*) used to monitor cyst expansion fused to sagittal T2 diagnostic MRI (*B*). The orange line depicts the prescription dose, which is compared to ensure that cyst expansion has not occurred nor falls outside the prescription dose for treatment.

and extracranial hemangiopericytoma), and carcinomas with perineural invasion (PNI).[24–36] PTs role is to limit moderate- and high-dose radiotherapy to adjacent sensitive neurovascular structures such as the brainstem, brain parenchyma, and optic apparatus.[37–46] Conventional dose regimens range from 50 to 78 GyRBE at 1.8 to 2 GyRBE and are summarized in **Table 2**.

Chordoma and Chondrosarcoma

Chordoma and chondrosarcoma are extradural osseous sarcomas with a long history of being treated with proton radiotherapy. Chordomas are remnant embryonic notochord tissues that form the nucleus pulposus. Histologically, they are most associated with Brachyury expression, and

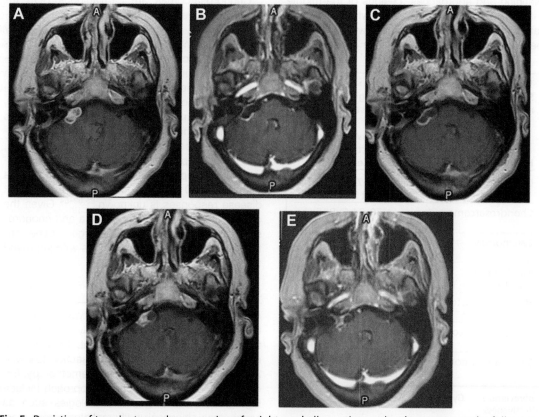

Fig. 5. Depiction of transient pseudoprogression of a right cerebellopontine angle schwannoma at the following time points: (*A*) preradiotherapy (*red arrow*); (*B*) 6 months; (*C*) 9 months; (*D*) 14 months; and (*E*) 18 months.

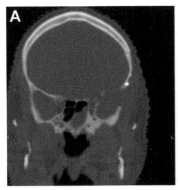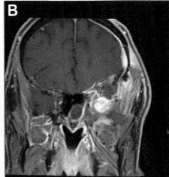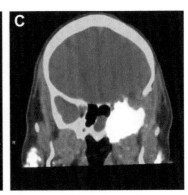

Fig. 6. Coronal planning CT (*A*) coregistered to a postoperative T1-enhanced MRI (*B*) and a gallium Ga 68-DOTA-TATE positron emission tomography (*C*). This helps identify residual disease in the infratemporal fossa (*red arrow*) and exclude the non-avid postoperative change (*blue arrow*) along the left lateral craniotomy postoperative resection change along the dura.

subtypes include conventional, dedifferentiated, and poorly differentiated. Maximal safe resection followed by radiotherapy is the initial treatment strategy except for poorly differentiated chordomas, for which induction chemotherapy is considered.[47] Anatomically, the clivus is divided into three segments (sellar, sphenoidal, and nasopharyngeal), which are used to determine surgical planning and approaches. Lesions of the middle third of the clivus are associated with the highest rates of gross total resection, followed by the upper and lower thirds. Lower third or craniocervical junction chordomas often present in a tent-like fashion both anteriorly and posteriorly to the dens (**Fig. 7**).[25–29,35,48,49,50] As chordomas are relatively radioresistant, studies have shown that dose escalation above 70 GyRBE and PT are associated with increased survival. Studies with high-dose conformal photon therapy have also been performed, including radiosurgery.[25,29,49,51]

Chondrosarcomas are cartilaginous BOS tumors. Compared with chordomas, which are typically midline, chondrosarcomas are usually paramedian and often arise from petroclival synchondrosis. A comparison of the radiographic features of chordoma is depicted in **Table 3**. Although the 10-year progression-free survival after radiotherapy for chordoma ranges from 50% to 65%, chondrosarcoma is generally over 85%. Studies have shown that radiotherapy may improve survival and decrease recurrence. In addition, although both pathologies are considered radioresistant with improvement in outcomes with doses greater than 70 Gy, the mechanism for the different disease responses is unknown.[25,52–54] Given the complexity of managing chordoma and chondrosarcoma, database studies from high-volume centers have also shown associations with improved survival.[25,49]

Table 2
Summary of fractionated dose regimens for malignant tumors of the skull-base

Histology	Conventional Fractionation Dose Regimens[a]
Chordoma	70–78 GyRBE at 1.8–2 GyRBE
Chondrosarcoma	70–74 GyRBE at 1.8–2 GyRBE
Carcinomas	60–70 GyRBE at 1.8–2 GyRBE
Meningioma (WHO grade II/III)	54–60 GyRBE at 1.8–2 GyRBE
Hemangioblastoma	50–55.8 GyRBE at 1.8–2 GyRBE
Soft tissue sarcoma	50–66 GyRBE at 1.8–2 GyRBE
Sinonasal tumors	50–70 GyRBE at 1.8–2 GyRBE

Abbreviation: GyRBE, gray relative biological effectiveness
[a] Dose ranges dependent on extent of residual disease and histology

Sinonasal

A wide range of distinct histologic types comprises this category, with treatment largely depending on the diagnosis and disease extent. Management often includes upfront surgical resection followed by radiotherapy with or without chemotherapy. Exceptions to an upfront surgical approach include high-grade, chemosensitive histologies such as lymphomas, sinonasal undifferentiated carcinomas, small cell carcinomas, or those that are

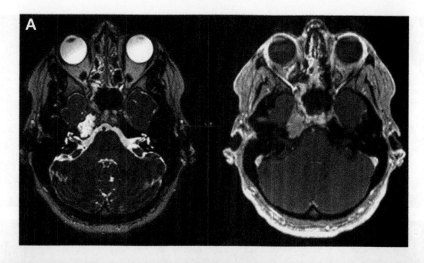

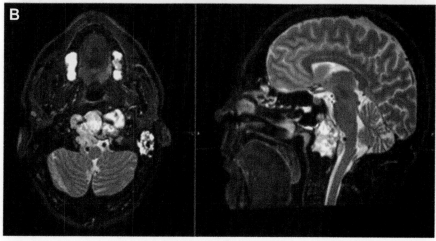

Fig. 7. Axial T2 CISS and enhanced T1 multiplanar reformation MRI of a right petroclival chondrosarcoma (*A*). Axial and sagittal images of a T2 SPACE MRI of a craniocervical junction chordoma (*B*).

Table 3
Summary of radiographic features comparing conventional chordoma and chondrosarcoma

Feature	Chondrosarcoma	Chordoma
Location	Paramedian	Midline
Calcifications	Intralesional calcifications common	No internal calcification
CT	Lytic lesions with a moth-eaten appearance and endosteal scalloping	Bony destruction
T1 signal intensity	low to intermediate	low to intermediate
T2 signal intensity	High	High
T1 + gadolinium	Heterogenous enhancement	Heterogenous enhancement
Diffusion-weighted Imaging	High ADC value Low to intermediate restriction	Low to intermediate ADC value Mild to moderate restriction

Abbreviations: ADC, apparent diffusion coefficient; CT, computed tomography.

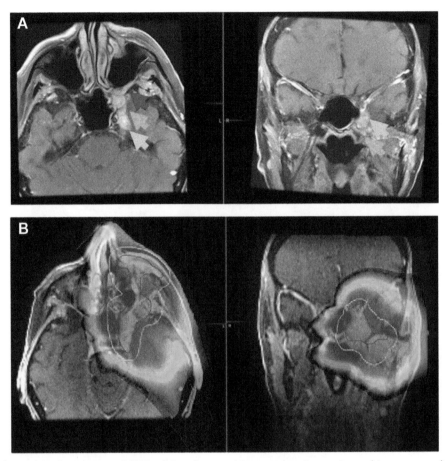

Fig. 8. Enhanced T1 fat-suppressed MRI axial and coronal images showing perineural tumor spread along V2, including inferior orbital fissure, the pterygopalatine fossa (*red arrow*), foramen rotundum (*blue arrow*), and cavernous sinus (*orange arrow*) (*A*). Colorwash dose distribution shows the gross tumor volume in red and the planning target volume in lime green (*B*).

inoperable.[30,55] Particle therapy is an emerging modality used to treat sinonasal malignancies, with the largest known systematic review and meta-analysis showing an association with improved locoregional control rates and disease-free survival rates in the proton subgroup.[31]

Carcinomas with Perineural Invasion (Salivary Gland or Skin)

High-grade carcinomas with PNI provide another indication for the use of PT.[30,32,33,52,53] Owing to the pattern of disease spread, which often involves nerves adjacent to the optic pathways, brainstem, spinal cord, temporal lobe, and auditory apparatus, the risk of treatment-related grade 3 or higher toxicity has historically ranged between 30% and 50% (**Fig. 8**). Although the initial proton therapies show that treatment complications remain high even with PT, high-dose conformality and biologic optimization improvements may improve the therapeutic ratio.[32,33]

COMPLICATION MITIGATION
Neurocognition

As PT limits the low- and moderate-dose bath to adjacent neural structures, there have been several promising dosimetric and outcomes studies regarding reducing the late effects of treatment. Most evidence for adult benefits comes from modeling and inferences from clinical outcomes from brain metastasis patients; literature shows that reducing dose to the temporal lobes, specifically the hippocampi, reduces the risks of neurocognitive decline.[54] In pediatric populations, however, there is concrete evidence of reduced neurocognitive declines in those treated with PT compared with photons.[56,57]

Second Malignancy

The most common secondary BOS tumors are meningiomas, and most can be successfully managed.[57] Database studies have shown that

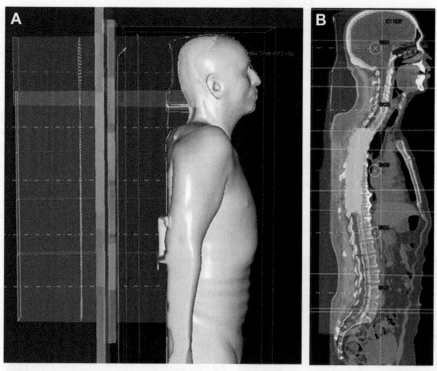

Fig. 9. Proton craniospinal irradiation (CSI) technique using a five-field posteriorly oriented pencil beam scanning technique showing the beam arrangement on a three-dimensional patient model (*A*) and colorwash dose distribution (*B*). Treatment is delivered in the supine positioning with plan robustness of 5 mm in all directions except anterior-posterior. A 3- to 4-cm overlap for field junction and dose gradient is used, and the position is verified daily. The red-shaded volume depicts the entire CSI field, and the green lattice distribution shows the individual spots from a single proton beam field.

PT can reduce the second-tumor hazard ratio by nearly one-third.[58] As shown in **Fig. 9**, craniospinal irradiation with proton radiation reduces the exit dose to all structures anterior to the vertebrae. Similarly, PT is used to reduce second malignancies in those with genetic predisposition syndromes (eg, neurofibromatosis type 1) or recurrent cancers that have been previously irradiated. These patients are more prone to developing second cancers from radiation; particle therapy reduces potential treatment overlap for future therapies.[8,58,59]

In addition to low- and moderate-dose reduction, PT can be used when dose-escalated radiotherapy is used for radioresistant BOS malignancies. However, despite the physical properties of protons, if the target is in direct contact with or a few millimeters from the avoidance structure, full-dose escalation is not always possible. Therefore, geometric optimization may precede PT (**Fig. 10**), in which a separation surgical debulking can create the physical distance needed between the organs-at-risk (OARs) and resection bed, allowing adjuvant PT that does not compromise target coverage. Although this

reduces the probability of complications, the high doses needed for some BOS tumors are not without some risk to the brainstem, optic apparatus, and temporal lobes.

Optic Pathway

Radiation injury to the optic pathway can occur among several mechanisms with the timing, severity, and treatment paradigm depending on the specific injury. Radiotherapy to anterior-based tumors can cause damage to the lens, cornea, retina, and treatment of posterior tumors, most commonly to the optic nerves, chiasm, and optic tracts. PT has been used to prevent corneal injury and damage to the intracranial pathway along the nerves, chiasm, and tracts. Although the risk of radiation-induced optic neuropathy (RION) is low, it ranges from 2% to 4% in high-risk scenarios.[38–40] **Fig. 11** illustrates the treatment of a patient with recurrent nasal cavity squamous cell carcinoma with extensive PNI and residual disease involving the clivus; the patient developed RION 2 years after therapy.

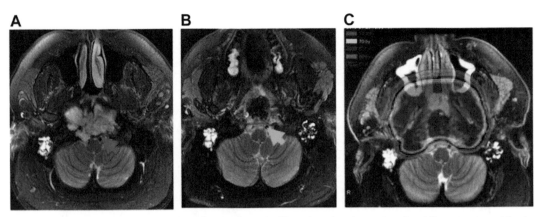

Fig. 10. Endoscopic endonasal resection of a craniocervical junction chordoma showing (*A*) pretreatment (*red arrow*) and (*B*) postsurgical extent of disease (*green arrow*) showing removal of disease in the premedullary cistern, registered to (*C*) a colorwash dose distribution.

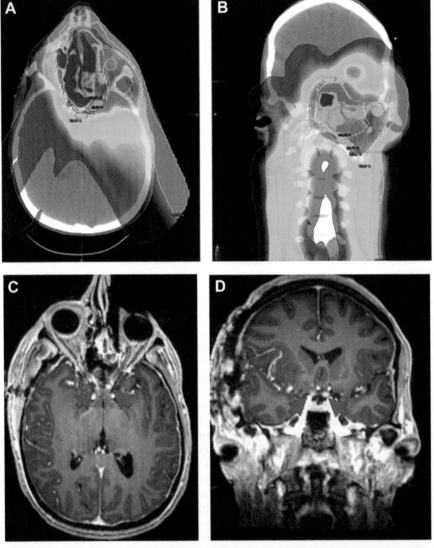

Fig. 11. (*A*) Axial and (*B*) coronal colorwash dose distributions at the time of treatment and posttreatment. MRI (*C*) axial and (*D*) coronal-enhanced T1-weighted images demonstrating bilateral radiation-induced optic neuropathy (*red arrows*). This area was immediately abutting areas of recurrent perineural tumor spread and the high-dose radiotherapy.

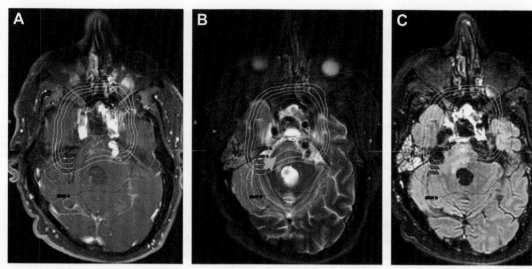

Fig. 12. Posttreatment brain MRI at the time of brainstem toxicity axial-enhanced T1-weighted fat-saturated (*A*), T2 fat sat (*B*), and fluid attenuated inversion recovery (FLAIR) (*C*) sequences coregistered to the isodose dose distribution at the time of initial radiotherapy. The 90% isodose line conformally wrapped around the surface of the brainstem, which is typical for high-dose skull-base treatment plans. Imaging findings suggestive of brainstem necrosis include T2 and FLAIR hyperintense signals (*blue arrows*), with enhancement and mass effect of affected tissue (*red arrow*).

Brainstem

Brainstem necrosis is another potential high-dose radiotherapy complication (**Fig. 12**). Fortunately, high-grade toxicity is rare in adults. In pediatrics, the risk of reported injury, even at lower doses, has been slightly higher, likely related to developing neural tissue, differences in chemotherapy regimens, and the extent and route of surgical procedures. There is no evidence that proton or photon radiotherapy has a more substantial risk of brainstem injury. Within PT planning, high prioritization is weighted to avoid brainstem injury. With PBS (**Fig. 13**), spot placement within 3 mm of the brainstem is largely avoided and does not include spots within the distal Bragg peak.[37,60,61]

Temporal Lobe

Temporal lobe radionecrosis is another potential toxicity following radiotherapy for skull-base tumors (**Fig. 14**). Most cases are asymptomatic and, if indicated, respond to vitamin E, pentoxifylline, and corticosteroids. The incidence of severe toxicity is generally 1% to 5%[62] in which bevacizumab, antiepileptics, or surgery are needed for refractory injury; the risk often varies widely based on the tumor location, the extent of disease, radiation dose and volume, and patient-specific risk factors.[42,43]

Controversies and Resource Allocation

The most controversial aspects of PT utilization relate to its geographic availability and cost. As a

high proportion of PT benefits involve late effects (with acute effects variably dependent on anatomic location), the therapeutic index may be drastically different for each patient when weighted to the person's specific OARs, health, and expected longevity.[63–65] From a clinical standpoint, PT has been allocated by different models because of the higher costs associated with treatment delivery. Cost–benefit analysis, treatment

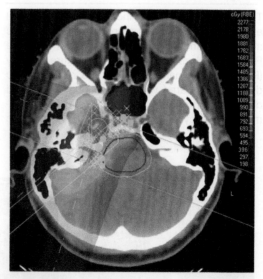

Fig. 13. Colorowash dose distribution with spot placement and weighting (*green x* and *circles*) of the three-field boost plan of skull-base chondrosarcoma treated with pencil beam scanning.

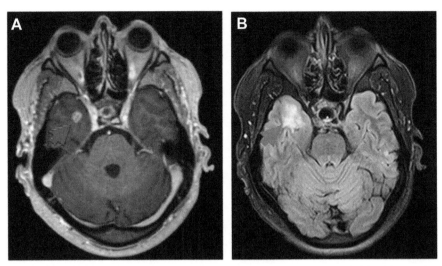

Fig. 14. Enhanced T1-weighted brain MRI demonstrating enhancement (*red arrow*) (*A*) with associated hyperintense FLAIR signal change (*blue arrow*) within the right temporal lobe (*B*).

utilization, and distribution of medical resources are country-, state-, and payer-dependent. In the United States, it is policy-dependent with specifically covered diagnoses, whereas other countries use normal tissue complication probability modeling (the Netherlands) or a commissioning policy (the United Kingdom). As machine maintenance and operational costs decline, these may change availability and disease site indications.[66–69,70]

Biologic Optimization and Future Directions

The future direction of PT includes further physical and engineering developments such as dynamic arc therapy and biologic optimization with variable RBE, FLASH, and proton boron capture therapy (PBCT).[71–78] Dynamic arc PT uses rotational arc delivery (compared with conventional static field delivery) to improve dose conformality and treatment efficiency (**Fig. 15**). Regarding the biologic

effects of proton radiotherapy, an area of continued evolution is the effect of RBE at the distal range.[73,74] PT has historically used an RBE of 1.1 for dose calculation; however, in vitro and emerging in vivo studies show that the dose at the distal range may be 20% to 30% higher. The RBE may also vary with tumor type and the OARs. This may mean that protons may have a differing biologic effect along the beam path and that an opportunity for biologic modulation exists when treating near critical OARs such as the skull-base.[77,78] Other areas of biologic optimization include FLASH, which is ultrarapid treatment delivery with a dose rate higher than 40 Gy/s. This can be done with electrons and protons, although electrons are limited to superficial malignancies because of the shallow beam profile.[75,76] Last, PBCT is emerging as a potential treatment method, using protons to generate alpha particles to bypass mechanisms for conventional radioresistance.[71,72]

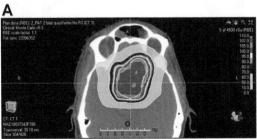
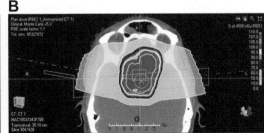

Fig. 15. Colorwash dose distribution using dynamic arc proton therapy. Proton dynamic arc therapy (*A*). Two-field intensity-modulated proton therapy (*B*).

SUMMARY

PT is widely used in skull-base tumors to limit normal nontargeted tissues for complication mitigation. Continued research with advancements in technical delivery and biologic optimization will provide additional avenues for clinical use beyond the physical properties of improved dosimetry.

CLINICS CARE POINTS

- When treating patients with craniopharyngioma, on-treatment verification imaging should be performed to monitor cyst dynamics.
- Transient treatment-related cystic expansion after radiation for craniopharyngioma and acoustic neuroma is a known phenomenon and should be clinically observed, particularly in the absence of new or worsening neurologic symptoms and do not meet the criteria for the definition of local progression.
- Maximal safe resection and geometric optimization before high-dose radiation for malignant skull-base tumors can improve target coverage and normal tissue sparing.
- Patients who undergo dose-escalated radiotherapy should be routinely monitored for treatment-related neurovascular complications.

CONFLICTS OF INTEREST

None.

REFERENCES

1. Berman AT, Plastaras JP, Vapiwala N. Radiation oncology: a primer for medical students. J Cancer Educ 2013;28(3):547–53.
2. Proton Therapy - Current Status and Future Directions. In: FitzGerald TJ, Bishop-Jodoin M, editors. IntechOpen 2021. https://doi.org/10.5772/intechopen.91072. Crossref.
3. Paganetti H. Proton Beam Therapy. IOP Publishing. 2017. https://dx.doi.org/10.1088/978-0-7503-1370-4.
4. Bradley JA, Indelicato DJ. Craniopharyngioma and Proton Therapy. International Journal of Particle Therapy 2014;1(2):386–98.
5. Koh ES, Nichol A, Millar BA, et al. Role of fractionated external beam radiotherapy in hemangioblastoma of the central nervous system. Int J Radiat Oncol Biol Phys 2007;69(5):1521–6.
6. Parekh AD, Amdur RJ, Mendenhall WM, et al. Long-term Tumor Control With Radiotherapy for Symptomatic Hemangioma of a Vertebral Body. Spine 2019; 44(12):E731–4.
7. Halasz LM, Bussiere MR, Dennis ER, et al. Proton stereotactic radiosurgery for the treatment of benign meningiomas. Int J Radiat Oncol Biol Phys 2011; 81(5):1428–35.
8. Weber DC, Bizzocchi N, Bolsi A, et al. Proton Therapy for Intracranial Meningioma for the Treatment of Primary/Recurrent Disease Including Re-Irradiation. Front Oncol 2020;10:558845.
9. Wattson DA, Tanguturi SK, Spiegel DY, et al. Outcomes of proton therapy for patients with functional pituitary adenomas. Int J Radiat Oncol Biol Phys 2014;90(3):532–9.
10. Koetsier KS, Hensen EF, Wiggenraad R, et al. Clinical outcomes and toxicity of proton radiotherapy for vestibular schwannomas: a systematic review. Journal of Radiation Oncology 2019;8(4):357–68.
11. Kennedy WR, Dagan R, Rotondo RL, et al. Proton therapy for pituitary adenoma. Appl Rad Oncol 2015. Available at. https://appliedradiationoncology.com/articles/proton-therapy-for-pituitary-adenoma. Accessed on Accessed April 6, 2022.
12. Rutenberg MS, Rotondo RL, Rao D, et al. Clinical outcomes following proton therapy for adult craniopharyngioma: a single-institution cohort study. J Neuro Oncol 2020;147(2):387–95.
13. Holtzman AL, Glassman GE, Dagan R, et al. Long-term outcomes of fractionated proton beam therapy for benign or radiographic intracranial meningioma. J Neurooncol 2023;161(3):481–9.
14. Zhu S, Rotondo R, Mendenhall WM, et al. Long-Term Outcomes of Fractionated Stereotactic Proton Therapy for Vestibular Schwannoma: A Case Series. Int J Part Ther. Spring 2018;4(4):37–46.
15. Russ S, Anastasopoulou C, Shafiq I. Pituitary Adenoma. In: StatPearls. StatPearls Publishing; 2022. Accessed November 3, 2022. http://www.ncbi.nlm.nih.gov/books/NBK554451/.
16. Jimenez RB, Ahmed S, Johnson A, et al. Proton Radiation Therapy for Pediatric Craniopharyngioma. Int J Radiat Oncol Biol Phys 2021;110(5):1480–7.
17. Merchant TE, Kun LE, Hua CH, et al. Disease control after reduced volume conformal and intensity modulated radiation therapy for childhood craniopharyngioma. Int J Radiat Oncol Biol Phys 2013;85(4):e187–92.
18. Rutenberg MS, Holtzman AL, Indelicato DJ, et al. Disease Control after Radiotherapy for Adult Craniopharyngioma: Clinical Outcomes from a Large Single-Institution Series. J Neuro Oncol 2022; 157(3):425–33.
19. Winkfield KM, Linsenmeier C, Yock TI, et al. Surveillance of craniopharyngioma cyst growth in children treated with proton radiotherapy. Int J Radiat Oncol Biol Phys 2009;73(3):716–21.

20. Leon J, Lehrer EJ, Peterson J, et al. Observation or stereotactic radiosurgery for newly diagnosed vestibular schwannomas: A systematic review and meta-analysis. J Radiosurg SBRT 2019;6(2):91–100.

21. Hayhurst C, Zadeh G. Tumor pseudoprogression following radiosurgery for vestibular schwannoma. Neuro Oncol 2012;14(1):87–92.

22. Adeberg S, Harrabi SB, Verma V, et al. Treatment of meningioma and glioma with protons and carbon ions. Radiat Oncol 2017;12(1):193.

23. Perlow HK, Siedow M, Gokun Y, et al. 68)Ga-DOTA-TATE PET-Based Radiation Contouring Creates More Precise Radiation Volumes for Patients With Meningioma. Int J Radiat Oncol Biol Phys 2022;113(4): 859–65.

24. Holtzman AL, Rotondo RL, Rutenberg MS, et al. Proton therapy for skull-base chondrosarcoma, a single-institution outcomes study. J Neuro Oncol 2019;142(3):557–63.

25. Holtzman AL, Bates JE, Morris CG, et al. Impact of Type of Treatment Center and Access to Care on Mortality and Survival for Skull Base Chordoma and Chondrosarcoma. J Neurol Surg B Skull Base 2022;83(3):328–38.

26. Holtzman AL, Rotondo RL, Rutenberg MS, et al. Clinical Outcomes Following Dose-Escalated Proton Therapy for Skull-Base Chordoma. Int J Part Ther. Summer 2021;8(1):179–88.

27. Indelicato DJ, Rotondo RL, Mailhot Vega RB, et al. Local Control After Proton Therapy for Pediatric Chordoma. Int J Radiat Oncol Biol Phys 2021; 109(5):1406–13.

28. Mercado CE, Holtzman AL, Rotondo R, et al. Proton therapy for skull base tumors: A review of clinical outcomes for chordomas and chondrosarcomas. Head Neck 2019;41(2):536–41.

29. Harsh IV, Vaz-Guimaraes F, editors. Chordomas and chondrosarcomas of the skull base and spine. 2nd Edition. Academic Press; 2017. https://doi.org/10.1016/C2015-0-00351-3. Accessed November 2, 2022.

30. Dagan R, Uezono H, Bryant C, et al. Long-term Outcomes from Proton Therapy for Sinonasal Cancers. Int J Part Ther. Summer 2021;8(1):200–12.

31. Patel SH, Wang Z, Wong WW, et al. Charged particle therapy versus photon therapy for paranasal sinus and nasal cavity malignant diseases: a systematic review and meta-analysis. Lancet Oncol 2014; 15(9):1027–38.

32. Bryant CM, Dagan R, Holtzman AL, et al. Passively Scattered Proton Therapy for Nonmelanoma Skin Cancer with Clinical Perineural Invasion. Int J Part Ther. Summer 2021;8(1):285–93.

33. Holtzman AL, Mendenhall WM. High-dose conformal proton therapy for clinical perineural invasion in cutaneous head and neck cancer. Oral Oncol 2020;100:104486.

34. Haas RL, Walraven I, Lecointe-Artzner E, et al. Radiation Therapy as Sole Management for Solitary Fibrous Tumors (SFT): A Retrospective Study From the Global SFT Initiative in Collaboration With the Sarcoma Patients EuroNet. Int J Radiat Oncol Biol Phys 2018;101(5):1226–33.

35. Fung V, Calugaru V, Bolle S, et al. Proton beam therapy for skull base chordomas in 106 patients: A dose adaptive radiation protocol. Radiother Oncol 2018;128(2):198–202.

36. Vern-Gross TZ, Indelicato DJ, Bradley JA, et al. Patterns of Failure in Pediatric Rhabdomyosarcoma After Proton Therapy. Int J Radiat Oncol Biol Phys 2016;96(5):1070–7.

37. Holtzman AL, Rutenberg MS, De Leo AN, et al. The incidence of brainstem toxicity following high-dose conformal proton therapy for adult skull-base malignancies. Acta Oncol 2022;61(8):1026–31.

38. De Leo AN, Holtzman AL, Ho MW, et al. Vision loss following high-dose proton-based radiotherapy for skull-base chordoma and chondrosarcoma. Radiother Oncol 2021;158:125–30.

39. Holliday EB, Esmaeli B, Pinckard J, et al. A Multidisciplinary Orbit-Sparing Treatment Approach That Includes Proton Therapy for Epithelial Tumors of the Orbit and Ocular Adnexa. Int J Radiat Oncol Biol Phys 2016;95(1):344–52.

40. Li PC, Liebsch NJ, Niemierko A, et al. Radiation tolerance of the optic pathway in patients treated with proton and photon radiotherapy. Radiother Oncol 2019;131:112–9.

41. Kountouri M, Pica A, Walser M, et al. Radiation-induced optic neuropathy after pencil beam scanning proton therapy for skull-base and head and neck tumours. Br J Radiol 2020;93(1107): 20190028.

42. Kitpanit S, Lee A, Pitter KL, et al. Temporal Lobe Necrosis in Head and Neck Cancer Patients after Proton Therapy to the Skull Base. Int J Part Ther. Spring 2020;6(4):17–28.

43. Zhang YY, Huo WL, Goldberg SI, et al. Brain-Specific Relative Biological Effectiveness of Protons Based on Long-term Outcome of Patients With Nasopharyngeal Carcinoma. Int J Radiat Oncol Biol Phys 2021;110(4):984–92.

44. Debus J, Hug EB, Liebsch NJ, et al. Brainstem tolerance to conformal radiotherapy of skull base tumors. Int J Radiat Oncol Biol Phys 1997;39(5):967–75.

45. Debus J, Hug EB, Liebsch NJ, et al. Dose-volume tolerance of the brainstem after high-dose radiotherapy. Front Radiat Ther Oncol 1999;33:305–14.

46. Mayo C, Yorke E, Merchant TE. Radiation associated brainstem injury. Int J Radiat Oncol Biol Phys 2010; 76(3 Suppl):S36–41.

47. Shih AR, Cote GM, Chebib I, et al. Clinicopathologic characteristics of poorly differentiated chordoma. Mod Pathol 2018;31(8):1237–45.

48. Soule E, Baig S, Fiester P, et al. Current Management and Image Review of Skull Base Chordoma: What the Radiologist Needs to Know. J Clin Imaging Sci 2021;11:46.

49. Palm RF, Oliver DE, Yang GQ, et al. The role of dose escalation and proton therapy in perioperative or definitive treatment of chondrosarcoma and chordoma: An analysis of the National Cancer Data Base. Cancer 2019;125(4):642–51.

50. Rice SR, Chhabra AM, Holtzman A, et al. Clinical outcomes and toxicities of 100 patients treated with proton therapy for chordoma on the Proton Collaborative Group Prospective Registry. Radiother Oncol 2023;20:109551.

51. Sahgal A, Chan MW, Atenafu EG, et al. Image-guided, intensity-modulated radiation therapy (IG-IMRT) for skull base chordoma and chondrosarcoma: preliminary outcomes. Neuro Oncol 2015; 17(6):889–94.

52. Hanania AN, Zhang X, Gunn GB, et al. Proton Therapy for Major Salivary Gland Cancer: Clinical Outcomes. Int J Part Ther 2021;8(1):261–72.

53. Rodriguez-Russo CA, Junn JC, Yom SS, et al. Radiation Therapy for Adenoid Cystic Carcinoma of the Head and Neck. Cancers 2021;13(24).

54. Brown PD, Gondi V, Pugh S, et al. Hippocampal Avoidance During Whole-Brain Radiotherapy Plus Memantine for Patients With Brain Metastases: Phase III Trial NRG Oncology CC001. J Clin Oncol 2020;38(10):1019–29.

55. Amit M, Abdelmeguid AS, Watcherporn T, et al. Induction Chemotherapy Response as a Guide for Treatment Optimization in Sinonasal Undifferentiated Carcinoma. J Clin Oncol 20 2019;37(6):504–12.

56. Kahalley LS, Peterson R, Ris MD, et al. Superior Intellectual Outcomes After Proton Radiotherapy Compared With Photon Radiotherapy for Pediatric Medulloblastoma. J Clin Oncol 2020;38(5):454–61.

57. Galloway TJ, Indelicato DJ, Amdur RJ, et al. Second tumors in pediatric patients treated with radiotherapy to the central nervous system. Am J Clin Oncol 2012;35(3):279–83.

58. Xiang M, Chang DT, Pollom EL. Second cancer risk after primary cancer treatment with three-dimensional conformal, intensity-modulated, or proton beam radiation therapy. Cancer 2020;126(15): 3560–8.

59. Indelicato DJ, Bates JE, Mailhot Vega RB, et al. Second tumor risk in children treated with proton therapy. Pediatr Blood Cancer 2021;68(7):e28941.

60. Haas-Kogan D, Indelicato D, Paganetti H, et al. National Cancer Institute Workshop on Proton Therapy for Children: Considerations Regarding Brainstem Injury. Int J Radiat Oncol Biol Phys 2018;101(1): 152–68.

61. Indelicato DJ, Flampouri S, Rotondo RL, et al. Incidence and dosimetric parameters of pediatric brainstem toxicity following proton therapy. Acta Oncol 2014;53(10):1298–304.

62. Niemierko A, Schuemann J, Niyazi M, et al. Brain Necrosis in Adult Patients After Proton Therapy: Is There Evidence for Dependency on Linear Energy Transfer? Int J Radiat Oncol Biol Phys 2021;109(1): 109–19.

63. Jones DA, Smith J, Mei XW, et al. A systematic review of health economic evaluations of proton beam therapy for adult cancer: Appraising methodology and quality. Clin Transl Radiat Oncol 2020;20: 19–26.

64. Mailhot Vega RB, Mohammadi H, Patel SI, et al. Establishing Cost-Effective Allocation of Proton Therapy for Patients With Mediastinal Hodgkin Lymphoma. Int J Radiat Oncol Biol Phys 2022; 112(1):158–66.

65. Mendenhall WM, Brooks ED, Smith S, et al. Insurance Approval for Definitive Proton Therapy for Prostate Cancer. Int J Part Ther. Winter 2022;8(3):36–42.

66. Crellin A. The Road Map for National Health Service Proton Beam Therapy. Clin Oncol 2018;30(5):277–9.

67. Langendijk JA, Hoebers FJP, de Jong MA, et al. National Protocol for Model-Based Selection for Proton Therapy in Head and Neck Cancer. Int J Part Ther. Summer 2021;8(1):354–65.

68. Lundkvist J, Ekman M, Ericsson SR, et al. Proton therapy of cancer: potential clinical advantages and cost-effectiveness. Acta Oncol 2005;44(8): 850–61.

69. Stieb S, Lee A, van Dijk LV, et al. NTCP Modeling of Late Effects for Head and Neck Cancer: A Systematic Review. Int J Part Ther. Summer 2021;8(1):95–107.

70. Gaito S, Hwang EJ, France A, et al. Outcomes of Patients Treated in the UK Proton Overseas Programme: Central Nervous System Group. Clin Oncol (R Coll Radiol) 2023. https://doi.org/10.1016/ j.clon.2023.01.024.

71. Blaha P, Feoli C, Agosteo S, et al. The Proton-Boron Reaction Increases the Radiobiological Effectiveness of Clinical Low- and High-Energy Proton Beams: Novel Experimental Evidence and Perspectives. Front Oncol 2021;11:682647.

72. Cirrone GAP, Manti L, Margarone D, et al. First experimental proof of Proton Boron Capture Therapy (PBCT) to enhance protontherapy effectiveness. Sci Rep 2018;8(1):1141.

73. Li X, Liu G, Janssens G, et al. The first prototype of spot-scanning proton arc treatment delivery. Radiother Oncol 2019;137:130–6.

74. Toussaint L, Indelicato DJ, Holgersen KS, et al. Towards proton arc therapy: physical and biologically equivalent doses with increasing number of beams in pediatric brain irradiation. Acta Oncol 2019; 58(10):1451–6.

75. Hughes JR, Parsons JL. FLASH Radiotherapy: Current Knowledge and Future Insights Using Proton-

Beam Therapy. Int J Mol Sci 2020;(18):21. https://doi.org/10.3390/ijms21186492.

76. Mascia AE, Daugherty EC, Zhang Y, et al. Proton FLASH Radiotherapy for the Treatment of Symptomatic Bone Metastases: The FAST-01 Nonrandomized Trial. JAMA Oncol 2023;9(1):62–9.

77. Deng W, Yang Y, Liu C, et al. A Critical Review of LET-Based Intensity-Modulated Proton Therapy Plan Evaluation and Optimization for Head and Neck Cancer Management. *Int J Part Ther*. Summer 2021;8(1):36–49.

78. Wang L, Fossati P, Paganetti H, et al. The Biological Basis for Enhanced Effects of Proton Radiation Therapy Relative to Photon Radiation Therapy for Head and Neck Squamous Cell Carcinoma. *Int J Part Ther*. Summer 2021;8(1):3–13.

Future Perspective
Carbon Ion Radiotherapy for Head and Neck and Skull Base Malignancies

Michael S. Rutenberg, MD, PhD*, Chris Beltran, PhD

KEYWORDS

- Carbon ion radiotherapy • Skull base malignancies • Head and neck cancer • Chordoma
- Chondrosarcoma • Adenoid cystic carcinoma • Particle therapy • Radiotherapy

KEY POINTS

- Carbon ion radiotherapy is a form of heavy particle therapy with biophysical characteristics particularly suited for treating head and neck and skull base malignancies to provide improved disease control outcomes with reduced radiotherapy-associated side effects.
- Carbon ion radiotherapy has dosimetric advantages compared with x-ray radiotherapy that can reduce the dose to normal surrounding tissues.
- Carbon ion radiotherapy has increased biological effectiveness against the target malignancy, which can improve the effectiveness of treatment, particularly for radioresistant or hypoxic tumors.
- Clinical trials are underway to establish the benefits of carbon ion radiotherapy compared with x-ray and proton radiotherapy.

INTRODUCTION

Carbon ion radiotherapy (CIRT) has unique biophysical characteristics that are particularly advantageous for head and neck and base of skull (BOS) malignancies. The physical properties of carbon ions provide dosimetric advantages over conventional photon-based radiotherapy that can reduce the radiation dose distribution to nearby surrounding organs at risk. This is particularly relevant for malignancies in areas dense with radiosensitive normal tissues. Additionally, carbon ion radiation has increased radiobiological effects on the target tissues to improve the treatment response for radioresistant histologies. Herein, we describe the history of carbon ion therapy, the physical and biological characteristics of CIRT, and clinical data utilizing CIRT in head and neck and skull base malignancies.

A BRIEF HISTORY OF CHARGED PARTICLES

Wilhelm Rontgen is credited with the discovery of x-rays in 1895 after he systematically analyzed and issued the first publication on the subject, describing x-rays as a new type of radiation. Rontgen identified the earliest medical use when he imaged his wife's hand on a photographic plate using x-rays. The discovery of radioisotopes by Antoine-Henri Becquerel and Marie and Pierre Curie led to the earliest uses of x-rays and radioactive elements to treat cancer and by 1902, radiation was being used for cancer therapy for a variety of malignancies. During the next half-century, the use of radiotherapy for the treatment of malignancies expanded and so did the understanding of the potential benefits and risks of such treatments. By 1956, the first medical linear accelerator in the Western Hemisphere was installed at Stanford Hospital in San Francisco. With advances in harnessing the potential radioactivity and the development of accelerators to energize and target radiation, interest increased in the use of varying forms of radiation, particularly particle therapy. Robert Wilson at The Lawrence Berkeley National Laboratory (LBL) first suggested the potential clinical benefits of particle therapy (protons) based on their favorable dose distribution

Department of Radiation Oncology, Mayo Clinic, 4500 San Pablo Road, Jacksonville, FL 32224, USA
* Corresponding author.
E-mail address: rutenberg.michael@mayo.edu

Oral Maxillofacial Surg Clin N Am 35 (2023) 485–492
https://doi.org/10.1016/j.coms.2023.02.009

characterized by relatively low entrance dose at shallow depths and high energy deposition and rapid fall-off at the end of the beam range (see "Bragg peak" below). The difference in physical properties between charged particles and x-rays/photons forms the basis of the dosimetric benefits of particle therapies. In short, particles deposit most of their energy at the end of the beam path via a spike in energy deposition as the particle decelerates. This spike in energy deposition is termed the "Bragg peak," after its discoverer, William Henry Bragg. Distal to the Bragg peak, there is little radiation dose deposition (exit dose). Upstream of the Bragg peak, there is relatively low-dose deposition. This is in contrast with electromagnetic radiation (x-rays and photons), which has no Bragg peak and deposit most of their dose outside of the intended target, including a significant dose upstream (entry dose) and downstream (exit dose) of the target. The LBL at the University of California, Berkeley, provided some of the earliest research and clinical experience with particle therapy. This included proton radiotherapy for intracranial targets beginning in the 1950s followed by helium ion therapy and additional charged particle therapy including neon, oxygen, nitrogen, and carbon from 1975 to 1992.[1] The LBL charged particle program was terminated in 1992. In 1994, the Heavy Ion Medical Accelerator in Chiba opened in Chiba, Japan, and began treatment with carbon radiotherapy. This was followed by another heavy ion center in Hyogo, Japan, HIBMC (Hyogo Ion Beam Medical Center) and then GSI (Gesellschaft fur Schwerionenforschung) in Darmstadt, Germany, in 1997. At the writing of this article, there are 13 active carbon ion treatment centers worldwide, 9 in Asia (2 China, 7 Japan), and 4 in Europe (1 Austria, 2 Germany, 1 Italy). There are no carbon ion treatment facilities yet in North America. A carbon ion facility at Mayo Clinic in Florida, United States is currently under construction with plans to begin treatment in 2027.

THE PHYSICAL AND RADIOBIOLOGICAL PROPERTIES OF CARBON

A major difference in physical behavior that imparts an advantage of charged particle radiotherapy over electromagnetic radiation (ie, photons/x-rays) is the nature of dose deposition by charged particles, including the "Bragg peak." All forms of radiation deposit energy along the beam path. Charged particles travel along their paths with energy deposition inversely related to the square of the velocity of the particle. Therefore, as the charged particle slows down in tissue, its energy deposition increases. Conversely, at shallow depths (ie, tissue surface) where the particle has its highest speed, there is relatively low energy deposition. As particles interact with tissue along their path, they slow down as they reach the end of their range and have a steep increase in energy deposition, resulting in an energy peak (ie, "Bragg peak") followed by a sharp dose falloff immediately beyond the Bragg peak. The practical implication of this phenomenon is that there is little or no exit dose from charged particles. **Fig. 1** shows radiation beam depth-dose profiles between photon and carbon ions and reveals differences between entrance doses and end of range doses between radiation sources. This difference in dose deposition between carbon and photons (x-rays) enables radiation delivery with reduced low and intermediate radiation dose to normal tissues surrounding the radiation target (via reduced entrance and exit dose). Although charged particles display generally similar dose distribution properties, there exist important differences between different particles, including the steepness of the Bragg peak and the steepness of the lateral dose falloff (ie, the amount lateral dose spread from the beam path). These differences between particles are due to differences in the particle mass and atomic number. The practical implication of this difference can be seen between 2 clinically useful particles—protons and carbon. Both are utilized in clinical practice and due to size and mass differences, they have different rates of distal and lateral dose fall-off (carbon has sharper dose falloff at both the distal and lateral beam edges).

Another significant difference between carbon and other types of radiation is the amount of energy deposited over the beam path. The term linear energy transfer (LET) quantifies the amount of radiation energy that is imparted over a distance in a medium (ie, tissue). Relative levels of LET are determined using gamma particles and x-rays as the reference. Carbon is a "high-LET" form of radiation and the LET of carbon is higher than that of protons, which is slightly higher than that of photons. High-LET radiation can have a higher impact on radioresistant tumors with increased cell killing. Additionally, high-LET radiation makes the biological impact of radiation less sensitive to cell cycle phase, tumor oxygenation, and radiation fractionation. Importantly, the LET of carbon is similar to photons along the flat portion of the dose deposition curve and only becomes high at the Bragg peak. This spares the normal tissues upstream of the intended radiation target from increased radiation treatment effect with high LET radiation and maximizes the impact of carbon radiotherapy on the target/tumor relative to normal tissues.[2]

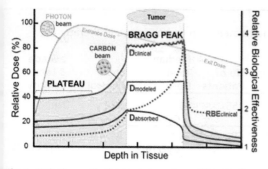

Fig 1. Relative radiotherapy dose deposition in tissue and relative biological effectiveness (RBE) curves between carbon ions and photons. Relative radiotherapy dose in the y-axis on the left indicates the amount of absorbed tissue dose with increasing depth in tissue (along the x-axis) for a carbon ion beam (top purple curve) compared with a photon beam (blue curve). The dose along each curves before and after the "tumor" represent dose deposited in normal tissue upstream (entrance dose) and downstream (exit dose) of the target (ie, tumor). The photon curve deposits significantly more dose before and after the tumor compared with the carbon curve. The RBE clinical curve represents the biological effectiveness of the dose deposited by the carbon ions. The RBE is relatively low along the "plateau" of the curve, however, increases in a nonuniform pattern along the Bragg Peak within the target.

Another potential benefit of carbon ion radiotherapy is seen in preclinical studies suggesting increased immune response with combined CIRT and immune checkpoint blockade.[3,4] Additionally, there are data suggesting enhanced suppression of cancer migration and cancer cell invasion with CIRT compared with x-ray radiotherapy.[5]

CLINICAL ROLE FOR CARBON ION RADIOTHERAPY IN THE HEAD AND NECK AND SKULL BASE

The most substantial expected benefits for CIRT include (1) the dosimetric advantages of sparing normal tissues from irradiation and (2) the increased biological effectiveness of carbon on the tumor. The dosimetric advantages of reduced normal tissue irradiation are particularly relevant in the head and neck/BOS areas where there is a density of radiosensitive normal tissues, including salivary glands, swallowing musculature, inner ear structures, optic apparatus, cranial nerves, brainstem, and cerebrum. These same structures render complete surgical resection of tumors in these areas difficult or impossible without significant morbidity. Therefore, radiotherapy is often necessary in the postoperative setting or even as part of definitive treatment. An additional

challenge in these anatomic sites is the presence of histologies that are less radiosensitive, including adenoid cystic carcinomas (ACCs), chordoma, and chondrosarcoma. The increased biological effectiveness of CIRT is especially relevant for these histologies especially when they are incompletely resected, as is often the case. The next section describes clinical data for several such histologies in the head and neck and BOS for which CIRT shows promise.

Head and Neck/Skull Base Soft-Tissue Sarcomas

Soft-tissue sarcomas (STSs) are among the most attractive malignancies for treatment with CIRT due to their relative radioresistance and their requirement for aggressive oncologic resections. These considerations are particularly relevant for head and neck/skull base sarcomas where en bloc and negative margin resections are difficult or impossible and achieving local control with radiotherapy requires high doses. Due to the rarity of STS, there are limited data available with the use of CIRT. The facility in Chiba, Japan, prospectively observed 27 patients with unresected sarcomas of mixed histologies, including soft-tissue (16 patients) and bone sarcomas (11 patients), treated with 70.4 GyE in 16 fractions.[6] With median follow-up of 37 months, 3-year local control was 91.8%. The local control rates for both STS and osteosarcoma in this study compared very favorably to historical controls at the same institution using lower doses of CIRT. Late radiation-related complications of Grade 3 or greater were observed in 23.1% of patients. Investigators at Gunma University Heavy Ion Center subsequently completed a prospective study including 10 patients with unresectable bone or STSs of the head and neck/BOS treated with 70.4 GyE in 16 fractions.[7] They reported a 3-year local control rate of 72.9%.

Chordoma

Due to the high radiotherapy dose requirements to achieve local control and difficulty in achieving adequate surgical resection, skull base chordoma has long been a disease with indications for the treatment with particle therapy.[8,9] Skull base chordoma has similarly been a major focus of carbon ion radiotherapy facilities, and despite its rarity, there are several large retrospective series and a single-arm prospective observation study (**Table 1**). Uhl and colleagues from the Heidelberg Ion Beam Therapy Center (HIT) retrospectively reviewed 155 patients with BOS chordoma treated with CIRT from 1998 to 2008. All patients had

Table 1
Select clinical outcomes series for skull base chordoma treated with carbon ion radiotherapy

Institute	Design	Histology	Dates	Median F/U	No of Patients	Median Total Dose	Local Control	≥Grade 3 Late Toxicity
HIT (Uhl, 2014)	Retro	Chordoma	1998–2008	72 mo	155	60 GyE/20fx	5/10 y 72%/54%	NR
CNAO (Iannalfi et al,[12] 2020)	Prospective	Chordoma	2011–2018	49 mo	65	70.4 GyE/16fx	5y 71%	3 y TFS 85%
HIT (Mattke, 2022)	Retro	Chordoma	2009–2014	52 mo	111	66 GyE/22fx	5y 65%	NR

Abbreviations: CRT, Heidelberg Ion Beam therapy center; Retro, retrospective; GyE, gray equivalent; NR, not reported; TFS, ≥Grade 3 toxicity free survival.

gross disease at the time of radiotherapy and received a median dose of 60 GyE in 20 fractions. With a median follow-up time of 72 months, they reported 5-year and 10-year local control rates of 72% and 54%, respectively.[10] Mattke reported a follow-up series including 111 patients treated at HIT from 2009 to 2014 with BOS chordoma.[11] Patients were treated to a median dose of 66 GyE in 22 fractions and with over 4 years median follow-up had 5-year local control of 65%. Toxicity outcomes have not yet been reported from this series. The carbon ion facility in Pavia, Italy prospectively observed 135 patients with BOS chordoma treated with 70.4 GyE in 16 fractions. With a median follow-up of 49 months, 5-year local control was 71% and 3-year grade 3 or greater toxicity-free survival was 85%.[12]

Chondrosarcoma

Though histologically and prognostically distinct from skull base chordomas, chondrosarcomas of BOS are often managed similarly. They are often incompletely resectable and require relatively high radiotherapy doses to achieve local control and are therefore an attractive target for particle therapy.[13,14] A study from Schulz-Ertner retrospectively reviewed the early outcomes from Heidelberg, Germany, including 54 patients with BOS chondrosarcoma treated from 1998 to 2005 treated with a median dose of 60 GyE in 20 fractions.[15] With median follow-up of 33 months, the 3-year local control was 96.2% and the rate of grade 3 or greater late radiotherapy complications was 1.9% (**Table 2**). A subsequent report from the same group with additional patients and longer follow-up (median 91 months) indicated 10-year local control rates of 88%.[16] Another retrospective

study included 79 patients treated with CIRT for BOS chondrosarcoma from 2009 to 2014. Patients received 60 GyE in 20 fractions. With a median follow-up time of 40 months, 4-year local control was 91%.[17]

Adenoid Cystic Carcinoma

ACC is a rare malignancy originating from salivary glands in the head and neck and often involving the paranasal sinuses. They have a propensity for perineural invasion with extension along cranial nerves to involve the skull base. Surgical resection remains the mainstay of treatment with radiotherapy often utilized in the postoperative setting for residual disease or high-risk features (perineural invasion, positive margins, T3/T4 disease) or for definitive treatment of unresectable disease. Although limited by the selection biases associated with retrospective reviews, most studies suggest decreased rates of locoregional control with radiotherapy alone compared with surgery ± postop RT, and therefore, definitive radiotherapy has been reserved for unresectable disease.[18,19] Due to the anatomic location and requirement for high dose radiation for effective disease control, carbon ion radiotherapy represents a promising treatment modality. The Heavy Ion Research Center (GSI) at Heidelberg initially published a 16 patient series with head and neck ACC with gross residual disease following subtotal resection (STR) or biopsy. Patients were treated with combined photon RT (45–54 GyE) and a carbon ion boost to a total dose of 72 GyE. With a median follow-up of 12 months, 1 and 3-year actuarial local control was 80.8% and 64.6%, respectively.[20] Researchers in at the National Institute of Radiological Sciences in Chiba, Japan,

Table 2
Select clinical outcomes series for skull base chondrosarcoma treated with carbon ion radiotherapy

Institute	Design	Histology	Dates	Median F/U	No of Patients	Median Total Dose	Local Control	≥Grade 3 Late Toxicity
GSI (Schulz-Ertner et al,[15] 2007)	Retro	Chs	1998–2005	33 mo	54	60 GyE/20fx	4y 90%	1.9%
GSI (Uhl, 2014)	Retro	Chs	1998–2008	91 mo	79	60 GyE/20fx	10 y 88%	NR
HIT (Mattke, 2018)	Retro	Chs	2009–2014	40 mo	79	60 GyE/20fx	4y 91%	NR

Abbreviations: GSI, Society for heavy Ion research (Darmstadt; Germany), HIT; Heidelberg Ion Beam therapy center, Retro; retrospective, GyE; gray equivalent, NR; not reported.

performed a dose escalation trial with head and neck cancers treated with CIRT.[21] Their study including mixed histologies of carcinomas, melanomas, and sarcomas, with a primary aim of determining safe dose and fractionation. They included doses from 52.8 to 64.8 GyE in 16 fractions and 48.6 to 70.2 GyE in 18 fractions. They concluded that 70.2 GyE in 18 fractions (over 6 weeks) or 64.0 GyE in 16 fractions (over 4 weeks) were the maximum tolerated dose for their fractionation schemes. The COSMIC trial was a prospective phase II single arm study from Heidelberg, which included patients with malignant salivary gland tumors with either R1/R2 resections or unresectable disease treated with combined photon/carbon radiotherapy including 50 GyE delivered with intensity-modulated ratdiotherapy(IMRT) (in 2 Gy per fraction) and 24 GyE delivered using CIRT (in 3 GyE per fraction).[22] Most patients included in the study (89%) had ACC. The 3-year local control for ACC was 81.9%, including 89.7% for patients with R1 resection, 86.9% with R2 resection, and 75.0% with unresectable disease. In 2016, the group at GSI published a follow-up series including 220 patients with head and neck ACC with gross disease following STR or biopsy.[23] Patients received combination x-ray therapy with a carbon ion boost, including a median dose of CIRT to 23.9 GyE (3 GyE per fraction) with photon RT to a median dose of 50 GyE (1.8–2 GyE per fraction). With a median follow-up of 34 months, 3-year local control was nearly 81% for patients with gross residual disease (either R2 resection or biopsy only). Local control at 5 years was just over 50%. These local control numbers are comparable to those published in a large series from the University of Florida using photon radiotherapy as definitive treatment of ACC.[8]

A large phase II single cohort study from Mizoe and colleagues at the Carbon Ion facility in Chiba included patients with locally advanced head and neck malignancies of various histologies treated with CIRT alone (without combining with x-rays).[24] Their study included 236 patients in total, including 69 patients with ACC, treated to a median dose of 57.6 GyE in 16 fractions. The response rate (partial and complete response) for the ACC cohort at 6 months was 63%, including 17% with a complete response. With a follow-up of more than 5 years for the ACC cohort, the 5-year actuarial local control was 73%. They reported no grade 3 or higher late treatment complications.

A combined multi-institutional series from the Japan Carbon-Ion Radiation Oncology Study Group reported outcomes from 289 patients who were treated with CIRT for head and neck ACC with gross disease.[24] The median dose was 64 GyE in 16 fractions. With a median follow-up time of 30 months, the 2-year and 5-year local control rates were 88% and 68%, respectively. Fifteen percent of patients experienced grade 3 or greater late toxicities, with osteoradionecrosis of the jaw (grade 3) being most common and 5% of patients experiencing vision toxicity. Two patients experienced grade 5 hemorrhage after being treated for T4 tumors of the nasopharynx involving the carotid arteries. The outcomes utilizing CIRT alone compare very favorably to the combined photon/carbon series and historical series reporting outcomes of photon radiotherapy alone for treatment of ACC with gross residual disease at the time of RT.[8,19,25]

Other Histologies

The histologies of the head and neck and BOS described in the sections above garner much of the interest for heavy particle therapy. However, the biophysical advantages of carbon ion radiotherapy can be leveraged to improve outcomes in the treatment of a variety of other malignant histologies in this anatomic site. High rates of local recurrence and treatment-associated toxicities are challenges in the treatment of HPV-negative mucosal carcinoma, esthesioneuroblastoma, and mucosal melanoma and are included in outcomes studies utilizing CIRT.[24,26]

Reirradiation

Patients who experience locoregional disease recurrence after earlier radiotherapy to the head and neck/BOS have a poor prognosis and limited treatment options with considerable morbidity from salvage treatments. Salvage surgery, when possible, is often indicated; however, they are often indications for postoperative radiotherapy (± chemotherapy).[27] However, curative salvage surgery is frequently not an option. In cases of reirradiation, risks of severe normal tissue injury, including grade 5 toxicities, can be unacceptably high. The dosimetric advantages of particle therapy, including CIRT, can be utilized to reduce the volume of overlapping dose, by reducing the volume of normal irradiated tissue. Despite this potential benefit in dose distribution for reirradiation, the areas of disease recurrence require high doses and minimizing risks of abutting tissue injury is often unavoidable, even with the use of particle therapy. Beyond the added risks of treatment complications with reirradiation, there are legitimate concerns regarding treatment futility in the setting of radioresistant disease that has recurred after prior radiotherapy. To mitigate some of the concerns of both normal tissue toxicity and radioresistant recurrent disease, when x-ray reirradiation is used, altered fractionation schemes are often used.[28,29] In addition to the dosimetric advantages of carbon ion radiotherapy, the increased radiobiological effectiveness of CIRT can provide improved tumor cell killing compared with other radiation modalities. This can be particularly important given the reduced sensitivity of CIRT to hypoxic conditions and treatment fractionation. Lack of high-quality comparative studies due to patient and disease heterogeneity has made significant advances in our understanding of how to best utilize reirradiation very difficult. Nonetheless, CIRT has been reported in relatively large retrospective series and provides a promising option that deserves further investigation.[30–32]

THE LIMITATIONS OF CARBON ION RADIOTHERAPY

Although the promise of carbon ion radiotherapy is immense, there are substantial limitations in its clinical implementation. The first and most obvious includes the massive cost requirements to construct a facility. The cost of constructing a new carbon ion facility for treatment approaches US$300 million, significantly more expensive than a proton facility (which is orders of magnitude more expensive than an x-ray radiotherapy center). Furthermore, in the United States, clinical treatment with CIRT will require FDA (U.S. Food and Drug Administration) authorization of the equipment and the establishment of a new system of billing codes and a treatment reimbursement system.[33]

Beyond the cost, however, there is substantial radiobiology and radiation physics research that is required to optimize the use of CIRT and maximize its potential benefits. These include refinement in the carbon ion modeling of the biological effectiveness in normal and target tissues and advances in beam delivery techniques and efficiency.[34–36]

Finally, the realization of whatever benefits of CIRT are achievable will only come through collaboration and cooperative efforts around the world. We have witnessed a proliferation of proton facilities across the world in the past 2 decades, yet we have limited high-level evidence on the actual benefits of proton radiotherapy compared with x-ray radiotherapy. The approach to the study and utilization of carbon ion radiotherapy should be much more thoughtful, deliberate, and cooperative.

SUMMARY

Carbon ion radiotherapy uses accelerated heavy ions to precisely target and kill cancer cells in tissue. The unique biophysical characteristics of CIRT can be particularly beneficial in the treatment of head and neck and skull base malignancies. This includes reduced dose to normal tissues surrounding the target, compared with other forms of radiotherapy (eg, x-rays and protons), potentially reducing treatment-related side effects. Additionally, because carbon ions are heavy particles, they have increased biological effectiveness in killing targeted cancer cells. CIRT has a reduced requirement for tissue oxygenation to be effective in tumor killing and therefore can be more effective in treating hypoxic tissues, including postoperative tissues or hypoxic areas within a tumor. Furthermore, because of the dosimetric and biologic advantages of CIRT, there is less need for treatment fractionation and the total treatment course can be delivered quicker compared with conventional radiotherapy. Because of the limited carbon ion radiotherapy facilities around the world, it is critically important that basic, translational, and clinical research is conducted in a collaborative and cooperative effort to maximize efficiency and expedite the advancement of this technology to realize its full potential to improve cancer treatment outcomes.

CLINICS CARE POINTS

- Carbon ion radiotherapy is a form of heavy particle radiotherapy that is not currently available in the United States. There are currently 13 active carbon ion centers in the world, all in Europe and Asia.
- Due to difficulties in achieving adequate oncologic resections, the high density of radiosensitive normal tissues, and the high radiation doses required for curative treatment, there is significant interest in carbon ion radiotherapy for head and neck and skull base malignancies.
- The benefits of carbon ion radiotherapy for cancer treatment comes from 2 main characteristics: (1) improved dose distribution with reduced dose to surrounding normal tissues and (2) improved cell killing within the target volume but not in areas outside the target.
- There are currently no randomized trials comparing carbon ion radiotherapy to x-ray or proton radiotherapy, however, several are currently underway.

REFERENCES

1. Castro JR. Results of heavy ion radiotherapy. Radiat Environ Biophys 1995;34(1):45–8.
2. Durante M, Loeffler JS. Charged particles in radiation oncology. Nat Rev Clin Oncol 2010;7(1):37–43.
3. Ando K, Fujita H, Hosoi A, et al. Intravenous dendritic cell administration enhances suppression of lung metastasis induced by carbon-ion irradiation. J Radiat Res 2017;58(4):446–55.
4. Helm A, Tinganelli W, Simoniello P, et al. Reduction of Lung Metastases in a Mouse Osteosarcoma Model Treated With Carbon Ions and Immune Checkpoint Inhibitors. Int J Radiat Oncol Biol Phys 2021;109(2):594–602.
5. Akino Y, Teshima T, Kihara A, et al. Carbon-ion beam irradiation effectively suppresses migration and invasion of human non-small-cell lung cancer cells. Int J Radiat Oncol Biol Phys 2009;75(2):475–81.
6. Jingu K, Tsuji H, Mizoe JE, et al. ,Carbon ion radiation therapy improves the prognosis of unresectable adult bone and soft-tissue sarcoma of the head and neck. Int J Radiat Oncol Biol Phys 2012;82(5):2125–31.
7. Musha A, Kubo N, Kawamura H, et al. Carbon-ion Radiotherapy for Inoperable Head and Neck Bone and Soft-tissue Sarcoma: Prospective Observational Study. Anticancer Res 2022;42(3):1439–46.
8. Mendenhall WM, Morris CG, Amdur RJ, et al. Radiotherapy alone or combined with surgery for salivary gland carcinoma. Cancer 2005;103(12):2544–50.
9. Mercado C.E., Holtzman A.L., Rotondo R., et al., Proton therapy for skull base tumors: A review of clinical outcomes for chordomas and chondrosarcomas, Head Neck, 41 (2), 2019, 536–541.
10. Uhl M, Mattke M, Welzel T, et al. Highly effective treatment of skull base chordoma with carbon ion irradiation using a raster scan technique in 155 patients: first long-term results. Cancer 2014;120(21):3410–7.
11. Mattke M, Ohlinger M, Bougatf N, et al. Proton and carbon ion beam treatment with active raster scanning method in 147 patients with skull base chordoma at the Heidelberg Ion Beam Therapy Center-a single-center experience. Strahlenther Onkol 2023;199(2):160–8.
12. Iannalfi A, D'Ippolito E, Riva G, et al. Proton and carbon ion radiotherapy in skull base chordomas: a prospective study based on a dual particle and a patient-customized treatment strategy. Neuro Oncol 2020;22(9):1348–58.
13. Holtzman AL, Rotondo RL, Rutenberg MS, et al. Proton therapy for skull-base chondrosarcoma, a single-institution outcomes study. J Neurooncol 2019;142(3):557–63.
14. Weber DC, Murray F, Combescure C, et al. Long term outcome of skull-base chondrosarcoma patients treated with high-dose proton therapy with or without conventional radiation therapy. Radiother Oncol 2018;129(3):520–6.
15. Schulz-Ertner D, Nikoghosyan A, Hof H, et al. Carbon ion radiotherapy of skull base chondrosarcomas. Int J Radiat Oncol Biol Phys 2007;67(1):171–7.
16. Uhl M, Mattke M, Welzel T, et al. High control rate in patients with chondrosarcoma of the skull base after carbon ion therapy: first report of long-term results. Cancer 2014;120(10):1579–85.
17. Mattke M, Vogt K, Bougatf N, et al. High control rates of proton- and carbon-ion-beam treatment with intensity-modulated active raster scanning in 101 patients with skull base chondrosarcoma at the Heidelberg Ion Beam Therapy Center. Cancer 2018;124(9):2036–44.
18. Mendenhall W.M., Morris C.G., Amdur R.J., et al., Radiotherapy alone or combined with surgery for adenoid cystic carcinoma of the head and neck. Head Neck, 26 (2), 2004, 154–162.
19. Balamucki CJ, Amdur RJ, Werning JW, et al. Adenoid cystic carcinoma of the head and neck. Am J Otolaryngol 2012;33(5):510–8.
20. Schulz-Ertner D, Nikoghosyan A, Jäkel O, et al. Feasibility and toxicity of combined photon and carbon ion radiotherapy for locally advanced adenoid cystic carcinomas. Int J Radiat Oncol Biol Phys 2003;56(2):391–8.

21. Mizoe JE, Tsujii H, Kamada T, et al. Dose escalation study of carbon ion radiotherapy for locally advanced head-and-neck cancer. Int J Radiat Oncol Biol Phys 2004;60(2):358–64.

22. Jensen AD, Nikoghosyan AV, Lossner K, et al. A Regimen of Intensity Modulated Radiation Therapy Plus Dose-Escalated, Raster-Scanned Carbon Ion Boost for Malignant Salivary Gland Tumors: Results of the Prospective Phase 2 Trial. Int J Radiat Oncol Biol Phys 2015;93(1):37–46.

23. Jensen AD, Poulakis M, Nikoghosyan AV, et al. High-LET radiotherapy for adenoid cystic carcinoma of the head and neck: 15 years' experience with raster-scanned carbon ion therapy. Radiother Oncol 2016;118(2):272–80.

24. Mizoe JE, Hasegawa A, Jingu K, et al. Results of carbon ion radiotherapy for head and neck cancer. Radiother Oncol 2012;103(1):32–7.

25. Miglianico L, Eschwege F, Marandas P, Wibault P. Cervico-facial adenoid cystic carcinoma: study of 102 cases. Influence of radiation therapy. Int J Radiat Oncol Biol Phys 1987;13(5):673–8.

26. Koto M, Demizu Y, Saitoh JI, et al. Definitive Carbon-Ion Radiation Therapy for Locally Advanced Sinonasal Malignant Tumors: Subgroup Analysis of a Multicenter Study by the Japan Carbon-Ion Radiation Oncology Study Group (J-CROS). Int J Radiat Oncol Biol Phys 2018;102(2):353–61.

27. Janot F., de Raucourt D., Benhamou E., et al., Randomized trial of postoperative reirradiation combined with chemotherapy after salvage surgery compared with salvage surgery alone in head and neck carcinoma. J Clin Oncol. 2008;26(34):5518-5523.

28. De Crevoisier R, Bourhis J, Domenge C, et al. Full-dose reirradiation for unresectable head and neck carcinoma: experience at the Gustave-Roussy Institute in a series of 169 patients. J Clin Oncol 1998;16(11):3556–62.

29. Vargo JA, Ward MC, Caudell JJ, et al. A Multi-institutional Comparison of SBRT and IMRT for Definitive Reirradiation of Recurrent or Second Primary Head and Neck Cancer. Int J Radiat Oncol Biol Phys 2018;100(3):595–605.

30. Held T, Windisch P, Akbaba S, et al. Carbon Ion Re-irradiation for Recurrent Head and Neck Cancer: A Single-Institutional Experience. Int J Radiat Oncol Biol Phys 2019;105(4):803–11.

31. Hayashi K, Koto M, Ikawa H, et al. Feasibility of Re-irradiation using carbon ions for recurrent head and neck malignancies after carbon-ion radiotherapy. Radiother Oncol 2019;136:148–53.

32. Bhattacharyya T, Koto M, Windisch P, et al. Emerging Role of Carbon Ion Radiotherapy in Reir-radiation of Recurrent Head and Neck Cancers: What Have We Achieved So Far? Front Oncol 2022;12:888446.

33. Pompos A, Foote RL, Koong AC, et al. National Effort to Re-Establish Heavy Ion Cancer Therapy in the United States. Front Oncol 2022;12:880712.

34. Grosshagauer S, Fossati P, Schafasand M, et al. Organs at risk dose constraints in carbon ion radiotherapy at MedAustron: Translations between LEM and MKM RBE models and preliminary clinical results. Radiother Oncol 2022;175:73–8.

35. Liang X, Liu C, Furutani KM, et al. Investigation of beam delivery time for synchrotron-based proton pencil beam scanning system with novel scanning mode. Phys Med Biol 2022;67(17):1–14.

36. Liang X, Beltran C, Liu C, et al. Investigation of the impact of machine operating parameters on beam delivery time and its correlation with treatment plan characteristics for synchrotron-based proton pencil beam spot scanning system. Front Oncol 2022;12:1036139.

Moving?

Make sure your subscription moves with you!

To notify us of your new address, find your **Clinics Account Number** (located on your mailing label above your name), and contact customer service at:

Email: journalscustomerservice-usa@elsevier.com

800-654-2452 (subscribers in the U.S. & Canada)
314-447-8871 (subscribers outside of the U.S. & Canada)

Fax number: 314-447-8029

Elsevier Health Sciences Division
Subscription Customer Service
3251 Riverport Lane
Maryland Heights, MO 63043

*To ensure uninterrupted delivery of your subscription, please notify us at least 4 weeks in advance of move.

Printed and bound by CPI Group (UK) Ltd, Croydon, CR0 4YY

08/05/2025

01864749-0013